D0912876

CRITICAL ISSUES
IN AMERICAN
PSYCHIATRY
AND THE
LAW

Volume 2

CRITICAL ISSUES IN AMERICAN PSYCHIATRY AND THE LAW

Volume 2

was edited for
THE AMERICAN ACADEMY OF PSYCHIATRY AND THE LAW
(TRI-STATE CHAPTER)

A Continuation Order Plan is available for this series. A continuation order will bring delivery of each new volume immediately upon publication. Volumes are billed only upon actual shipment. For further information please contact the publisher.

CRITICAL ISSUES
IN AMERICAN
PSYCHIATRY
AND THE
LAW

Volume 2

Edited by

Richard Rosner, M.D.

Diplomate in Forensic Psychiatry
Clinical Associate Professor
Department of Psychiatry
School of Medicine
New York University
and Medical Director
Forensic Psychiatric Clinic for the New York Criminal
and Supreme Courts
(First Judicial District)
New York, New York

PLENUM PRESS • NEW YORK AND LONDON

Library of Congress Cataloging in Publication Data

Main entry under title:

Critical issues in American psychiatry and the law.

(American lectures series: publication no. 1047)
"Collected papers, revised . . . given at the annual series of postgraduate medical education programs in New York City by the regional membership of the American Academy of Psychiatry and the Law"—Introd. v. 1.
"A monograph in the Bannerstone Division of behavioral science and law"—Vol. 1.
Vol. 2, published by Plenum Press.
Includes bibliographical references.
Includes indexes.
    1. Forensic psychiatry—United States—Addresses, essays, lectures. I. Rosner, Richard. II. American Academy of Psychiatry and the Law. [DNLM: 1. Forensic psychiatry. W 740 C934]
KF8922.C75   1982   614'.1   81-9059
ISBN 0-306-41954-8

© 1985 Plenum Press, New York
A Division of Plenum Publishing Corporation
233 Spring Street, New York, N.Y. 10013

Printed in the United States of America

To the memory of
Henry J. Rosner, C.P.A.,
my father

Contributors

Richard Garmise • Family Court Mental Health Services, City of New York; Institute of Advanced Psychological Studies, Adelphi University, Garden City, New York

Robert Lloyd Goldstein • Department of Psychiatry, The College of Physicians and Surgeons, Columbia University, New York, New York; Member of the New York State Bar

Peter D. Guggenheim • Family Court Mental Health Services, City of New York; Department of Psychiatry, School of Medicine, New York University, New York, New York

Morris Herman • Department of Psychiatry, School of Medicine, New York University, New York, New York

Graham Hughes • School of Law, New York University, New York, New York

Brian E. Lynch • Canadian Security Intelligence Service, Ottawa, Ontario, Canada

Ruth Macklin • Department of Epidemiology and Social Medicine, Albert Einstein College of Medicine, Bronx, New York

Martin T. Orne • Unit for Experimental Psychiatry, The Institute of Pennsylvania Hospital, University of Pennsylvania, Philadelphia, Pennsylvania

Jacques M. Quen • Payne Whitney Clinic, New York Hospital, New York, New York; School of Medicine, Cornell University, Ithaca, New York

Jonas R. Rappeport • School of Medicine, University of Maryland, College Park, Maryland; School of Medicine, Johns Hopkins University, Baltimore, Maryland; Medical Service of the Circuit Court, Baltimore, Maryland

Richard Rosner • Forensic Psychiatry Clinic for the New York Criminal and Supreme Courts (First Judicial Department) of the Department of Mental Health, Mental Retardation and Alcoholism Services of The City of New York; Department of Psychiatry, School of Medicine, New York University, New York, New York

Robert L. Sadoff • Center for Studies in Social-Legal Psychiatry, School of Medicine, University of Pennsylvania, Philadelphia, Pennsylvania; School of Law, Villanova University, Philadelphia, Pennsylvania

Daniel W. Schwartz • Department of Psychiatry, Downstate Medical Center, State University of New York, Brooklyn, New York; Forensic Psychiatry Service, Kings County Hospital Center, Brooklyn, New York

Bertram Slaff • The Mount Sinai Medical Center, New York, New York; Department of Psychiatry, The Mount Sinai School of Medicine, The City University of New York, New York

Alan J. Tuckman • Department of Psychiatry, School of Medicine, New York University, New York, New York

Norman Weiss • Department of Psychiatry, New York Medical College, Valhalla, New York; Diplomate in Forensic Psychiatry

Foreword

As President of the American Academy of Psychiatry and the Law (AAPL), it is a pleasure to write this foreword. Dr. Richard Rosner deserves full credit for helping AAPL pursue its educational goals by publishing a series of books.

Consumerism and the civil rights movement have dramatically changed the practice of American psychiatry over the last 2 decades. Extensive legal regulation now makes it necessary for both general and forensic psychiatrists to keep abreast of changing laws. The contents of Volume II of *Critical Issues in American Psychiatry and the Law* demonstrate Dr. Rosner's gift for selecting and editing important theoretical and practical articles.

This volume addresses a broad range of forensic issues. The pendulum-like swings of laws regarding civil commitment and insanity are clearly illuminated by Dr. Quen's contribution, "Violence, Psychiatry, and the Law." A review of historical psychiatric testimony supporting insanity defenses on the bases of homicidal mania, moral insanity, and phrenological evidence should make modern forensic psychiatrists humble. However, some of our colleagues continue to testify that defendants were unable to refrain from criminal conduct because of CT evidence of schizophrenia, pathological gambling, or the effects of junk food.

Excellent theoretical discussions are presented by Dr. Macklin ("A Philosophical Perspective on Ethics and Forensic Psychiatry") and Mr. Hughes ("Legal Aspects of Predicting Dangerousness"). These chapters present thorough, up-to-date, scholarly analyses of complex issues from the vantage point of nonpsychiatrists.

The section on scientific truth detection covers amytal, polygraphy, and hypnosis. Dr. Orne's chapter, "The Use and Misuse of Hypnosis in Court," is the definitive work on the subject.

Drs. Sadoff and Tuckman address psychiatric malpractice from the perspective of expert witnesses employed by the plaintiff and defendant.

In addition to providing practical advice for the forensic psychiatrist, the authors remain sensitive to transference issues and the emotional distress of the defendant psychiatrist. Additional chapters cover a rich variety of topics that are useful for both the novice and the experienced forensic psychiatrist.

On behalf of the Academy, I congratulate Dr. Rosner and his contributors for an excellent addition to the literature on psychiatry and the law.

PHILLIP J. RESNICK

Introduction

This second volume in the series *Critical Issues in American Psychiatry and the Law* has been designed as a self-contained collection of essays that complements the first volume but is not dependent on it. Readers who are familiar with the initial book, published by Charles C Thomas Company in 1982, will find completely new material for their consideration here. Those who have not read Volume I will be able to appreciate the contents of this book without feeling unprepared.

These chapters draw on a range of resources within the extended training programs of the Tri-State Chapter of The American Academy of Psychiatry and the Law. The annual meetings of the Tri-State Chapter have recently focused on the themes of ethical issues in forensic psychiatry, violence and dangerousness, and psychiatric malpractice; six of the essays draw on materials that were presented at those annual meetings. In conjunction with the Post-Graduate School of Medicine of New York University, senior members of the Tri-State Chapter organized and participated in a program on scientific truth detection that provided the foundation for three of our essays. A joint project of the Tri-State Chapter, the national organization of The American Academy of Psychiatry and the Law, and The American Society for Adolescent Psychiatry resulted in a program on adolescent psychiatry for forensic psychiatrists and inspired two of the essays in this collection. A recent program on assessment of psychiatric disability for civil law purposes was the foundation for two chapters. Finally, based on our ongoing series of weekly seminars in forensic psychiatry, four topics were regarded as meriting special attention and resulted in contributions to this book.

As a result of the range of educational sources from which these papers have been drawn, there is no overall unifying theme to this collection of essays. Rather, there is a representation of the broad scope of interests in the membership of the Tri-State Chapter: All of our educational programs are designed in response to the expressed educational concerns of our membership. Thus, this book may be viewed as an introduction to the diversity of professional interests among contemporary forensic psychiatrists.

The great bulk of these chapters was originally designed for oral presentation. It was expected that the authors would vigorously present their own views and that the audience would have an ample opportunity to question them afterward. In many instances, here represented only by the pair of essays on malpractice, each view presented was answered by an equally vigorous statement from an alternative perspective. It is not possible to present the intellectual excitement of those lively discussions, disputes, and occasional confrontations through the format of a book. Rather, the reader is invited to challenge the content of these essays himself, to actively engage in a learning process in which these papers are seen as efforts to stimulate thought about important issues. As in the adversary system in American law, each of the contributors should be seen as an honest advocate for the position that is being made. The reader is cast in the role of the judge, whose task it is to evaluate the quality of the data being submitted, the interpretations being made of that data, and the conclusions that are being urged. The goal of these essays is *not* to provide definitive answers, but to stimulate each reader to think and arrive at his or her own conclusions.

RICHARD ROSNER

Contents

I

Fundamental Considerations

Legal Regulation of Psychiatry and Forensic Psychiatry
Clarifying Categories for Clinicians

RICHARD ROSNER

MENTAL HEALTH AND LAW IN PSYCHIATRY

There are two major areas in which a psychiatric clinician must have a general understanding of the relationship of mental health to American law. The first devolves from the legal regulation of psychiatric practice. The second entails the field of forensic psychiatry. As both of these areas of concern are changing as the law itself changes, it is more important to understand how to think about problems related to mental health and law than to memorize specific statutes, cases, and administrative codes (although such specific data may be relevant to the resolution of one or another problem that may arise for the psychiatrist's consideration). This chapter reviews approaches to thinking about problems in mental health and the law.

Legal Regulation of Psychiatry

There are several sources of lawful power in the United States. Ultimately, all lawful power is derived from the people of this nation, according to our legal philosophy. That original power was specified and delimited in the constitution of the United States and in the fifty

---

RICHARD ROSNER • Department of Psychiatry, School of Medicine, New York University, New York, New York 10016.

constitutions of the individual states that comprise the union; thus, there are 51 sources of constitutional law that are simultaneously operative in various areas of America, any one of which may be predominant in a given law suit at a given moment. In accordance with these 51 sources of lawful power, there are 51 legislatures that have made 51 sets of laws for the nation; there are 51 judicial systems that have interpreted the 51 sets of legislated statutes to produce 51 sets of judge-made "case law." It is not possible to set forth any single series of guidelines for the psychiatrist in the area of the legal regulation of psychiatry because of this multiplicity of constitutions, legislated statutes, and case-law interpretations.

In each instance, however, the laws of the state in which the psychiatrist is licensed will address the general practice of medicine and, often, the specific practice of psychiatry and the allied mental health professions. In the State of New York, for example, a large proportion of the relevant laws will be included in the Mental Hygiene Law of the state. Other parts of the law, for example, the Criminal Procedure Law, will often contain regulations that are of interest to the clinician. It is difficult to find, between the covers of any one book, even in a sir gle state, all the laws that are relevant to the regulation of psychiatry. There is no way for the psychiatrist to function as his own attorney; it is essential to work cooperatively with a lawyer to find and understand the laws that are applicable to psychiatric practice in one's own locale.

The importance of law as the source of legitimate authority is often not fully understood by physicians. Doctors may think that they have some autonomous authority, as doctors, to act on behalf of their patients. However, all the authority that physicians possess is ultimately derived from the lawful and delimited power of the legally established federal and state governments. The most obvious example of this delegation of power is that the license to practice medicine is given by the government, not by the National Board of Medical Examiners. On a more sophisticated level, a surgeon who opens a patient's abdomen is not committed to the custody of the police on a charge of assault and battery because he has (wittingly or unwittingly) complied with the laws that govern doctor–patient relationships; if he has not complied with those laws, he may face a civil suit for malpractice or even the criminal charges mentioned earlier.

The question occasionally asked by an insensed physician, as to who the lawyers think they are to tell doctors how to practice, is based on a misunderstanding. The doctors know how to act; that is not the issue. The lawyers tell the doctors what actions are lawful, permissible in our society, consistent with the fundamental principles of our nation; that is the vital issue. The power of the physician is granted by law. The extent and the limits of the physician's power is also set forth in law. How one may practice, on whom one may practice, when one may practice, where one may practice and what one may practice, all are delegated by law and defined by law. The right to practice medicine is a conditional right; those conditions may be changed by law, and the clinician who does not understand this reality will have great difficulty in functioning effectively.

In general, legal regulation of psychiatry will address such matters as under what conditions may a doctor–patient relationship be said to exist; what are a doctor's legal obligations to his patients; under what conditions may a doctor treat a patient; under what conditions may a doctor not treat a patient; under what conditions may a doctor be held liable for injuries sustained by a patient in the course of medical treatment; under what conditions may a patient be treated against his/her will; under what conditions may a child or an unconscious person or an adjudicated incompetent be treated; under what conditions must a doctor keep secrets confided by a patient; under what conditions must a doctor reveal secrets confided by a patient. It should be clear that these are not questions that relate to the science and art of medical therapy and technology but rather to the conditions under which medical expertise may be lawfully practiced. Medical expertise may be determined by physicians; the lawful practice of medicine is determined by the power of the people of America as delegated to their representatives in legislatures, their governmental administrators in the executive branch and their decision makers in the judiciary.

Most doctors do not think of themselves as agents of government. However, every time that a doctor acts in accordance with the power delegated to him by law, as a result of having been admitted to practice by the laws of a particular jurisdiction, the doctor is using powers granted by the law and is in that sense a governmental agent. All governmental agents act within prescribed boundaries, so do physicians. The legal regulation of medical practice is, in principle, no different from the legal regulation of any other profession, skilled trade, or business. This is particularly evident when a doctor is obligated to act against the wishes of a patient, for example, in an involuntary hospitalization procedure. By what right does a doctor deprive a citizen of liberty and confine him/her to a mental hospital? The power is not inherent in the individual doctor, nor derivative from the profession of medicine; rather, it is granted by law and must be implemented by procedures specified by law.

There are two grounds for the restriction of individual liberty that are recognized in American law. One of these is the *police power* of government, the right of the government to protect its citizens from harm. Thus, one criteria for involuntary hospitalization may be that a person is judged to be a clear and present danger to others, that he is mentally ill, and that the mental illness is causing the dangerousness. When local community groups complain that deinstitutionalized psychiatric patients are unsightly, odoriferous, and a nuisance, the psychiatrist may want to point out that being ugly, smelly and in-the-way may not be a legal criteria for involuntary hospitalization. Only those who meet the legal criteria may be admitted against their will.

The second ground for the restriction of personal liberty that is well-founded is the *parens patriae* power of government, the right of the government to care for those who are legally not entitled to care for themselves; for example, orphaned children, persons adjudicated incompetent by the courts and mentally ill persons who meet legal criteria for intervention into their privacy. Thus, another criteria for involuntary hospitalization in a mental institution may be that a person is gravely disabled by mental illness and cannot function safely outside of a hospital setting. Although this is a criteria that many doctors favor, it is not one that is highly regarded by civil rights lawyers. To return to our earlier example of deinstitutionalized psychiatric patients, many of them are able to function safely outside of a hospital, even though they live in a manner that the average citizen disparages. It is not obvious that they are gravely disabled by their own atypical standards.

Legal regulation of psychiatry is designed, among other purposes, to insure that psychiatrists exercise their lawfully delegated power in ways that are consistent with constitutional guarantee that no person may be deprived of life, liberty or property without due process of law. For example, a doctor may believe that a patient has become incompetent to consent to treatment, but the person remains legally competent until he has been adjudicated incompetent by a court. (The analogy is that a person may have ceased to live, but he is not legally "dead" until declared *dead* in accordance with law.) The doctor merely expresses an opinion regarding the patient's competence; the real decision is made by a judge.

Why should a judge decide? The answer is based on the balance of powers concept that influenced the framers of the United States' constitution. It was felt that power was less likely to be abused if it was distributed among separate branches of the government. One branch would make law, one branch would execute/implement law, one branch would adjudicate disputes about legal rights and duties. The judge, as a representative of the judicial branch, is the person vested with constitutional authority to make decisions when legal disputes arise. In our example, the dispute is between the patient who regards himself as competent and the medical staff member who believes the patient incompetent. The judge will hear both sides to the dispute and provide a legally binding decision as to which of the two differing parties is right. The judge is the legally designated decision maker; the doctor does not have the authority to decide the issue. It is a general principle that a party to a dispute may not be the judge of the dispute.

It may seem ridiculous to a doctor that a disagreement between a physician and a patient should be resolved by a judge. Doctors are not accustomed to being in an adversary relationship with persons they regard as their patients. Many physicians are used to the adage "Doctor knows best." One of the important tasks of a forensic psychiatrist may be to assist medical staff in obtaining a more realistic understanding of the limits of a physician's authority.

In New York State, for example, there is a governmental agency, known as the Mental Health Information Service, that must be advised of the involuntary hospitalization of psychiatric patients and that is charged with the legal representation of the patient's interests, often against the recommendations of the psychiatric staff of the mental institution. In other states, the Public Defender or Public Advocate may have a special division devoted to the representation of the rights of involuntary mental patients. Typical cases may include

- the patient who wants to leave the hospital against medical advice, but the psychiatric staff believes that the patient should be involuntarily hospitalized for further treatment; and
- the patient who does not want to take any medications, but the psychiatric staff believes that neuroleptics are essential for the treatment of the patient's psychosis and urges that the patient be involuntarily medicated.

The thrust of this section is to remind the psychiatric clinician of the fact that medicine is practiced in a social context, that the profession of medicine is increasingly being treated as merely one of many special interests groups, that medical authority was always derivative from the source of all lawful power in America, and that the legal regulation of psychiatric practice must be understood so as to make the continuance of that practice feasible.

Without attempting a lengthy exploration of this subject, I believe it is vital to understand that a conflict of values is at the root of much of the disagreement between physicians and lawyers. Doctors are trained to regard *health* as a principal value, whereas lawyers are trained to regard *liberty* as a principal value. For a physician, a person who has the freedom to remain sick (a mentally ill patient who refuses treatment because he enjoys being manic and gets a lawyer to sue for his release from a hospital) is a problem in medical management, not a case study in civil liberties. For a lawyer, when the price of health is involuntary hospitalization, it may be preferable to be free and ill. There are no villains in this context. Liberty and health are both major values. Under our system, conflicts between those values will be part of the social policy decisions to be considered by the American people. In discussions between attorneys and doctors, it may be useful to recognize that disagreements may be less about the facts of a particular case and more about the evaluation of those facts in the context of health-centered or liberty-centered principles. At times the psychiatric clinician has to understand moral philosophy.

Forensic Psychiatry

One of the more accepted definitions of forensic psychiatry is that it is the application of psychiatric expertise to legal ends (as contrasted to the application of psychiatric expertise for therapeutic ends, which is clinical psychiatry). Whereas the legal regulation of psychiatry encompasses all of clinical psychiatry, forensic psychiatry is an entirely different field. The legal regulation of practice will deal with those situations that arise between doctors and their patients. Forensic psychiatry will deal with problems of concern to lawyers and judges, problems in which the doctor will be evaluating someone who is frequently not a patient. It becomes extremely important for the doctor to understand, in advance, and to advise the person he is examining, whether or not a doctor–patient relationship exists between them. In a doctor–patient relationship, the patient may reasonably expect that what is discussed will be kept confidential, that the information exchanged will be used for the patient's benefit. In the different relationship that exists between a forensic psychiatrist and the person he is evaluating, it is not automatic that information will be held confidential; further, the information may be used against the interests of the person being examined. This change of customary expectations is so shocking to some doctors that they prefer not to work in forensic psychiatry. How is one to understand this special type of psychiatric work?

One of the best examples is the role of the military psychiatrist. The psychiatrist in the Armed Forces is expected to put the interests of the nation-as-a-whole above the interests of the individual patient. The military psychiatrist must help someone get well enough to go back into the war zone, for example, and risk death. It would be inconsistent with the military physician's loyalty to the country to help the soldier escape active duty, on the grounds that it was better for the soldier's health to stay far away from bullets and shrapnel. Further, confidentiality in such a setting would not exist, as the doctor's duty would be to help his country win the war, not to shield malingerers. While the role of the military physician is a special one, it is an instance of the general class of conditions in which a doctor must apply his skills on behalf of some larger interest than just the well-being of the particular person he is examining.

In forensic psychiatry, that larger interest is the integrity of the national system of law, which has need for psychiatric expertise in a variety of civil and criminal law matters. The forensic psychiatrist, like the military psychiatrist, has a higher allegiance to serve than the interests of a particular individual who is being evaluated. Problems arise because the same doctor may function as a clinical psychiatrist in some settings and as a forensic psychiatrist in other settings. The doctor may not always be as clear in his own mind as might be wished as to what role he is playing, and may not clarify that role properly for the person he is examining. One of the first rules of forensic psychiatry is to know whether one is wearing one's "forensic hat" or one's "clinical hat" and to be sure to share that role definition with the person being evaluated.

Among the types of nonclinical, nontherapeutic roles that call for a forensic psychiatrist are

- evaluating whether a defendant in a criminal case is competent to stand trial;
- determining if a Social Security disability claimant is truly disabled or merely feigning illness to get extra money;
- assessing whether a patient in a hospital, who was acquitted by reason of legal insanity, is likely to be dangerous if released;
- attempting to determine which of two competing parents would be the better custodian of their child, during a divorce case;
- reconstructing the mental state of a dead person around the time he signed a last will and testament, to develop an opinion as to the competence of the person to make a will; and
- reviewing records to assist the police in the development of a psychological profile on a murderer who has not been found and is likely to strike again.

In each of these examples, the person who is the focus of the psychiatrist's expertise is not the person on whose behalf the psychiatrist is working. In fact, there is an excellent likelihood that the person being evaluated (directly or indirectly) might have opposed any such evaluation being done at all. To emphasize that the focus of evaluation is *not* a patient, forensic psychiatrists tend to refer to such persons as defendants, claimants, testators, plaintiffs, purported perpetrators, etc. This is not just a linguistic subterfuge, it is a way of clarifying for all parties that the doctor is using his skills for forensic, not clinical, purposes.

Is forensic psychiatry ethical? To forensic psychiatrists, the answer is clear: yes. They point out that they are not functioning in a doctor–patient relationship with the persons they examine, and are thus not doing anything inconsistent with the principles of ethical medical practice. Further, they point out that some of the larger societal tasks would be significantly impaired without psychiatric experts to assist the legal system; the refusal of psychiatrists to assist the legal administration of American justice would be unethical. Although these arguments can be countered, the fact remains that the practice of forensic psychiatry is not inconsistent with the Code of Ethics of the American Medical Association, and it is not inconsistent with the Annotations for Psychiatrists of that AMA Code that was developed with the assistance of the American Psychiatric Association. A doctor is not obliged to have the same relationships with all persons as those he has with his patients. A doctor can bargain with a car dealer, without being concerned for the best interests of the automobile salesman. A doctor may seek his own advantage in filing his tax return with the Internal Revenue Service, rather than trying to pay extra to help support the Medicare program. The Oath of Hippocrates is not applicable in all of a doctor's human interactions, only in those with his patients. So long as the forensic psychiatrist is clear, in his own mind, as to his nontherapeutic role, and so long as he makes it clear to the people he is asked to evaluate that he is not acting as their doctor, then he is functioning ethically, but outside of his role as physician. The point is valid: A psychiatrist may ethically use the skills he has acquired in the course of clinical training for ends that are not clinical, so long as all parties understand his nonmedical function.

Although the psychiatric clinician will have more direct interest in the legal regulation of clinical psychiatry than in the subspecialty of forensic psychiatry, the clinician will encounter forensic psychiatrists in the courtroom. Whenever an issue in the legal regulation of psychiatric practice requires testimony before a judge, there is a likelihood that a forensic psychiatrist may be called to testify, rather than a clinical psychiatrist. It becomes important to understand how forensic psychiatrists analyze a psychiatric-legal problem, if only to make the best use of their services. Often a forensic psychiatrist may make a better witness *for* the psychiatric clinician than will a clinical psychiatrist. Under some circumstances, each side in a legal contest will be represented by its forensic psychiatrist, rather than by its therapeutic staff psychiatrist. This should come as no surprise: Just as one would want a clinician to deal with a clinical problem, one would want a forensic expert to deal with a legal problem.

In general, all psychiatric-legal problems can be understood in terms of a four-step analysis, and it is this approach that the forensic psychiatrist is most likely to utilize. The steps are

1. What is the psychiatric-legal issue(s)?
2. What is the legal criteria that will be used to decide the issue(s)?
3. What is the relevant clinical data?
4. What is the reasoning that can apply the relevant data to the legal criteria in order to generate an opinion on the issue(s)?

It is important to understand that a single clinical case may be the basis for several psychiatric-legal issues. For example, if a person assaults another person, among the issues may be whether the assaultive person is a suitable candidate for involuntary psychiatric hospitalization, whether the assaultive person was not criminally responsible for the assaultive behavior because of legal insanity, and whether the assaultive person is not currently competent to stand trial. A forensic psychiatrist may be particularly adept at delineating the various psychiatric-legal issues to be addressed; alternatively, one can obtain an even surer analysis by consulting an attorney regarding the various issues raised by a single case.

For each psychiatric-legal issue, there will be a separate set of legal criteria on which the issue will be decided. To illustrate this point by analogy, for each psychiatric diagnosis there is a separate listing of psychiatric criteria that must be met. If the issue is whether the patient has schizophrenia, paranoid type, the criteria to be met are found in DSM-III. Analagously, if the issue is whether the patient is competent to stand trial, the criteria are to be found in the law. The psychiatric-legal issue is a question to be answered "yes" or "no." The legal criteria to determine the issue may be brief, lengthy, precise, vague, recent, old, but are the lawful guidelines that must be used to evaluate the data. Although some forensic psychiatrists are familiar with the legal criteria that govern the psychiatric-legal issues under consideration, it is wisest to obtain this information from an attorney, as it is the attorney who will be representing the clinician's interests at the legal hearings in court.

The collection of relevant clinical data is different from the collection of all clinical data. *Relevant* data is that which is germane to the legal criteria that will determine the issue. It may be confusing to the judge or jury to present all the information that the clinician possesses about a case. Further, it may be that the information that the clinician possesses does not relate pertinently to the legal criteria that the judge or jury must use in reaching a decision about the psychiatric-legal issue. To take a simple example, based on the assault case mentioned above, the issue of criminal responsibility will require information about the assaultive person's mental condition at the time of the offense, information about the past, about what *was* going on in his mind. The issue of current competence to stand trial, however, will require information about the assaultive person's present mental abilities, about what is *now* going on in his mind. If irrelevant information is provided to the court, the psychiatrist may find that the case has been lost.

The presentation of the reasoning process by means of which one moves from the relevant clinical data to their application to the legal criteria, to an opinion regarding the specific issue, is the special province of forensic psychiatry. Clinicians often have difficulty explaining their reasoning processes to the court, so that some judges have despaired of ever being able to make effective use of psychiatric testimony. Part of this is due to the anxiety of clinicians when called to testify in court; it is difficult to think clearly and speak cogently when nervous. Another problem is that one of the lawyers, the one on the opposing side, is obliged to challenge the testimony the clincian is trying to present; it is disconcerting for many doctors to have to prove their assertions. It is particularly important to work closely with the attorney on your side to prepare to present your reasoning processes effectively.

This four-step process (issue, criteria, data, reasoning) can be applied to each instance in which the psychiatric clinician finds that a court case is at hand. It will help clarify the psychiatrist's thinking and assist in making the best use of both legal services and forensic psychiatric experts. The clinician does not have to be a forensic psychiatrist, but it may be useful to know how to think like one.

As a practical matter, the clinician may want to know how to find a forensic psychiatrist. The best source is The American Board of Forensic Psychiatry, at 1211 Cathedral Street, Baltimore, Maryland 21201, which can provide a list of those physicians who have been certified in the subspecialty. Alternatively, one can contact The American Academy of Psychiatry and the Law, at the same address, to get the much larger list of noncertified forensic psychiatrists. At the present time, there are only about 200 certified forensic psychiatrists, but there are nearly one thousand noncertified forensic psychiatrists. Another supplementary source of information is The American Academy of Forensic Sciences, which has a listing of forensic psychiatrists, forensic pathologists, forensic odontologists, forensic anthropologists, as well as specialists in criminalistics, engineering, toxicology, questioned documents and jurisprudence; the AAFS address is 205 South Academy Boulevard, Colorado Springs, Colorado 80901. Under some circumstances, a forensic psychologist may be useful and a list may be obtained from the American Board of Forensic Psychology or from the American Psychology–Law

Society; the addresses of these organizations change with the officers who are elected to lead them.

Practical Problems and Potential Solutions

The following examples are designed to illustrate some of the practical problems that clinicians and administrators may encounter in the practice of psychiatry in a general hospital. Although the specific details are fictitious, to protect the identities of the persons who are the bases of these vignettes, the problems are real. It is hoped that the approach used in developing potential solutions will prove useful.

CASE 1: A QUIET EVENING IN THE EMERGENCY ROOM

Fifteen minutes into a good novel, on a rainy Saturday evening in March, the psychiatric consultant to the emergency room received an urgent call. Reportedly, an agitated woman had brought in a comatose man; the medical intern was concerned that a suicide had been attempted and was requesting assistance. Upon questioning, the woman (who was indeed agitated) related that she and her boyfriend had recently broken up and that she found him stuporous when she came by the apartment to pick up some of her belongings. The man, responding to medical treatment, had regained consciousness, but was evasive about what had happened, claiming that it was only an accident, that he had been having trouble sleeping, that he took "a couple of shots" of Scotch to relax and, when the alcohol did not help sufficiently, took some sleeping pills. He denied suicidal intent. The girlfriend was terrified and guilt ridden, concerned that he might try to kill himself as soon as he was released. The medical intern indicated that the man was not in need of admission for his medical condition, but insisted on obtaining "psychiatric clearance" before the man could be permitted to leave the Emergency Room. What to do?

SOLUTION 1

The psychiatric-legal issue was whether or not the man met the legal criteria for involuntary hospitalization. In New York State, there are two possible routes: (a) the Involuntary Hospitalization procedure, which requires a certification by two physicians to the effect that a patient is in need of care and treatment in a hospital *and* that he is suffering from a defect of judgement (due to his mental illness) that prevents him from recognizing that need; and (b) the Emergency Hospitalization procedure, which requires a certification by only one physician to the effect that a patient is in need of care and treatment in a hospital because he is dangerous to himself or others (as a result of his mental illness). The psychiatric consultant attempted to collect data that would be relevant to the two potential legal criteria. As a practical matter, as the consultant's own hospital did not accept nonvoluntary psychiatric patients, it would be necessary to arrange for an interinstitutional transfer of the patient if it was established that he was a candidate for either legal procedure. Similarly practical was the consultant's awareness that the potential receiving hospital for nonvoluntary patients would be reluctant to accept a nonemergency case on Saturday night.

The consultant engaged in a clinical interview with the patient, attempting to establish rapport as well as to gather data. The man was not psychotic, although he was unhappy with his work and with his "failure" to satisfy his girlfriend. He was thought to be having an "Adjustment Disorder" with depressed mood, superimposed on a "Mixed Personality Disorder," with histrionic, dependent and passive-aggressive features. The consultant was aware of the fact that, in his area, courts were extremely reluctant to support nonvoluntary retention of nonpsychotic patients. The conclusion was that the patient was neither a candidate for Involuntary nor for Emergency psychiatric hospitalization. The girlfriend agreed to spend the weekend with the man, to insure his safety, and to assuage her guilt, and he was permitted to depart.

CASE 2: AUNT MINNA WANTS TO GO HOME

The Gastroenterologist called because his patient, an 87 year old lady, was refusing to take her medications and insisting on leaving the hospital. He wondered if she was competent to refuse treatment and if she might be a candidate for a guardianship proceeding. The liaison psychiatrist was asked to evaluate the matter. He found the patient with her bags packed, next to her niece, who explained that "Aunt Minna wants to go home."

SOLUTION 2

The liaison psychiatrist was aware of the fact that America is dedicated to personal freedom, that each citizen has the right to make mistakes, that no one can be protected from the responsibility for their own lives, if they are competent. In New York State, generally, there are two types of guardianships. One, a conservatorship, is for persons who can not manage their finances responsibly, although they are otherwise competent. The other, a committee, is for persons who are globally incompetent to cope with the world they live in. Did Aunt Minna fit into either of these two potential legal categories?

Aunt Minna had been losing weight for the past 2 months. Her appetite was poor, she was restless and irritable, she had constipation chronicly, along with nausea and vomiting during the past week. Initial laboratory data included a positive guaiac test for occult blood in her stool. The gastroenterologist was concerned about a bowel obstruction, perhaps due to a malignancy: Waiting were the usual panoply of radiological examinations, colonoscopy, and a surgical consultation. Aunt Minna would have to consent to all of these procedures, if she was competent to do so.

The patient was oriented to time, place, and person. She could do serial 7 subtractions from 100. She knew the names of the United States presidents from Reagan back to Hoover. She could spell five letter words forwards and backwards. She could recite the days of the week in reverse. She could add 98 + 26 = 124 and she could subtract 98 − 26 = 72. Aunt Minna had worked as a bookkeeper, she read the New York Times daily, and she did not have an organic mental syndrome. She had cats. Apparently, this childless lady had adopted the cats of her neighborhood and made it her personal mission to see that they were fed in winter. If she was in the hospital, "her" cats might starve and suffer.

With the help of the niece, arrangements were made to have the cats fed while Aunt Minna was in the hospital. The patient agreed to stay, was concerned to get the best possible care, was cooperative: After all, if anything happened to her, the cats would suffer. Aunt Minna's reasons for wanting to leave were unusual, but she was not psychotic and, if she had insisted on leaving, there would have been no good legal grounds to stop her. Fortunately, a negotiated solution was arranged and an impasse was avoided.

CASE 3: BLOOD IN THE GUTTERS

Recently fired from his job, the middle-aged man was disappointed, frustrated, furious at his boss, threatening to kill him as soon as he left the emergency room. He had been brought in by his wife, who reported that he had been excited, irritable, talkative, and filled with "plans for the future." The psychiatric consultant was called by the resident psychiatrist because of the concern that the patient might hurt his former boss, to determine if there was a duty to warn the former employer that the patient was threatening that there would be "blood in the gutters."

SOLUTION 3

The resident was advised that there was no clear "duty to warn" potential victims of dangerous patients, as yet, in the State of New York. Rather, if the resident felt that the patient was a "clear and present danger" to the boss, that the patient could be offered admission to the hospital as a voluntary patient (with constant companioning by orderlies while waiting for psychotropic medications to become effective). Alternatively, if the patient refused voluntary admission, he was an excellent candidate for Emergency psychiatric hospitalization. If the patient was hospitalized, he was not going to be dangerous to the boss (who was far from the hospital). If the treatment was successful, the patient would be safe when he was well enough to be discharged. However, the consultant noted that a good after-care plan was particularly important, to insure that future risks would be minimal.

These three case examples demonstrate some of the common problems encountered in the general hospital by practitioners and by administrators: assessment of suicidal risk, involuntary hospitalization, com-

petence to refuse treatment, need for guardianship proceedings, dangerousness to others. In each case, there is a blend of clinical and forensic
considerations. Often, by careful clinical intervention and by the use of
such old-time skills as taking an accurate history, making a diagnosis,
treating the patient as a person rather than as a case, there may be no need
to utilize the powers that the law holds in reserve. However, it is important
to know what those powers are, and to be familiar with both their scope
and their limitations, in order to decide if they are applicable in difficult
cases.

The good forensic psychiatrist is also, fundamentally, a good clinical
psychiatrist. Without a solid grounding in clinical psychiatry, the tactical
and logical skills of the forensic psychiatrist will be of no avail. Just as the
clinician and administrator must know how to use the forensic psychiatric
consultant, so that consultant must appreciate and build on the therapeutic
and managerial skills of those who seek his help. Without such cooperation, cases such as those described here might have had much less desirable
outcomes.

CONCLUDING CONSIDERATIONS

As this chapter has sought to suggest, the specific laws relating to
the legal regulation of psychiatric practice are in continual evolution, so
that no succinct statement of what to do and what to avoid can be
regarded as of lasting value. Similarly, the nontherapeutic psychiatric
interface with the law, as represented by forensic psychiatry, presents a
wide range of issues, variable legal criteria, an absence of any fixed
examination format or data collection model, and the burden of close
reasoning. Faced with this flux, the psychiatric clinician is better advised
to learn how to understand the derivation of legal control over psychiatry and how to utilize the services of a lawyer or of a forensic psychiatrist
than to learn a long list of arbitrary rules, regulations and procedures. It
is more important to know how to think about these matters, how to
conceptualize the problems, than to try to recall a specific response that
may be outdated by the time that this book is published. For those who
insist on a having firm guidelines, this will continue to be a difficult area
in psychiatry because the law changes, medical science changes, and no
fixed answers can be obtained.

BIBLIOGRAPHY

Allen, R, Ferster, E, and Rubin, J: *Readings in Law and Psychiatry*, rev ed. Baltimore, Johns
    Hopkins Univ Press, 1975.

Brooks, A: *Law, Psychiatry and the Mental Health System.* Boston, Little, Brown, 1974, with a 1980 Supplement to the book.

Gutheil, T, and Appelbaum, P: *Clinical Handbook of Psychiatry and the Law.* Hightstown, NJ, McGraw-Hill, 1982.

Rosner, R: *Critical Issues in American Psychiatry and the Law.* Springfield, Illinois, Charles C Thomas, 1982.

Sadoff, R: Forensic psychiatry, *Psychiatric Clinics of North America,* Vol. 6, N. 4, December 1983.

Slovenko, R: *Psychiatry and Law,* Boston, Little, Brown, 1973.

2

A Philosophical Perspective on Ethics in Forensic Psychiatry

RUTH MACKLIN

THE PHILOSOPHICAL ENTERPRISE

Philosophy has traditionally sought to understand and explain all manner of cosmic and human phenomena. Yet to characterize philosophy in this way fails to distinguish it from scientific investigation and from other forms of humanistic inquiry. By the very nature of its activity, philosophy is a critical inquiry, seeking to provide standards for correct reasoning, for proper conduct, and for adequate evidence in support of every type of belief. In all these pursuits, different philosophical approaches—and there are many—are guided by principles. In offering standards for correct reasoning, philosophers use principles of deductive and inductive logic. In an effort to develop standards for proper conduct, philosophers have proposed moral principles, which are usually embedded in a larger ethical theory. And in asking what counts as adequate evidence in support of beliefs or claims to knowledge, philosophers employ epistemological principles that rest on a theory of knowledge: empiricism, rationalism, intuitionism, or some combination of these. Accordingly, a philosophical perspective on ethics in forensic psychiatry cannot be limited to moral concerns. It must also address modes

RUTH MACKLIN • Department of Epidemiology and Social Medicine, Albert Einstein College of Medicine, 1300 Morris Park Avenue, Bronx, New York 10461.

of reasoning and standards of evidence accepted and employed by psychiatrists practicing in the forensic arena.

As a critical enterprise, the task of philosophy is to leave no premise unexamined, to take no assumptions for granted, and to accept no argument without thorough scrutiny. The objective is to gain as much clarity as the subject under examination will allow and to arrive at as much certainty as is humanly possible. Indeed, a fundamental philosophical question that underlies the field of epistemology asks just how much certainty is humanly possible. Achieving these objectives enables philosophy to provide sound justifications for beliefs, principles, theories, policies, and practices. Thus, philosophical inquiry into forensic psychiatry, as in any other area, demands a critical assessment of the premises that underlie the enterprise as a whole, as well as a detailed examination of particular practices and activities that constitute the parts.

EXTERNAL AND INTERNAL QUESTIONS

A distinction can be made between two kinds of critical questions philosophers have posed about a wide variety of activities or practices. (For the purposes of this essay, I will refer loosely to forensic psychiatry as an activity or practice.) This distinction sorts questions into external and internal ones. *External* questions explore the very nature and legitimacy of an enterprise, whereas *internal* questions typically accept the basic premises underlying an activity but seek justifications for specific practices, rules, roles, or judgments. An illustration from another field should clarify this distinction.

Philosophers have long inquired into the nature and functions of government: the proper role of the state, the acceptable scope of its power, the source of its authority. External questions probe the legitimacy of the state itself: What considerations can succeed in justifying the existence of a sovereign power with the authority to make rules that prescribe or proscribe certain types of conduct and to punish people who violate those rules by removing their liberty or exacting money from them?

Internal questions are typically related to those external questions, but the former presuppose that the latter have been or can be satisfactorily answered. Some internal questions, resting on the assumption that government is a legitimate institution whose general authority and power can be justified, are the following: Which form of government (representative democracy, monarchy, oligarchy) is best, and why? How wide a scope of governmental activities is permissible or desirable? Ought the state attempt to legislate morality? Should it engage in forms of censorship? Is government paternalism justified at all, and if so, over what activities and behaviors may it be imposed? If the state may legitimately punish individuals for transgressing its laws, can it justify not only removing their liberty but also taking their lives?

These are only a few of the many internal questions about the nature, scope, and legitimacy of the state raised by philosophers and political theorists over the centuries. That inquiry goes back to the writings of Plato and Aristotle, through the accounts by Locke, Hobbes, and Rousseau to Karl Marx and contemporary theorists. Analogous sets of questions, external as well as internal, have been directed at other familiar human endeavors: religious beliefs and practices, science and technology, and untold numbers of subdisciplines and pursuits ranging from astrology to parapsychology, from chiropractic to psychoanalysis. Undoubtedly well known to readers of this volume are the debates that have raged over the years concerning the theory and practice of psychiatry: the legitimacy of its claims to knowledge, the efficacy of its various modes of practice, and the proper scope and limits of both theory and practice. Several features of that more general debate about psychiatry reappear in questions raised about forensic psychiatry.

External and internal questions are often closely linked; it is easier to draw a sharp distinction analytically than it is in practice. A telling example that bears on forensic psychiatry is its acceptance of and reliance on the *parens patriae* doctrine, about which both internal and external questions are forthcoming. The questions and proposed answers constitute a blend of moral, political, psychiatric, legal, and social concerns. Under its *parens patriae* power, the state is authorized to protect the interests of those who are deemed incompetent to act on their own behalf. Such persons have typically included the mentally retarded, the mentally ill, and minors in cases where they have no parents or guardians or where their parents or guardians decide or act in ways held to be contrary to the minors' best interests. The doctrine has been used to justify a variety of coercive intrusions by the state into the lives of its citizens: sterilizing mentally retarded young women; ordering blood transfusions for Jehovah's Witness patients who refuse consent for this procedure; supervening parental decisions regarding treatment for their minor children; and providing grounds for involuntary commitment for persons judged dangerous to self, to name only the more prominent.

A broad external question addresses the legitimacy of the doctrine itself: Should the state, at any level of government, be granted the power and authority vested in it by the *parens patriae* doctrine? With the exception of anarchists, who deny the legitimacy of government as an institution, and libertarians, who accept only a minimalist state, it is widely agreed that the *parens patriae* doctrine embodies a legitimate function of the state. The justification for this function is essentially a moral one, which can be expressed in several ways. It can derive from the duty of benevolence, a general moral duty that may rest with any agent in a position to protect or help those in need. It can stem from a humanitarian concern for mentally incapacitated or otherwise disabled individuals who may suffer or perish if left uncared for. It may be thought of in utilitarian terms, holding that the government, like any moral agent, should strive to bring about "the greatest happiness for the greatest number of people," or an alternative formulation of the "principle of utility" originally propounded by the British philosophers, Jeremy Bentham[1] and John Stuart Mill.[2]

But even if an acceptable moral justification can be offered for the *parens patriae* doctrine, as a general concept embodied in statutes and in judicial decisions, numerous internal questions remain: With what justification can this doctrine be invoked to override another cherished moral value—individual liberty—when these two values come into conflict? In what situations or for what purposes may the state supervene parental decisions, presumably made in the "best interest" of their children, since this represents an intrusion into family privacy and autonomy? How incapacitated, and in what specific ways, must a person be in order to be a candidate for intervention under the doctrine? Should there be different standards or tests of competency for different purposes, and if so, what principles can be used to justify setting the standard high or low? These are only a few internal questions about the *parens patriae* doctrine, once its overall legitimacy has been accepted. These questions arise repeatedly in the form of ethical dilemmas in several areas in which forensic psychiatry relies on the doctrine: child custody proceedings, involuntary commitment cases, mental patients' refusal of treatment, and the need to determine competency for various purposes.

The challenge posed by internal questions may be as great as that arising from external questions. Often, it is hard to pinpoint a question as *internal* or *external,* especially when the issue involves fundamental values rooted in our moral and political heritage. Consider again the practice of civil commitment. It has been asserted that "involuntary confinement is the most serious deprivation of individual liberty that a society may impose."[3] This opening sentence of an article examining the justifications for civil commitment can be read either as a critical challenge to the legal and psychiatric mechanisms permitting the involuntary incarceration of persons who have committed no crime or as an internal question probing the particular circumstances and evidential bases that render such mechanisms morally permissible. In fact, the article seeks to do both, demonstrating that internal and external questions are sometimes hard to disentangle.

Or take another example, one that addresses the "best interest" doctrine as it pertains to children. Joseph Goldstein has posed a series of external questions about the meaning and utility of the best interest "doctrine."[4,5] He asserts that "as *parens patriae* the state is too crude an instrument to become an adequate substitute for parents."[6] (p. 160) Yet, after noting that parents may place their children at unwarranted risk rather than promote their survival to adulthood, Goldstein contends that "That danger justifies a policy of *minimum* state intervention rather than one of *no* state intervention."[6] (p. 161) With that acknowledgment, even this staunch opponent of state intrusion into family autonomy grants the legitimacy of *some* state intervention, thereby shifting the inquiry to an internal one: Under what precise circumstances may the state invoke its *parens patriae* powers to protect children from the decisions and actions of their parents?

External Questions about Forensic Psychiatry

To raise fundamental external questions about forensic psychiatry is to cast doubts on the legitimacy of the enterprise. Because I will end by trying to dispel many of these doubts, it is appropriate to begin with a hard critical look at the assumptions on which the activity rests. A tentative formulation of three such questions might look like this.

(1) Is not forensic psychiatry an ethically questionable activity, as placing psychiatrists in the legal arena forces them to compromise or abandon their primary professional responsibility: duties and obligations to patients?

(2) Is not forensic psychiatry an ethically questionable activity, as it presupposes the acceptability of morally controversial laws, such as ones permitting involuntary commitment, and it forces practitioners to intrude on individual rights, such as rights to liberty, rights of confidentiality, and family rights of privacy and autonomy?

(3) Is not forensic psychiatry an ethically questionable activity, because the legal requirements call on psychiatrists to make assessments, judgments, and official statements that go beyond their professional expertise?

Question (1) criticizes the enterprise on the grounds that it contains a structural moral defect; why erect such a system, with built-in ethical flaws? This external question focuses on the role responsibilities of forensic psychiatrists and assumes that the responsibilities that inhere in the psychiatrist's typical therapeutic role are identical to those in forensic practice. There is reason to question that assumption.

Question (2) raises doubts about the ideological premises on which laws and doctrines that underlie the practice of forensic psychiatry rest. If the forensic psychiatrist helps to implement morally controversial laws, or is forced into choosing among conflicting ethical and legal principles, grounds for ethical doubts about the morality of the enterprise have been established. Because there is no settled hierarchy of ethical principles, and because courts are frequently called upon to engage in "balancing" when two legal doctrines or precepts come into conflict, to impose that burden of moral choice on individual forensic psychiatrists is to cast them in a role for which they are ill prepared.

The moral force behind question (3) lies in the presumption that honesty and integrity are compromised by the demands of the law, demands that compel psychiatrists to rely on disputed facts or theories or to make judgments having considerable prognostic uncertainty. A somewhat attenuated form of this same external question applies to forensic medicine generally, because there, too, probabilistic and evidential uncertainty infects much of the material expert witnesses must testify about. Physicians from other medical specialties face the same conflicting demands: Legal proceedings require a degree of epistemic certainty that most clinicians are understandably reluctant to assert. The chief reason the problem is more severe in forensic psychiatry lies in the fact that considerably greater skepticism prevails about psychiatric theory and practice than is usually the case regarding organic medicine. This skepticism is voiced by psychiatrists themselves, as well as by "outsiders." At one extreme are the frontal attacks by critics such as Thomas Szasz[7,8] and by E. Fuller Torrey[9]—both psychiatrists. Severe critics among outsiders include civil libertarian lawyers such as Bruce Ennis.[10,11] More moderate challenges are posed by several contributors to Volume I of *Critical Issues in American Psychiatry and the Law*[12,13] and by Jonas Robitscher in his compelling book, *The Powers of Psychiatry*.[14]

I will not attempt to answer questions (1) to (3) directly. Instead, let us look first at the two chief sources that give rise to these and related external questions about forensic psychiatry. These sources are (a) the laws and judicial practices that both enable and require psychiatrists to perform in the forensic arena; and (b) the scientific status of psychiatric theory and the particular claims to knowledge on which psychiatrists base their judgments and testimonies.

Laws and Judicial Practices. Embodied in our legal system in a number of different ways are features that enable psychiatrists to legitimately enter the legal arena in a special role. Those same enabling factors also require that individuals with presumed psychiatric expertise make evaluations and offer testimony, because without that presumed expertise, the laws could not be properly executed. The *parens patriae* doctrine, the insanity defense in criminal law, the notion of the best interest of the child, the legal concept of competency (as used in competency to stand trial, to make a will, to grant or refuse informed consent for biomedical treatment or research, and competency to manage one's financial affairs), and adoption of the rehabilitative model in the penal system are the major legal features that enable and typically require psychiatrists to take on a role quite different from that of therapist, healer, counselor, or researcher. By the very act of taking on that additional role, a forensic psychiatrist confronts an array of potential moral dilemmas, some of which arise also in other psychiatric contexts and in the medical setting generally. But in forensic psychiatry, the potential conflicts abound, and they cut deeply.

Conflicts of duty or obligation and conflicts of loyalty, a pair of conflicts often placed under the heading *problems of double agency*,[15,16] are in the forefront. A classic example is the conflict between the duty to keep confidentiality, especially strong in psychiatric practice, and the duty to disclose when required by law. Furthermore, as is true of many situations people face in everyday life, forensic psychiatrists confront conflicts between moral principles, any one of which may be perfectly sound taken by itself, but all of which cannot simultaneously be followed.

A typical conflict between moral principles arises in cases of involuntary commitment justified by judgments of dangerousness to self. The ethical principle known as *"respect for persons"*[17] places the highest value on individual autonomy. A related ethical precept is couched in the language of rights: rights of freedom or liberty, the right to self-determination, the right to control one's body. In direct conflict with this precept is a different ethical principle, the principle of beneficence.[17] It requires people to choose actions that maximize benefits and minimize harms. Unless one rejects altogether either of these moral principles— respect for persons or the principle of beneficence—dilemmas resulting from their conflict are bound to arise. To opt for involuntary commitment is to risk violating a presumptive right to liberty. To act in defense of that right is to risk harm or even death to the person permitted to remain at liberty.

A second feature of the laws and judicial practices enabling psychiatrists to enter the forensic arena gives rise to another recurring moral dilemma: the need for psychiatrists to reply to questions and to make determinations that go beyond their professional training and expertise. A related problem, one that derives from the standards of evidence in judicial proceedings, is the need in that context for psychiatrists to respond to queries with more certainty than their professional judgment would otherwise allow. Forthright honesty calls for one decision or action, and maximizing the chances for a good outcome in the case often pulls in the opposite direction. This points to an irony in the psychiatrist's role in the forensic setting. The court's reliance on psychiatric expertise in making its judicial determination poses a genuine dilemma for the psychiatrist who possesses both expertise and integrity. As an expert in his field, the psychiatrist not only has knowledge that the nonexpert lacks; but also, a crucial aspect of that expertise is the knowledge of what he does not and cannot know, what he cannot predict, and his awareness of an irreducible uncertainty that pervades psychiatric judgments, evaluations, and prognoses. This dimension of expertise— knowing what one does not know and cannot know in the nature of the case—when conjoined with the virtue of integrity, gives rise to an external question that casts doubt on the legitimacy of forensic psychiatry. It may go even farther, creating an aura of skepticism about the morality of forensic psychiatry as a societal institution.

A topic of ongoing controversy, the debate over whether psychiatrists can and should engage in predicting dangerousness, cuts across these separate yet related external questions. The debate reflects disagreements both about facts and about values. Factual disagreements center around the accuracy with which psychiatrists are capable of predicting dangerousness and the question of what methods or assessment tools work best for this purpose. Value disagreements include the fundamental moral controversy that surrounds removal of a persons's right to liberty when that person has not (yet) violated the law, pitted against the potential harm that may befall innocent victims. Which moral value should take precedence: the individual's right to liberty? Or the duty to prevent harm whenever possible?

I have not attempted to provide an ethical analysis of the issues raised by laws and judicial practices that enable psychiatrists to play a role in the forensic arena. Instead, I have described some of the moral conflicts and dilemmas inherent in that role, and have indicated why those moral conflicts give rise to a number of external questions about the legitimacy of forensic psychiatry. The demands of the role adopted by the forensic psychiatrist depart from those of the psychiatrist practicing under the traditional medical model and create built-in conflicts of responsibility, obligation, and loyalty. This intrinsic potential for moral conflict forms the locus on one critical attack. It is a species of a larger genre: problems of double agency. Institutional psychiatry, prison psychiatry, and mental health workers in schools, the military, and industry all face similar conflicts in their professional setting. There is, moreover, a different source of external questions about forensic psychiatry: the scientific status of psychiatric theory and the knowledge base on which particular judgments rest.

Scientific Status and Data Base of Psychiatry. It lies well beyond the scope of this essay to review the controversy surrounding the scientific status of psychiatry, the global warfare waged by the various factions that comprise the antipsychiatry movement, and the many skirmishes in the internecine conflicts among competing schools within psychiatry and among psychiatry, psychology, and other mental health disciplines. It should suffice to note that even if the extremist attack on psychiatry (as represented by Thomas Szasz and his followers) is disregarded, there remains a central core of concern about the scientific status of psychiatry and about the knowledge base for at least some of the judgments forensic psychiatrists are called on to make. Probably more than any other medical specialty, psychiatry continues to abound with multiple, coexisting theories and therapies, from organic and biochemical approaches, now on the rise, to social, behavioral, and cognitive schools, to the still-entrenched psychoanalytic wing of the profession. Correctly or incorrectly, justifiably or not, it appears to the outsider (hence, external questions) that psychiatry as a whole suffers from an absence of a well-confirmed general theory of human behavior and psychopathology, and from a lack of agreement on a wide variety of topics among large numbers of professional practitioners.

Although these features need not be grounds for rejecting the entire enterprise of psychiatry in its therapeutic role, they nonetheless present a serious challenge to the activity of forensic psychiatry. How can there be expert witnesses and expert testimony for legal purposes, the objection runs, when there is such widespread disagreement among alleged experts on fundamental matters of theory, etiology, preferred treatment approaches, the definition of success in therapy, and the rest?

If the requisite level of expertise in the legal arena is impossible for the discipline of psychiatry to meet, then forensic psychiatry violates a basic ethical presupposition: *Ought implies can.* Simply put, before moral obligations, duties, or responsibilities are ascribed, it must be possible for those to whom they are ascribed to fulfill them. If psychiatrists lack the requisite expertise to make judgments and assessments for legal purposes, then there ought not exist a system or mechanism that both enables and requires them to do so. The "ought implies can" maxim, a general ethical presupposition, has clear application to forensic psychiatry. External questions about the legitimacy of forensic psychiatry and the validity of its underlying assumptions constitute grounds for moral skepticism about the nature of the activity.

Family Law: A Paradigm Case. Family law offers a paradigm case in which the several considerations that give rise to external questions come together. All three of the tentatively formulated questions posed earlier apply to this area of forensic psychiatry. To begin examination of this illustrative paradigm, recall first the viewpoint of Joseph Goldstein and his collaborators, who deny all but the most minimal role to the state in exercising its *parens patriae* power regarding children. That viewpoint is rooted in a particular theoretical orientation in psychiatry—a strong interpretation of psychoanalytic theory—and it also reveals a wide-spread but dubious metaethical presupposition known as *ethical relativism*.

From his preferred theoretical perspective, Goldstein argues that

> the right of parents to raise their children as they think best, free of coercive intervention, comports . . . with each child's biological and psychological need for unthreatened and unbroken continuity of care by his parents. . . . There is little doubt that . . . breaches in the familial bond will be detrimental to a child's well-being.[6] (p. 159)

As general psychological claims, these statements cannot be faulted. But when they are invoked in order to rebut state supervention of parental refusal of medical treatments recommended for their children, and when they are used to deny categorically the appropriateness of joint custody following a divorce, these theory-laden judgments assume the air of ideology.

This strong theoretical bias, in the absence of confirming evidence in the form of "well-designed longitudinal studies of the growth and development of statistically significant numbers of children,"[12] (p. 167) leaves Goldstein and his colleagues open to critical attack:

> In these books, psychoanalytic theory is applied to family court issues and numerous specific recommendations are presented for consideration and implementation. . . . As serious research or as reports of serious research, they are worse than valueless—they are dangerous. The firm beliefs of the authors color their interpretations of their clinical data, and their convictions overpower their critical judgment.[12] (p. 167)

But it is not only Goldstein's psychoanalytic bias that opens him to critical attack; it is also his adherence to a radical form of ethical relativism. A widely held metaethical view, ethical relativism denies that there is any objective basis for making moral judgments: What is right for one person, or culture, or time, or place may be wrong for another. That is a potentially pernicious thesis about ethics. It is possible that Goldstein would not embrace ethical relativism as a general metaethical position, but he certainly expresses one version of it in his rejection of the "best interest" doctrine as it pertains to the role of the law in parenting. Addressing the situation in which parents refuse medical treatment for a child, Goldstein writes:

> how can parents in such situations give the wrong answer since there is no way of knowing the right answer? . . . Precisely because there is no objectively wrong or right answer, the burden must be on the state to establish *wrong*, not on the parent to establish that what is *right* for them is necessarily *right* for others.[6] (pp. 166–67)

In contrast to Goldstein's almost dogmatic adherence to psychoanalytic theory, at one extreme, is his skepticism regarding the objectivity of moral judgments, at the other.

There remain other, more general sources of external questions about psychiatric expertise and family law. In addition to the problems just discussed, the theoretical biases of psychiatrists and the lack of adequate clinical data, further areas of uncertainty and conflict are the ambiguous role responsibilities and divided loyalties psychiatrists face in the forensic setting. These problems of double-agency are aptly characterized by Rosner:

> If the case entails functioning as a friend of the court, as *amicus curiae*, many forensic psychiatrists believe that the ethical commitment is to the family law/juvenile justice system rather than to the individual child or adolescent. This may entail advising the court about data that will lead to an outcome inconsistent with the wishes of the child, the adolescent, and his parents. The forensic psychiatrist in that setting has a loyalty to society as a whole as embodied in the judicial system rather than to the person he has examined.[12] (p. 162)

Rosner is unequivocal in stating that

> in such settings, a doctor–patient relationship does not exist. It is essential for the forensic psychiatrist to understand this nontherapeutic role from the beginning and to advise the child, the adolescent, and the parents that the materials that they provide will *not* be held in confidence.[12] (p. 162)

This view is seconded by a number of commentators on problems of double agency in psychiatry,[16] most of whom concur that the obligations and loyalties psychiatrists owe to their patients in the prototypical private practice situation are largely if not entirely absent in institutional and forensic settings.

Internal Questions

Even if satisfactory responses to the external questions can be offered, there remain a host of internal questions to contend with. The line between external and internal questions is not a bright one. This is because acceptance of the fundamental legitimacy of forensic psychiatry does not guarantee satisfactory answers to specific questions regarding psychiatric expertise in the various areas covered by forensic psychiatry. Also, an overall acceptance of the enterprise still leaves room for critical doubts in cases in which lack of intersubjective agreement persists.

Specific questions about forensic psychiatry may fall into one of several categories. A rough schema is as follows.

Epistemic Questions. Put generally, is the theoretical or evidential base sufficiently valid or well-confirmed to warrant the use of psychiatrists as experts in particular areas of forensic psychiatry?

Examples. Is enough known and agreed on concerning good or adequate parenting to warrant a reliance on psychiatric judgments in child custody proceedings?

Is there a theoretical or clinical basis (other than evidence from past behavior of a particular person) for making sufficiently accurate predictions of dangerousness to justify psychiatric testimony leading to involuntary commitment?

Is there a sufficiently well-confirmed theory about the causes of and remedies for aggressive or violent behavior to warrant the acceptance of psychiatric assessments regarding the "rehabilitation" of violent offenders?

These epistemic questions arise as well in specific cases in which psychiatric judgments or testimonies are called for. Whether or not the general questions can be answered in the affirmative, it is likely that in some cases the evidence will be insufficient or intersubjective disagreement so pervasive as to cast doubt on the appropriateness of settling the matter by an appeal to the expertise of forensic psychiatry. The "ought implies can" precept applies directly to these situations.

Value Questions. (1) Setting standards. What moral presumptions should underlie the setting of standards for certain psychiatric assessments in the forensic context?

Example. Should tests of competency (to stand trial, to make a will, to grant informed consent) be set high, thus compromising the subject's rights of self-determination for the sake of other values? Or should tests of competency be set low, maximizing the subject's freedom and autonomy, yet carrying the risk that his decisions and actions will fail to serve his other interests (physical health or financial well being, for instance)?[18-20]

(2) Conflicts of loyalty. How should inevitable conflicts of loyalty or duty on the part of forensic psychiatrists be resolved? Should a general presumption lie in favor of the patient or client? Should there be no general presumption in favor of one side or the other when obligations or loyalties conflict, but instead, should priorities be determined for each particular conflict?

Examples. Should a psychiatrist who has been treating a patient and who has grounds to suspect that patient may pose a danger to others owe primary loyalty to the patient? Or does the obligation to protect innocent members of society render it the psychiatrist's higher duty to break confidentiality and disclose information to the authorities or to specific persons thought to be in danger?

Can a prison psychiatrist make legitimate promises of confidentiality to a prisoner who appears to pose no threat of violence? Or does the role of prison psychiatrist demand overriding loyalty to the employing institution?

This schema divides questions somewhat artificially into epistemic and value questions. But it should be clear that the way in which the epistemic questions are answered has ethical implications, and the value questions, in turn, rest on deeper epistemological foundations. Moral dilemmas in forensic psychiatry, as elsewhere in applied ethics, can frequently be traced to a conflict of moral principles: paradigmatically, respect for the rights of the individual versus protection of the interests of others. But a broader underlying conflict stems from two fundamentally different ethical perspectives drawn from two prominent philosophical traditions: the consequentialist moral perspective and the deontological approach to ethics. A brief look at these classic philosophical approaches should make it clear why the roots of moral conflict are often deep.

Consequentialism.   Briefly stated, *consequentialism* is the theoretical perspective in ethics that makes results, outcomes, or consequences the morally relevant features of actions or practices. It is the approach explicitly or implicitly embodied in medical practice, expressed in simplistic maxims such as "do no harm". And it underlies the more complex task of making risk–benefit assessments in the conduct of biomedical treatment and research. The basic moral principle that lies at the heart of consequentialism has a number of different formulations. For our purposes here, the version referred to earlier as *"the principle of beneficence"* is most suitable: Maximize possible benefits and minimize possible harms.

Applications of the principle of beneficence in the realm of forensic psychiatry are numerous. They include the "best interest" doctrine in child custody proceedings, a doctrine whose aim is to ensure the best outcomes for a child's character development, psychological adjustment, and overall mental health. Another application is the justification for civil commitment, as noted earlier in discussing the clash between respecting an individual's rights and seeking to protect his interests. That conflict of moral principles not only arises when the grounds for commitment are dangerousness to self; it occurs just as intractably when the basis for commitment is dangerousness to others. In the latter case, however, it is not the *parens patriae* doctrine that underlies the state's authority to limit the rights of its citizens; rather, it is the state's interest in protecting its members from harm at the hands of internal or external aggressors.

The principle of beneficence can serve as a moral justification for setting a high standard of competency for psychiatric evaluations for testamentary and informed consent purposes. If a person exhibits uncertain mental capacity, it is frequently assumed that the best consequences for that person and perhaps others, such as relatives who stand to be affected by that person's actions, will come about if psychiatrists adopt a high standard for judging competency.

Consequentialism, as a moral perspective, also underlies the rehabilitative model in the criminal justice system. An alternative to the retributive model of punishment, the rehabilitative model rests on the assumption that offenders have a mental or emotional condition that can be cured, ameliorated, or modified by prison programs and therapeutic interventions. As a result of such rehabilitation, the consequences both for offenders themselves and for society are believed to be better than those that would result if prison were limited to confinement and punishment.

To point out the justificatory role of the principle of beneficence or other formulations of consequentialism for acts or existing practices in forensic psychiatry is not to beg the question of whether they actually succeed in bringing about better consequences than would alternative acts or practices. That conclusion could only be drawn after sufficient empirical observations and confirmation. Consequentialism can be properly applied only when there is adequate evidence, prospectively or retrospectively, that practices such as civil commitment do, in fact, result in better consequences for the individual or society than the abandonment of the practice altogether would be likely to bring about. Perhaps more than any other moral principle, the consequentialist approach must be based on solid evidential foundations in order to provide a legitimate moral justification for limiting individual liberty.

Deontologism. Failure to recognize the relevance or legitimacy of a competing moral perspective, deontologism, has led many physicians to be puzzled if not disdainful when confronted with appeals to patients' autonomy, their rights of self-determination, privacy, and liberty. Typical expressions of this attitude can be seen in the spate of responses to recent court cases granting institutionalized mental patients the right to refuse psychoactive drugs.[21-25] Yet opposition to this trend is understandable, given the salient value in medical practice of bringing about good outcomes. The predominant ethos in medicine over the centuries has been paternalistic, leading physicians to act in their patients' best interests, even when patients have disagreed about what those best interests are. The deontological moral perspective, expressed in the "respect for persons" principle noted earlier, has its philosophical roots in the ethical theory of Immanual Kant and his followers. Central to this moral perspective is the notion that individuals should be treated as autonomous agents, where "an autonomous person is an individual capable of deliberation about personal goals and of acting under the direction of such deliberation"[17] (p. 4).

However, the fact that not every individual is fully capable of self-determination gives rise to a related moral requirement: that those with diminished autonomy stand in need of protection. If full autonomy presupposes the capacity to deliberate about personal goals and to act under the direction of such deliberation, it is evident that some individuals lack this capacity. "The principle of respect for persons thus divides into two separate moral requirements: the requirement to acknowledge autonomy and the requirement to protect those with diminished autonomy"[17] (p. 4).

This second requirement serves to legitimate a form of paternalism that has been termed *"weak paternalism"*: limitations of individual liberty in circumstances where conduct is substantially nonvoluntary or when temporary intervention is necessary to establish whether it is voluntary or not.[26] Some commentators argue that this should not be classified as paternalism at all, and that the term should be confined to limitations of the liberty of fully autonomous agents.[26,27] Semantic quibbles aside, the task is to arrive at a suitable set of criteria for making determinations of an individual's autonomy, or capacity for rational deliberation. This is the task psychiatrists are frequently called upon to undertake when they evaluate people in order to determine their competency.[18–20, 28–30]

Determining Competency. Competency determinations have a technical aspect and a value aspect. The technical aspect requires psychiatric expertise, experience, and clinical judgment. But determinations of competency also have an irreducible value component: the need to set the level of competency high or low for the purpose at hand. This is where a balance must be struck between the two ethical requirements of deontologism, the requirement to acknowledge autonomy, and the requirement to protect those with diminished autonomy. It takes more than technical, psychiatric expertise to arrive at a suitable balance between these two moral requirements. How that balance is struck typically rests on a number of factors: the purpose for which the competency evaluation is made; the prevailing ideological currents of the time and place; the subjective biases of the psychiatrist making the evaluation; and perhaps other features of the situation. This is one of the areas of forensic psychiatry in which ethical considerations provoke a series of internal questions: Is it better to err on the side of acknowledging autonomy or in the direction of protecting diminished autonomy? For what purposes should a standard for determining competency be set high, and for what purposes should the presumption lie in favor of a lower standard of competency? Should the profession strive to develop a uniform set of criteria, or should things remain essentially as they are now, leaving the standard for making evaluations largely up to the individual psychiatrist?

Answers to these and other internal questions about forensic psychiatry can be informed by an ethical analysis, but no clear, unequivocal answer can be forthcoming by an appeal to moral principles. The reason should be obvious by now: competing ethical principles are at work here, and the quest for a resolution of those conflicts of principle is rooted in the foundations of ethics. No satisfactory resolution of the conflict between the competing moral perspectives embodied in deontologism and consequentialism has been forthcoming, despite long-standing efforts by untold numbers of philosophers and others grappling with the problem. The pragmatic necessity that confronts forensic psychiatrists in their ongoing work cannot await the solution to this intractable theoretical dispute. It would be demanding more than moral philosophy could possibly deliver to ask for a clear mandate from ethical theory when moral problems in applied or professional ethics can be traced to conflicts of principle.

THE VALUE OF PHILOSOPHICAL ANALYSIS

If moral philosophy cannot provide answers when confronted with ethical dilemmas traceable to conflicts of principle, what, then, is its value? Is the application of ethical theory to a field such as forensic psychiatry anything but a source of intellectual stimulation for underlaborers with a philosophical background? These questions demand some response, along the following lines.

The first point to note is the circumscribed area in which philosophy stops short of the hoped-for goal of resolving ethical problems in practice. The area in which applied ethics can provide no solutions is that in which the moral problems stem from a conflict of fundamental ethical principles—principles that lie at the heart of leading moral theories. Such conflicts of fundamental principles comprise a distinct minority of the overall concerns of ethics. Although they command a great deal of attention on the part of philosophers and professionals from a variety of disciplines interested in ethics, the incidence and prevalence of insoluble dilemmas are considerably lower than might be indicated by the attention they receive. A bit of reflection reveals that the majority of ethical problems can be satisfactorily addressed through careful understanding and analysis of the facts and values they embody, and by appeal to an appropriate moral principle that is applicable to the case and does not clash with a competing principle.

A second point to recall is that philosophical analysis, even when focused primarily on ethical concerns, is rarely limited to those concerns. Conceptual analysis and epistemological inquiry are part and parcel of any philosophical enterprise and can go a long way toward attaining clarity and reaching closure on a problematic issue. An example referred to earlier in this essay is the confusion surrounding the "best interest" doctrine. A phrase like "the best interest of the patient" is frequently invoked without an adequate explication of its meaning. This is not to suggest that professionals working in their own disciplines are incapable of such explication, or that the task must be left entirely to philosophers. It is generally true, however, that the meanings of concepts are assumed rather than spelled out by those who use them most often. Misunderstandings and talking at cross-purposes are likely to result from the vagueness and ambiguity of terms having wide currency but lacking in precision. Because of their training in conceptual analysis and their skill in detecting ambiguity and vagueness, philosophers stand to contribute in ways that can lead to a resolution of practical problems involving value considerations.

The role philosophers play in identifying ethical dimensions, structuring the issues, and clarifying the nature of problems in applied contexts is one about which professionals in those fields have expressed gratitude. Physicians unschooled in philosophical analysis sometimes recognize their own inability to grapple with ethical problems; at other times, they contend that there exists no special expertise regarding ethics. A demonstration of what philosophical inquiry can do to foster an understanding and promote a resolution of perplexing practical problems does much to dispel doubts about the kind of expertise necessary for approaching ethical issues in a systematic way.

Because of the premium placed on logical reasoning and correct modes of inference, philosophy is well-suited to pointing out inconsistencies and contradictions in thought and practice. Although the value of philosophical analysis is not limited to its ability to detect informal fallacies as well as glaring errors in logic, it represents still another area in which philosophical expertise is desirable. Consequentialist reasoning is the dominant mode in psychiatry and in medical decision making, yet outside their own professional practice, physicians adhere to deontological as well as to other values. It may come as a surprise to those who act paternalistically in their professional setting, and indeed, defend their own paternalistic behavior and that of their colleagues, to learn that such behavior is inconsistent with general principles they apply to themselves and others outside their professional context. Recognition of such inconsistencies of belief and action may not result in a change in those beliefs and actions, but an honest appraisal demands an acknowledgement of these contradictions.

Finally, and most importantly, philosophers possess the analytic tools, the skills of argumentation, and the knowledge of ethical theory and principles to provide justifications for behavior. In the forensic arena, where intraprofessional and interprofessional disagreement abounds, parties to a dispute may be reduced to name-calling, to *ad hominem* arguments, or to uttering the useless phrase, "That's your opinion," in the absence of being able to provide a sound justification for their own position. Psychiatrists and others who listen and learn from philosophers in this regard stand to gain much that can aid in providing a solid defense for their past or prospective actions or for their firmly held beliefs. It is surely better to be able to defend one's views by rational argument, perhaps even to persuade others of the correctness of those views, than to take refuge in the claim that "We all have our own ethics," or that "All ethics has its roots in religious beliefs, so there's nothing to discuss." Both statements, and their variants, are not only unhelpful; they are also largely false. The skills required for providing rational justifications enable philosophers to contribute to ongoing debates within and about psychiatry, with psychiatrists acknowledging their indebtedness.

Despite the inability of philosophers to resolve the intractable ethical dilemmas that stem from a conflict of fundamental principles, they nonetheless can confer a range of benefits. Identifying ethical issues, structuring those issues in a systematic way, teasing out the moral principles that underlie practical problems and dilemmas, introducing clarity and precision, and providing rational justifications for beliefs and actions are the chief contributions that philosophy can make in its applications to other disciplines. These contributions stand to be illuminating in theory and helpful in practice to professionals who are willing to allow outsiders to engage in critical scrutiny of their own enterprise.

CONCLUSION: FORENSIC PSYCHIATRY DEFENDED

In light of the critical scrutiny philosophy brings to its every object of inquiry, how can doubts about forensic psychiatry, such as those raised in this essay, be dispelled? Are there satisfactory replies to the external questions posed here and elsewhere? Are challenges in the form of internal questions any easier to answer? It is probably impossible, if not unwise, to try to dispel all skeptical doubts about forensic psychiatry, since some of those doubts are warranted. An adequate defense of the overall enterprise can only succeed if it takes the form of a consequentialist justification. That justification requires detailed, systematic answers to two broad questions: (a) Is society as a whole benefited more than it is harmed? and (b) Are the outcomes better, for all those who are affected by forensic psychiatry, than they would be if the practice did not exist at all?

These questions are value-laden, but an attempt to answer them requires adequate empirical evidence as well as an appeal to the underlying moral principle of utility. The best way to gather the empirical evidence would be to conduct a controlled social experiment comparing two large groups in society: one in which forensic psychiatry operated, and one in which the activity was absent. This methodology offers the only valid scientific means of gathering data for the comparison needed to provide a consequentialist justification. It would be much less satisfactory methodologically to make a historical or cross-cultural comparison, as "observation in nature" methodology fails to control for too many crucial variables. However, practical, legal, and probably also ethical barriers stand in the way of mounting such a social experiment. The only method remaining is a *gedanken* experiment, a rational reconstruction of the likely consequences of eliminating the practice of forensic psychiatry from our medical-legal system. The thought experiment is left to the reader. But the canons of inquiry should be made clear, and the philosophical methodology must be rigorous. The criteria for what is to count as "good" and "bad" consequences need to be spelled out. There should be a procedure for determining when good consequences outweigh bad ones, or the reverse, in each individual case. Ethical premises and value priorities have to be acknowledged and spelled out: Should individual liberty, autonomy, and rights be introduced into the consequentialist calculations? If so, how can these two philosophical approaches be made commensurable? How are medical and treatment needs to be balanced against a patient's or subject's own informed, quality-of-life choices and decisions? Can acts or practices by forensic psychiatrists, sanctioned by paternalistic laws, be justified by their actual or probable good consequences? Could the judgment that they are so justified be tested empirically with results that could produce intersubjective agreement?

Having conducted this thought experiment, I conclude, with provision, that medical patients, mental patients, criminally insane defendants, and possibly also prisoners not diagnosed as having a mental disorder are better off with forensic psychiatry in the picture than they would be without it. An attempt at a consequentialist justification, whether by social experiment in the real world or by thought experiment in the realm of ideas, is the only way to reply to the broad external questions about forensic psychiatry posed in this essay. The internal questions need to be addressed one at a time, and in each case the epistemic as well as the value questions must be answered satisfactorily. It might turn out, for example, that a considerable number of situations in family law cannot bear the scrutiny of a critical inquiry into the role of forensic psychiatry. Could adequate evidence be marshalled to support the conclusion that child custody decisions following divorce require psychiatric expertise to ensure that the child's best interest is served? When neither divorcing parent suffers from gross psychopathology, the realm of psychiatric expertise is narrowed to the point where judgments about adequate or optimal parenting can be readily contested. Neither an actual social experiment nor a thought experiment is likely to yield clear enough conclusions to warrant confidence in the role forensic psychiatrists have assumed in child custody determinations. Perhaps the same can be said for other areas of family law in which psychiatrists play a legally sanctioned role.

To engage in armchair speculations on the outcomes of hypothetical research, however tempting, is bad science and bad ethics. There is no adequate substitute for rigorous inquiry, whether philosophical or empirical. Forensic psychiatry could be better served by subjecting itself to ongoing critical scrutiny, including a study of the myriad norms and values that permeate the practice, than by offering defensive replies to polemical attacks.

REFERENCES

[1]Bentham, J: *An Introduction to the Principles of Morals and Legislation.* New York, Hafner, 1948.

[2]Mill, JS: *Utilitarianism.* New York, Bobbs-Merrill, 1957.

[3]Livermore, JM, Malmquist, CP, and Meehl, PE: On the justifications for civil commitment, 117 *U. PA. L. REV. 75* (1968).

[4]Goldstein, J, Freud A, and Solnit, A: *Beyond the Best Interests of the Child.* New York, The Free Press, 1973.

[5]Goldstein, J, Freud A, and Solnit, A: *Before the Best Interests of the Child.* New York, The Free Press, 1979.

[6]Goldstein, J: Medical care for the child at risk: On state supervention of parental autonomy, in Gaylin, W. and Macklin, R. (Eds.): *Who Speaks for the Child: The Problems of Proxy Consent.* New York, Plenum Press, 1982.

[7]Szasz, TS: *The Myth of Mental Illness.* New York, Hoeber-Harper, 1961.

[8]Szasz, TS: *Law, Liberty and Psychiatry: An Inquiry into the Social Uses of Mental Health Practices.* New York, Macmillan, 1963.

[9]Torrey, EF: *The Death of Psychiatry.* Radnor, Pennsylvania, Chilton, 1974.

[10]Ennis, BJ, and Litwack, TR: Psychiatry and the presumption of expertise: Flipping coins in the courtroom, 62 *Cal. L. Rev. 693* (1974).

[11]Ennis, BJ: Civil liberties and mental illness, 7 *Crim. Law Bull. 101* (1971).

[12]Rosner, R: Misguided loyalty, therapeutic grandiosity, and scientific ignorance: Limitations on psychiatric contributions to family law and juvenile justice, in Rosner, R (ed): *Critical Issues in American Psychiatry and the Law.* Springfield, IL, Charles C Thomas, 1982.

[13]Gorovitz, S: Could Oliver Wendell Holmes, Jr., and Sigmund Freud work together if Socrates were watching? in Rosner, R (ed): *Critical Issues in American Psychiatry and the Law.* Springfield, IL, Charles C Thomas, 1982.

[14]Robitscher, J: *The Powers of Psychiatry.* Boston, Houghton Mifflin, 1980.

[15]Halleck, SL: *The Politics of Therapy.* New York, Harper & Row, 1971.

[16]*In the service of the state: The psychiatrist as double agent,* Hastings Center Report 8, Special Supplement, 1978.

[17]National Commission for the Protection of Human Subjects: *The Belmont Report: Ethical*

Principles and Guidelines for the Protection of Human Subjects of Research. Washington, DC, U.S. Department of Health, Education & Welfare, 1979.

[18]Roth, LH, Meisel, A, and Lidz, CW: Tests of competency to consent to treatment. *Am J Psychiatry 134*:279–284, 1977.

[19]Appelbaum, PS, and Roth, LH: Competency to consent to research: A psychiatric overview. *Arch Gen Psychiatry 39*:951–958, 1982.

[20]Freedman, B: Competence, marginal and otherwise. *Int J Law Psychiatry 4*:53–72, 1981.

[21]Appelbaum, PS, and Gutheil, TG: Drug refusal: A study of psychiatric inpatients. *Am J Psychiatry 137*:340–346, 1980.

[22]Appelbaum, PS, and Gutheil, TG: Rotting with their rights on: Constitutional theory and clinical reality in drug refusal by psychiatric patients. *Bull AAPL 7*:306–315, 1980.

[23]Appelbaum, PS, and Gutheil, TG: The Boston state hospital case: "Involuntary mind control," the constitution and the "right to rot." *Am J Psychiatry 137*:720–723, 1980.

[24]Shwed, H: Social policy and the rights of the mentally ill: time for the re-examination. *J Health Politics Policy Law 5*:193–198, 1980.

[25]Tancredi, LR: The rights of mental patients: Weighing the interests. *J Health Politics Policy Law 5*:199–204, 1980.

[26]Feinberg, J: Legal paternalism. *Canadian J Phil 1*:105–124, 1971.

[27]Beauchamp, TL: Paternalism and bio-behavioral control, in Beauchamp, TL, Walters, L (eds.): *Contemporary Issues in Bioethics.* Encino, CA, Dickenson, 1978, pp 522–529.

[28]Macklin, R: Problems of informed consent with the cognitively impaired, in Pfaff, DW (ed.): *Ethical Questions in Brain and Behavior.* New York, Springer-Verlag, 1983.

[29]Macklin, R: Treatment refusals: Autonomy, paternalism, and the "best interest" of the patient, in Pfaff DW (ed): *Ethical Questions in Brain and Behavior.* New York, Springer-Verlag, 1983.

[30]Miller, BL: *Autonomy and the refusal of lifesaving treatment, Hastings Center Report 11*:22–28, 2981.

II

Violence and Dangerousness

3

Violence, Psychiatry, and the Law
A Historical Perspective

JACQUES M. QUEN

The *Oxford English Dictionary* requires seven and a half columns, or more than two pages, to define violence and violent. The first definition is "The exercise of physical force so as to inflict injury on, or cause damage to, persons or property; action or conduct characterized by this; treatment or usage tending to cause bodily injury or forcibly interfering with personal freedom." It also includes examples of violence to feelings and conscience.[1]

For those who consider this definition too "nonlegal," we can look at a classic American legal dictionary, more than 100 years old. It defines violence as

> The abuse of force. . . . That force which is employed against the common right, against the laws, and against public liberty . . . violence is not confined to an actual assault of the person, by beating, knocking down, or forcibly wresting from him; on the contrary, whatever goes to intimidate or overawe, by the apprehension of personal violence or by fear of life, with a view to compel . . . equally falls within its limits.[2]

One might consider the definition of violence that John Monohan uses in his monograph *The Clinical Prediction of Violent Behavior*. "Acts

---

JACQUES M. QUEN • Payne Whitney Clinic, New York Hospital, 525 East 68th Street, New York, New York 10021.
Read at the Annual Symposium of the Tri-State Chapter of the American Academy of Psychiatry and the Law, at the New York University Medical Center, 23 January 1982.

characterized by the application or overt threat of force which is likely to result in injury to people." Monohan elaborates this by adding that "*injury*" shall be taken to mean physical injury; that the notion of "*threat*" is included so that the definition will encompass armed robbery or other situations in which injury is threatened but not accomplished; and that the notion "*likely*" is included so that shooting at someone will be considered violent even if the bullets miss.[3] Unfortunately, this definition implicitly excludes violence to one's self, such as self-mutilation and suicide.

One should include, in any consideration of violence, the implied, inferred, or perceived nonexplicit threat, including menacing behavior, as sensed or experienced by the "reasonable individual." One should also consider the inflicting of pain, without physical damage, in order to compel, punish, or intimidate as, a form of violence. Without such an addition, many ancient and modern coercive tortures or punishments would be eliminated from consideration. Furthermore, the constricting of the concept of violence to physical harm only seems to involve a radical disregard of the concerns and values of the eighteenth century American revolutionaries and the framers of their Constitution. I think we can agree that the definitions of violence are complicated, varied, and context dependent. Unless explicitly defined at the time people discuss it, the concept of violence will mean different things to each person.

In considering the history of violence, psychiatry, and the law, I shall skip over the striking example of the violence attributed to the first human born of humans as described in the Bible.[4] I shall begin, rather, with the findings of a study of homicide in late medieval England (the fourteenth and fifteenth centuries). "So common was violent death from homicide that in medieval London . . . , the man in the street ran more of a risk from dying at the hands of a fellow citizen than he did from an accident. There were 43% more deaths by homicide than by misadventure [accident]." Ninety-three percent of the accused murderers were men and seven per cent were women. Ninety percent of the victims were men and 10% were women. Twenty-five percent to 31% of the homicides occurred in the course of burglary or robbery. This was an effective way of diminishing the number of witnesses.[5]

In this study, Barbara Hannawalt considered the important issue of society's response and judgement of the relative acceptability of different kinds of violence. She found that juries were more inclined to condemn damage to property than homicide. This was not a function of the punishment, as both were capital crimes.

What were the findings relative to the insane? In one rural area, out of a total of 347 homicides, 1 was attributed to insanity. In London, of a total of 112 homicides, none were attributed to insanity. Hannawalt reported that, generally, the cases in which the medieval juries assigned insanity as the motivation for homicide were those of parents (usually the mother) who killed their children. This sort of case usually involved an attempted suicide in addition to the murder of the children. One mother came home after a suicide attempt and stabbed her 2-year-old daughter with a knife and forced her 4-year-old to sit on the flames in the hearth.[5]

Another case of insane violence, 3 centuries later, was that of Edward Arnold, known to his neighbors as "Crazy Ned" and tried in 1724 for the attempted murder of Lord Onslow. Arnold believed that Lord Onslow had sent demons and "bolleroys" into his body to plague him. It was at Arnold's trial that Judge Tracy charged the jury with what later came to be known, unfortunately, as the "Wild Beast" test:

> It is not every kind of frantic humour, or something unaccountable in a man's actions, that points him out to be such a madman, as is exempted from punishment: it must be a man, that is totally deprived of his understanding and memory, and doth not know what he is doing, no more than an infant, than a brute, or a wild beast, such a one is never the object of punishment.

Arnold was convicted and sentenced to hang. The recovered Lord Onslow interceded and Arnold's sentence was commuted to life imprisonment.[6]

The legal criteria for exculpable insanity were not well defined. Lord Mathew Hale, a leading British judge who died in 1695, offered as his rule that only perfect, as opposed to partial, insanity would exculpate for criminal acts. Although many have insisted that Hale meant some bizarre, near-decerebrate state, those who finished reading the rest of that sentence know that Hale explained that he meant a state in which the understanding was less than that *ordinarily possessed by the ordinary 14-year-old.*[7]

Philippe Pinel, in his *Treatise on Insanity* (1801),[8] described a condition he called *manie sans délire*, an insanity that was characterized by episodes of homicidal fury in an individual who otherwise spoke and behaved in a sane fashion. Initially greeted with scepticism and disbelief, it was later confirmed by Esquirol of France, Heinroth of Germany, Prichard of England, and Isaac Ray in America. There was vehement objection expressed by the public and by some psychiatrists to the acknowledging of a disease whose only manifestation appeared to be criminal behavior and that would encourage the depraved and criminal element in society to commit crimes with a protective medical shield. *Manie sans délire* later became grouped with the concepts of monomania, moral insanity, affective psychoses, alcoholism, pyromania, kleptomania, and most recently with the DSM-III 312.34 and 312.35 (intermittent explosive disorder and isolated explosive disorder).

In 1800, James Hadfield, a former soldier who had received obvious head wounds in battle, fired a shot in the direction of King George III. Hadfield had the delusion that God was going to destroy mankind, but that the destruction could be averted by the sacrifice of his own life. He did not want to commit the sin of suicide, and he knew that attempted regicide was a capital crime. Hadfield's subsequent acquittal on the ground of insanity was responsible for the first English statute authorizing the detention of those acquitted of felonies on the basis of insanity, as well as the form of the verdict (Not Guilty by Reason of Insanity, NGRI). It was also at the Hadfield trial that the burden of proof of sanity was assigned to the prosecution, and that the jury was instructed that if the scales "hung anything like even," to throw in "an extra portion of mercy for the party."[9]

The next major trial for criminal violence by an insane person was that of John Bellingham, in 1812, for the murder of Lord Spencer Perceval, First Lord of the Exchequer and Prime Minister. The homicide occurred on Monday, May 11th; the defense attorneys were notified of their appointment on Thursday evening, May 14th; and the trial began on Friday morning, May 15th. Ignoring the Hadfield case, including any precedents established in it, Judge Mansfield charged the jury with judging the knowledge of right and wrong as the *only* relevant issue in determining Bellingham's mental state and culpability. That afternoon, the jury brought in its verdict of guilty, at which time Lord Chief Justice Mansfield pronounced sentence; on Monday, May 18th, Bellingham, although very likely insane, was hung and dissected. It would be difficult to find a more flagrant case of judicial murder.[10] The Bellingham case is also distinguished by being the only insanity trial of the last 2 centuries in which the verdict was protested by significant members of the public as blatantly unjust to the defendant.[11] It was also explicitly rejected, in 1840, as having any precedential authority for English law, because of the shameful judicial conduct of the case.[12]

In 1843, a Glasgow wood turner, Daniel M'Naghten, shot and killed Edward Drummond, private secretary to Sir Robert Peel, Prime Minister of England. Careful reading of the trial transcript and the newspaper reports of the time makes it abundantly clear that the origins of the myth that M'Naghten intended to shoot Sir Robert Peel probably lie in the wish of the prosecution to convert an insane act into a reasoned, political crime. All medical testimony at the trial was agreed that M'Naghten was insane. He was acquitted and there was a great newspaper and establishment outcry. That this was an outcry of the general public has been asserted but not proven and must be questioned, since the country was in a state of great civil and socioeconomic turmoil, with much violence, unrest, and major public dissatisfaction with the government.

The House of Lords convened the 15 judges of the Queen's Bench, the legal equivalent in status of our Federal Supreme Court justices, and asked them to answer five questions designed to clarify the law of criminal insanity. The judges combined two of the questions and gave their four answers with much hesitancy, concerned that their answers were likely to receive too much weight and thus freeze the proper flexibility and development of the common law. Their concern was justified. Their answers represented a regressive interpretation of the law, which excluded many earlier interpretations that gave the juries greater latitude in their deliberations and allowed for more legal safeguards for the defendant.[13]

To some degree, the cases of Hadfield and M'Naghten exemplify the general pattern of the legal response to violence by the insane. When little or no damage is caused, the offenders are treated with regard and concern for maximizing their legal protections. When significant or threatening damage is done by somebody who is probably insane, the laws are recast (or loud calls for such recasting are made) in order to minimize or prevent any leniency or judicial regard for the legal safeguards for the defendant. It is curious that it is mostly the legal profession and the legislatures (composed largely of lawyers) who call for such changes, although the newspapers almost invariably lead the campaign. There is a palpable demand to reject consideration of any exculpatory insanity.

Historically, psychiatrists and the psychiatric profession are also subject to this behavior. In America, prior to the Hinckley trial for the attempted assassination of President Reagan, one of the most embarassing illustrations of this phenomenon could be found in the trial of Charles Guiteau for the assassination of President Garfield.[14]

When I first made the observation of this correlation between the nature and degree of the damage and the response, I had not seen earlier reference to it in the psychiatric literature.[15] Later I read *Two Hard Cases* by W. W. Godding, Superintendent of St. Elizabeths Hospital and a psychiatrist for the defense in the Guiteau trial. In the book Godding observed, after the shooting and before Garfield's death:

> If the President dies, no plea of insanity can save this man from the gallows; if the President lives, no Commission of Lunacy will fail to find him insane and he will end his days in an asylum, for the tidal wave of public opinion in this case will be irresistible.[16]

The outcome of that trial may well be one of the most telling indictments of the functioning of our legal system and of the organized medical and psychiatric professions. In fact, it should be a matter of concern to all that no successful presidential assassin has escaped violent death in the history of America, no matter how insane they were.

There are, of course, exceptions to and variations of this pattern that appear to be important ones. One such exception is homicide by women of their infants and of their seducers. In 1865, Mary Harris was tried for the murder of Adoniram J. Burroughs, in Washington, D.C. Thomas McDade summarized the case:

> Burroughs was, by any standards, a cad who tried to entice his fiancee to a house of assignation for the purpose of compromising her and breaking off the engagement. He married another and Miss Harris followed him to Washington and shot him. . . . Mrs. Abraham Lincoln sent flowers to Miss Harris while she was in jail. She was acquitted.[17]

The public reaction to this prompted Isaac Ray, a founder of the Association of Medical Superintendents of American Institutions for the Insane (AMSAII), later the American Psychiatric Association (APA), to comment:

> The acquittal of Mary Harris, lately tried in Washington, has greatly exercised the public mind, and given rise to an unusual amount of objurgation. And the leading facts of the case, superficially considered, seemed to warrant this state of feeling. A young woman, smarting under the loss of her lover, provides herself with weapons, travels hundreds of miles to find him, watches patiently for a suitable opportunity, and at last deliberately shoots him dead. . . . She is then tried with the sympathies of the court, jury, and audience, all in her favor, acquitted on the plea of insanity, under a more liberal rule of law on this subject than was ever admitted before in any English or American court, and immediately, . . . is set at large. Thus regarded, . . . the result seems to have been but a mockery of justice, worthy of the severest condemnation. But for all that, the girl may have been insane, and therefore very properly acquitted; for there was nothing in the case incompatible with the phenomena of insanity. Among the medical witnesses who thought her insane was Dr. Nichols, Superintendent of the Government Hospital for the Insane.[18]

Some have reported that members of minority groups may elicit a different consideration from society in the courts. A case in point is that of William Freeman, an insane black who killed several white people one night, in Auburn, N.Y., in 1848. He was defended by former Governor William Seward (later Lincoln's cabinet officer responsible for the purchase of Alaska, "Seward's Folly"). Seward was a man with strong anti-black prejudices, who persisted in defending Freeman, despite the physical abuse and danger to himself and his family, in order to ensure that the law was applied impartially and properly, extending its safeguards to the black Freeman. Freeman died in jail while awaiting a court-ordered retrial.[19]

Another group, those with a record of prior arrests and convictions, generally are seen as criminals only. If they should plead insanity, they are accused of trying to escape justice, on the assumption that one cannot be both "bad" and "mad." It is not only journalists and the general public who express apprehension that somebody will "get away with something" by way of the insanity plea: many psychiatrists share this fear.

The response to the discharge of a defendant in an apparently uncomplicated criminal trial because of a legal procedural technicality seems to result in praise of our legal system because it is designed to insure that 10 guilty ones go free rather than one innocent be convicted. Let somebody plead insanity, rather than procedural error, however, and even psychiatrists will prejudge and become incensed, claiming that the plea is "phony" and abused and that it should be abolished. The cry then becomes that it is far better that 10 insane innocents be found guilty and sentenced to prison, rather than allow the risk of one sane criminal to be found not guilty by reason of insanity.

Related to the general topic of violence, psychiatry, and the law is the question of violence that may be directed against the insane or their civil rights when the issue of involuntary hospital treatment is considered. One must consider, also, the violence done to the insane when they are denied needed treatment because the nature of their mental illness prevents them from perceiving their need or from requesting it in "sane" or conventional language.

Nor should we ignore the uncontrolled violence that too many of our patients are subjected to, by other patients and staff, in our more mismanaged and impoverished state hospitals.

> On November 17, 1977, plaintiff reported that evening shift attendants beat him with sticks while he was tied to a bed. The next day he pointed out the sticks, which were hidden at the nurse's station. The investigation that followed resulted in the suspension of one employee for three days. Plaintiff and the attendant remained together in the same ward.[20]

Prior to the development of the insane asylum and hospital systems in America, most of the insane were housed in community facilities called almshouses, poor houses, and poor farms. The rest were either cared for at home or received no care. In some cases, paupers (sane and insane) were auctioned to the highest bidder, who cared for them and for whom they, in turn, worked. Some of these insane were treated well, many were not. Dorothea L. Dix spent her years as a social reformer exposing some of the inhumane practices of these methods of care, including maintaining the insane, frequently near naked, covered with excrement, in open sheds, in the severe New England winters.[21]

In 1838, Isaac Ray noted that

> in confining the insane, we have in view one or more of the following objects; first, their own restoration to health; secondly, their comfort and well-being

merely, with little or no expectation of their cure; thirdly, the security of society.[22]

By this time, Massachusetts had a statute requiring the confinement of all lunatics "so furiously mad as to render it manifestly dangerous to the peace and safety of the community, that they should be at large."[23] The raison d'être for this statute was the third purpose enumerated by Ray, not an unreasonable one. In 1836, Massachusetts passed a statute to allow for the confinement of the nondangerous "idiot or lunatic or insane person."[24] The raisons d'être for this statute were Ray's first and second reasons, because for most of these insane, life was far more dangerous and cruel than for most of our present day "bag people" or "skid row bums."

The AMSAII (now the APA) proposed, in 1868, a model code for the legal relations of the insane, drafted by Isaac Ray and modified by the membership sitting as a Committee of the Whole. Few psychiatrists are aware of the existence of this model code; an unfortunate indicator of how little we know of what our profession has done or tried to do in the past.

This code proposed regulation

> by statutory enactments calculated to secure their [the insane's] rights and also the rights of those entrusted with their care, or connected with them by ties of relationship or friendship, as well as to promote the ends of justice, and enforce the claims of an enlightened humanity.

It allowed for the placement of insane people in an asylum or hospital by a legal guardian or, absent such guardian, by relatives or friends, in every case accompanied by a certificate signed by a physician who had examined the patient within the week prior to admission. They could also be hospitalized by a magistrate who, in conjunction with a medical certificate, had determined that the individual was "dangerous to themselves or others, or require[d] hospital care and treatment." On receiving a written statement "that a certain person is insane and that the welfare of himself, or others requires his restraint [confinement]," a judge could appoint a commission of 3 or 4, including 1 physician and 1 lawyer, to investigate and recommend action. "The party involved is to have seasonable notice of the proceedings," and the judge was authorized to have him placed in suitable confinement while the inquiry was pending.[25]

Nineteenth century American psychiatrists were generally agreed that many of the insane were dangerous to themselves, if only by virtue of their mental disease making them incompetent to deal with the "hazards of liberty" (including our society's predators), or dangerous to others. Today, commitment laws usually do not address themselves to questions of welfare of the individuals or others—perhaps fortunately, perhaps unfortunately—but only to questions of danger. Over a period of time, the courts have narrowed the meaning of *danger* to physical harm or injury only, excluding danger to the peace, danger to other individuals' freedoms, and danger in a psychological or nonmaterial sense.

Researchers, in an effort to make an exceedingly difficult task easier, have restricted their definition of danger further, to include only those acts of physical violence which are confirmed by police arrest, arraignment, and, in some instances, criminal trial and conviction, or by judicial hearing and involuntary hospital commitment. They have also designated an identification of dangerousness as a *prediction* of police identified and recorded violent behavior. Anyone previously designated as dangerous, who is not arrested or committed to a psychiatric hospital on the basis of a court hearing, is classified, for research purposes, as a *false positive* and *proof* of an invalid prediction.

Danger refers to a state of potential and to a relative probability of realization. In identifying objects, situations, or people, as dangerous, we are referring to their potential for harm and to the relative probability of that harm being realized. Whether or not a probability is realized is not a simple function of correct or incorrect. It is not probative of validity or invalidity.

The fact that a drunk driver has driven an automobile a given number of miles without an accident does not invalidate the perception that during that trip that driver was a dangerous driver. It would be ludicrous to claim that because many drunk drivers have driven many miles without accidents, that there are many false positives of identifying drunk drivers as dangerous. A loaded gun in the hands of an infant is dangerous whether or not it is discharged and whether or not the discharged bullet is spent without inflicting any damage. A truck loaded with nitroglycerine is carrying a dangerous cargo, whether or not that cargo explodes on that trip. Undoubtedly, there have been many trips, adding up to thousands or millions of miles, of trucks carrying explosives without causing an explosion. I doubt that any reasonable jurist would argue that therefore all statutory restrictions on the free movement of such trucks should be eliminated, as there were so many "false positives."

The research use of the term *false positives,* in this regard, is misleading, and properly qualified researchers should be expected to acknowledge this explicitly. Weather reports of the probability of rain are not false positives if it doesn't rain. The fact that an individual has survived a particular surgical procedure that the surgeon considered dangerous does not mean that the procedure was not dangerous. Our political system and our moral standards do not allow the kind of research techniques that would validate relative probabilities in this area, nor for controlling relevant variables, nor for constant observation of the individual at liberty.

There is also relatively little basis for the assertion that psychiatrists have no experience or education in evaluating the dangerousness of particular individuals with particular mental states and behaviors. Psychiatrists and psychiatric residents responsible for inpatient ward care have much experience with people who may be dangerous to themselves or others because of their mental illness. With the professional obligation to anticipate danger and physical violence (neither prematurely nor too late), there is persistent pressure for the examination and reexamination of possibly relevant factors preceding all violent and dangerous incidents on the wards.

Changes in medications, application of mechanical restraints, withdrawal of off-ward passes, use of seclusion rooms, and the order for "suicidal precautions" or "M.O." (maximum observation) are frequently the expression of such anticipations. Many of these measures impose some increase of psychological stress on the ward staff. Consequently, there is a built-in motivation for reevaluating these measures for excessive or insufficient use in specific instances. That is, in the case of realized violence on the ward, what other measures might have been taken? In the absence of realized violence, was the ordering of preventive measures in a particular case successful or were these measures unnecessary?

Psychiatrists generally do not have experience with armed robbery, murder, or rape, but they do have experience with the possible loss of impulse control and violent behavior caused by mental illness in the here and now and in the immediate future, on the part of those who are mentally ill. The ability to identify such possibility is one of the factors that enter into our evaluation of clinical skill. With the passing of time, after the last evaluation, and the occurrence of unanticipated and unknowable future life experiences, these identifications becomes less reliable than they were at the time that they were made. Less reliability in the future does not invalidate present reliability.

Arrest rates as an instrument of research can be useful as a comparative measure of social behavior between selected populations. There has been interest in the comparative arrest rates of the insane and the general population, as an indicator of potential for violence, for many decades. Findings in the past have tended to be inconsistent. More recent studies show higher arrest rates for some mental hospital patients for some crimes. Rabkin found that "mental patients are more likely to be arrested for assaultive and sometimes lethal behavior than are other people."[26] A study done in France indicated that "paranoids, paranoid schizophrenics, and undifferentiated schizophrenics . . . were hospitalized much more often for violent crimes than the [hospitalized] population with other psychiatric diagnoses."[27]

It is important to remember that most of these studies involved a small subset of a large universe of mentally ill people. Unfortunately, this area of research has become an emotionally charged one. So much so, that one study that found higher arrest rates in a population of hospitalized mentally ill than in a nonmentally ill population[28] provoked one prominent lawyer to make an implied threat of suing the researchers.

Historically, there is an area of violence that has been of major interest in the past but has not been satisfactorily investigated. I am referring to the question of contagion of violent behavior. On November 4, 1825, a 27-year-old French maid, Henriette Cornier, decapitated a neighbor's infant and threw her head out the window into the street. Her mental status was unclear, despite prolonged study. She was tried, found guilty, and sentenced to hard labor for life.[29] There were several killings and near-killings following the reporting of this widely publicized case, which were attributed to it as the triggering cause.[30]

There have been many instances of sensational and distinctive acts which were widely publicized and followed by an "epidemic" of similar acts. Several years ago a Buddhist monk poured gasoline over his body and ignited it as a form of protest. This grisly act was publicized the world over. In the following months, many similar acts of self-immolation occurred in widely separated areas of the world. Many have wondered about the apparent contagious effects of such acts and news stories. Studies have been made of suicide and murder rates during newspaper strikes and they generally show some drop in suicide rates, indicating the probability of some suggestion or contagion effect.[31] However, we still know very little about this phenomenon and the nature of the special relationship, if any, it has to the mentally ill population.

Another area of violence that is of interest is that of the psychological and symbolic relationship between the motivations for murder and suicide. These have been thought to be different facets of the same basic mental condition, with different targets. Although a few individual reported case histories appear to support this view, there have been few large population studies supporting it.

In summary, it is clear that in the development of Western culture, and more specifically, Anglo-American culture, there has been believed to be a relationship between violence and the mentally ill. The reality of this relationship, as well as its nature, is an unclear one, with apparently inconsistent findings, fraught with remarkably intense emotional prejudgements on the part of research investigators, the psychiatric profession, the legal profession, the courts, law making bodies and society (as manifested by the labile social support for the identification and treatment of those violent individuals with mental disease).

REFERENCES

[1]*The Compact Edition of the Oxford English Dictionary.* New York, Oxford Univ. Press, 1971.

[2]Bouvier, J: *A Law Dictionary Adapted to the Constitution and Laws of the United States of America, etc.,* ed. 12. Philadelphia, George W. Childs, 1868.

[3]Monohan, J: *The Clinical Prediction of Violent Behavior.* Rockville, MD, U.S. Department of Health and Human Services, DHHS Publication No. (ADM)81-921, 1981, p. 5.

[4]Genesis. 4:8, in American Revision Committee (ed): *The Holy Bible,* King James Version, New York, Thomas Nelson & Sons, 1929.

[5]Hanawalt, BA: Violent death in fourteenth- and early fifteenth-century England. *Comp Studies in Society and Hist,* 1976, *18*:297–320.

[6]Arnold, E (Trial of): In Howell, TB (compiler): *A Complete Collection of State Trials and Proceedings for High Treason and Other Crimes and Misdemeanors. 1722–1725.* London, T. C. Hansard, 1812, Vol. 16, N. 465.

[7]Hale, M: *The History of the Pleas of the Crown.* London: E. R. Nutt & R. Gosling, 1736.

[8]Pinel, P: *A Treatise on Insanity.* Trans. DD Davis, M.D. London, Cadell & Davies, 1806, Facsimile edition, New York, Hafner Publishing, 1962.

[9]Hadfield, James (Trial of) in Howell, TB, & Howell, TJ, (Compilers): *A Complete Collection of State Trials and Proceedings for High Treason and Other Crimes and Misdemeanors. 1798–1800.* London, TC Hansard, 1820. Vol. 27. N. 646. See also Quen, JM: James Hadfield and the medical jurisprudence of insanity. *NY State J Med,* 1967, *69*:1221–1226.

[10]Bellingham, John (Trial of): In Collinson, GD: *A Treatise on the Law Concerning Idiots, Lunatics, and Other Persons Non Compotes Mentis.* London, W. Reed, 1812, Vol. I, p. 236.

[11]Junius, Jun: *Bellingham. The Defence Defended; or, the Trial Re-tried.* London, M. Jones, 1812.

[12]Regina v Oxford. In: *The English Reports.* Vol. 173. Moody & Malkin, Edinburgh, 1928.

[13]Quen, JM: Psychiatry and the law: Historical relevance to today. In Freedman, LZ (ed): *By Reason of Insanity: Essays of Psychiatry and the Law.* Wilmington, Delaware, Scholarly Resources, 1983, pp. 153–166.

[14]Quen, JM: An historical view of the M'Naghten trial, *Bull. Hist. Med.,* 1968, *42*:43–51.

[15]Rosenberg, CE: *The Trial of the Assassin Guiteau: Psychiatry and Law in the Gilded Age.* Chicago, Chicago Univ Press, 1968.

[16]Godding, WW: *Two Hard Cases.* Boston, Houghton, Mifflin & Co, 1882, pp. 37–38.

[17]McDade, TM: *The Annals of Murder.* Norman, Oklahoma, Univ of Oklahoma Press, 1961 No. 445, p. 132.

[18]Ray, I: The insanity of seduced or deserted women, reprinted in Ray, I: *Contributions to Mental Pathology.* Boston, Little, Brown, 1873 pp. 282–293.

[19]Hall, BF: *The Trial of William Freeman, for the Murder of John G. Van Nest, Including the Evidence etc. etc.* Reported by Benjamin, F Hall, Auburn, NY, Derby, Miller, 1848.

[20]Rennie v Klein, 653 F.2d 836 (1981).

[21]Dix, DL: *Memorial to the Legislature of Massachusetts.* np, 1843.

[22]Ray, I: *A Treatise on the Medical Jurisprudence of Insanity.* Boston, Charles C. Little & James Brown, 1838, p. 472, sec. 362.

[23]Mass. Revised Statutes (1836), Chapter 136, Paragraph 15.

[24]Ray, I: *A Treatise on the Medical Jurisprudence of Insanity.* Boston, Charles C. Little & James Brown, 1838, p. 475, fn. 1.

[25]*Project for a Law Regulating the Legal Relations of the Insane.* Boston, Association of Medical Superintendents of American Institutions for the Insane, 1868.

[26]Rabkin, JG: Criminal behavior of discharged mental patients: A critical appraisal of the research, *Psychol Bull*, 1979, *86*:1–27.

[27]Benezech, M, Bourgeois, M, & Yesavage, M: Violence in the mentally ill. A study of 547 patients at a French hospital for the criminally insane, *J Nerv Ment Dis*, 1980, *168*:698–700.

[28]Zitrin, A, Hardesty, A, Burdock, E, *et al*: Crime and violence among mental patients, *Am J Psychiatry*, 1976, *133*:142–149.

[29]Ray, I: *A Treatise on the Medical Jurisprudence of Insanity.* Boston, Charles C. Little & James Brown, 1838, p. 218, sec. 155.

[30]Ray, I: *A Treatise on the Medical Jurisprudence of Insanity.* p. 202, sec. 140, p. 207, sec. 146, p. 209, sec. 148.

[31]Motto, JA: Newspaper influence on suicide: A controlled study, *Arch Gen Psychiatry*, 1970, *23*:143–148.

4

Legal Aspects of Predicting Dangerousness

GRAHAM HUGHES

INTRODUCTION

It is difficult to imagine a rational legal system refraining entirely from making dispositions that rest, at least in part, on the anticipation of violent or otherwise dangerous behavior. For example, one justification for warrantless arrest is that the arrested person is by his criminal conduct posing an immediate threat to others. The granting or denial of bail depends sometimes on such an assessment. But, although we cannot shun the business of making these decisions, there are times when the process bristles with social and moral conundrums. The legal system must try to solve these in the light of its deepest level of principle.

A large area of difficulty (which is not a principal subject of this chapter) is the process of civil commitment. Here the theory of the law is that we may not commit people simply because they are in some way mentally ill nor simply because they might be identified as in some way dangerous, but only if they are found to be both mentally ill and dangerous to others or to themselves. Why do we demand this double assurance? One reason is surely that we view mental illness as a condition that can be identified with reasonable certitude so that it provides a sufficiently definite foundation to permit us to move on to the more elusive second-stage inquiry as to dangerousness. We are no doubt comforted too by the belief that mental illness is often curable. This per-

GRAHAM HUGHES • School of Law, New York University, New York, New York 10012.

suades us that we can endeavor to help people and at the same time protect them from themselves or protect others from them. Mental illness also comprises a set of conditions that is traditionally assigned to the special jurisdiction of a group of experts–doctors, psychiatrists and psychologists of the abnormal. Perhaps we are becoming skeptical of the special expertise of these professionals to predict dangerousness in the general population, but we retain our faith in their discernment when it comes to dubbing people as significantly mentally or emotionally abnormal. For these reasons the field of civil commitment seems (perhaps deceivingly) to offer the shelter of benevolent aims combined with identifications that have a working degree of reliability.

In the criminal justice area (the principal topic of this chapter), there are two reasons why reliance on predictions of dangerousness is rightly perceived as involving a more difficult and uneasy judgment. In the first place, our criminal justice aims are benevolent only in the widest social sense. Setting aside the presently unfashionable pursuit of rehabilitation, we do not for the most part consider criminals as people for whom we must care, but rather as persons deserving of censure or sanction. It is morally harder to justify doing unpleasant things to people then to justify curing them, though the difference in what is done to them in each case has seemed less than conspicuous to some observers. Second, there can no longer be any claim that we are dealing with a special subpopulation of mentally ill people. Although criminals and delinquents (or some segments of them) may in some important sense constitute definable subgroups, they do not do so in a way that elicits the same responses in our culture as the mentally ill. A leading question that soon protrudes, therefore, is whether a finding of criminal behavior can bestow the same warrant for inquiries into future dangerousness as a finding of mental illness does.

Even if we conclude that this finding does confer such a warrant then we run into a second difficulty, for we can no longer so comfortably lean on our experts. Psychiatrists and allied professionals are supposed to be in the business of telling us what kinds of things mentally ill people are likely to do. But are they any better than judges and juries who have heard the evidence in a criminal case at telling how a convicted defendant is likely to behave in the future? Are they, indeed, any better than any other person who has been given sufficient information about the defendant's history and circumstances and an adequate supply of data bases from which to work? In other words, is psychiatry as such a discipline of any particular relevance here? And is anybody, psychiatrist or not, good enough at such predictions to justify our taking any action on the basis of any assessment of this kind?

These are some of the plaguing questions that must be confronted.

I

Attention to estimates of dangerousness in individuals figures in the decisions of officials of the criminal justice system in a wide variety of contexts and with wide variations in the degree of structure and formality of the decision making. At one extreme of informality, we have the discretion that police executives must exercise in deciding how to allocate their resources. We can all understand why more effort would be devoted to tracking down a gang of bank robbers who have been in the habit of shooting and killing in the course of their raids than to pursuing a fugitive individual who has peacefully embezzled a sum of money, even a large amount. And we would all readily agree that this extra effort is justified not only because the bank robbers are more deserving of very serious punishment for what they have done in the past but also because we judge that they are an acute source of danger for the future. The allocation remains justifiable even though there is a possibility that this judgment might be wrong because the gang may have made enough money and may now be dissolving to seek retirement in softer climates. The police may properly deal in probabilities.

The decision may be more subtle as when more of an effort is made to catch murder suspect x than murder suspect y. Recently, the exercise of this branch of police discretion has become more sophisticated as efforts are made to identify career criminals. If the police have reason to believe that a suspect not yet apprehended has committed a string of serious robberies, they may reasonably concentrate resources on his capture that they would not devote to the suspect who is linked only with a single robbery. Again, this is surely not only due to a heightened sense of the gravity of what has been done but also to common sense and a heightened appreciation of the greater future danger of the one individual as compared with the other. Reduction in crime and protection of the public can only be achieved by the most efficient use of police resources, and this in turn calls for some estimate of the dangerousness of particular offenders, whether it be done by rough common sense or with the aid of baselines and computers.

The law remains for the most part untroubled by such exercises of discretion. Nobody has seriously argued that the equal protection rights of the workaholic robber are violated because he is pursued more zealously than his lazy confrere who ventures out only occasionally. But (and this links up with subtler questions that we must raise later) a police decision to pursue only black robbers and to ignore white ones would be much more difficult (probably impossible) to defend constitutionally even if it could be incontrovertibly demonstrated that by and large black robbers are much more active at their trade than are white ones. Some data bases may legally amount to inherently suspect classifications that the Constitution will not countenance.

Even more visible than at the police level is the discretion exercised by prosecutors. Inundated with business in a market where the supply (of crime) hugely exceeds the demand, prosecutors have to make decisions at many levels about the allocation of resources. Most notably this occurs in the context of plea bargaining, in deciding what concessions will be made, or indeed whether any concessions at all can be granted, in return for a plea. But there are other important instances of discretion, as in decisions on what resources to put into working up particular cases. More experienced attorneys may be assigned, collaboration with the police may be more intense, and the use of investigators from the prosecutor's office may be ordered to try to strengthen the case against the defendant. In decisions of this kind, there can be no doubt that prosecutors' offices have always taken as one of their rough guides some estimate of the threat posed by the defendant to the public. Today, these policies are often more articulate and rely in a more sophisticated way on statistical tables.

This exercise of discretion is not free from the possibility of constitutional attack. Selective or discriminatory prosecution is a well enough known objection in the lexicon of criminal defense, though it is equally well known to be a frail reed on which a defendant should not place much reliance. Constitutional rights have always in American history contended with the deference afforded to executive discretion. Although some continental European observers react with astonishment to our exclusionary rule, they are no less taken aback by the discretion enjoyed by our police and prosecutors. Courts are, for example, reluctant to interfere with prosecutorial discretion in entering into plea bargains, even though this may involve relentless prosecution of some members of a group of criminals, whereas other members for one reason or another go quite free or escape with nominal convictions. The defendant who protests that he is prosecuted to the limit of the law while those around him are going free will have to make a very positive showing of an impermissible motive, perhaps one stemming from a constitutionally prohibited classification, before his objection will have any chance of succeeding.

In this way, at the earliest (but often the most decisive) levels of the criminal justice process, judgments are made daily in very large numbers that ensure very different dispositions for suspects or defendants when the particular crimes for which they are charged or suspected are very similar. Often this is based on rough or refined estimates by police and/or prosecutor of the future dangerousness of the individual. Psychiatrists and other mental health professionals play no immediate part in these decisions except in the attenuated sense that some of the information and data bases or other techniques for constructing relevant profiles may owe something to information and theories developed in the past by the work of these professionals.

II

It is naturally in the field of dispositions of convicts that estimates of dangerousness, whether they be inarticulate assessments or allegedly refined predictions, play their most important and controversial role. In some form or another, this practice is no doubt as old as the whole institution of criminal punishment. In spite of the adjurations of the "desert" school that sentencers should look only to the acts for which the defendant has been found guilty, so severely blinkered a perspective will surely be difficult to attain if not actually undesirable. *Desert theory,* in its strongest form, invites us to accept the unreal and stultifying propostion that people are to be thought of only as they have been and not in terms of what we expect them to be or do. This surely falsifies human experience. Our judgments of people are colored by expectation as much as by historical review. The notion that a person has a "serious problem" is much like the notion that he has a "serious illness"; it incorporates both observation of past and present symptoms or behavior with an implicit evaluation of likely developments in the future. If we decide to have nothing to do with a person, it is usually at least in part because our experience of the person in the past leads us to expect unacceptable behavior in the future.

Suppose that *x* has committed three serious assaults at intervals of 3 years, having spent most of his intervening periods in prison serving time for the assaults. If he now commits a fourth serious assault, an extreme form of desert theory will recommend that he receive the same sentence as the one imposed for the first assault providing that this first sentence was justly proportionate. This outcome is not only unlikely in any real system but would be wrong in principle. Setting aside the possibility of mental illness, we certainly think of *x* as a "worse" person than someone who committed one assault, has served his sentence and lived peacefully since. But what is the nature of the judgment that *x* is "worse"? It is surely a combination of a heightened condemnation of his whole past life with a deepened apprehension of the life that he will lead in the future.

People are not (or should not be) sentenced for their acts alone but for the character of their acts, which in an important sense means for the character of the person. Moderate desert theorists sometimes concede this, being willing to say that an act deserves more punishment if it follows on previous bad acts, as it is thereby characterized as a worse offense than a first violation would be. But it seems difficult to make this admission and at the same time deny that sentencing is in any way properly based on expectations of the future, because in the practical and everyday business of judging people past actions are not only relevant for what they are but also for what they indicate and point to. And surely a sharper apprehension for the future is the most natural companion of the observation of a repetition of violent offenses.

The practice of sentencing has at any rate surely always proceeded along these lines. Most of the time, it has been informal though not always tacit. As modern sentencing practices developed in the nineteenth century, with the fading away of fixed penalties and the growth of judicial discretion, judges frequently made references in sentencing statements to the need to impose a severe sentence because the defendant had shown himself to be a menace. Such estimates, unscientific and uncontaminated by data bases, were, in conjunction with the broad tariff provided by the sentencing statutes, probably the main components of sentencing dispositions. If forced to a moral justification, the judicial response would no doubt have been eclectic. First, the defendant who has committed repeated violent offenses has shown himself to be unrepentant and hardened in evil ways and so has called down a larger dose of retribution. Second, such persons have not been deterred by previous sentences and so a greater sentence is called for in the hope of hitting the deterrence button. Third, the longer sentence will protect the public for a longer time by incapacitating the defendant.

If this is so, the practice of enhancing sentences has ancient roots and is not to be explained solely in terms of the now fashionable prominence of the incapacitation theory. It draws sustenance from retribution and deterrence theory as well, though the justifications are somewhat different. Retribution looks preeminently to the past, though, as we have suggested above, it is very difficult in practice to disentangle it from estimates of future danger. Deterrence theory has a utilitarian foundation but a different one from incapacitation for it assumes that the defendant is still corrigible and may be influenced into giving up his criminal ways. Incapacitation theory is avowedly not concerned with such issues. It is willing to assume that the convict is incorrigible; indeed, it reaches its strongest expression in such cases, for the protection of society from the incorrigible is the purest form of incapacitation. But, whereas these strands can be analytically distinguished, it is likely that in practice they have been closely woven together so that the enhancement of a sentence has almost always entailed the justification that society is being protected for an additional period from one who has indicated his special dangerousness.

The indeterminate sentence and the parole system (in recent times past their heyday and the target of sharp attacks) were embodiments of the mixed criteria described here. With its avowed emphasis on rehabilitation, the parole system certainly downgraded retribution (though probably more in theory than in practice) but at the same time was perfectly consonant with deterrence and incapacitation aims. A judgment that a prisoner is rehabilitated suggests that deterrence has worked and that incapacitation is no longer necessary. On the other hand, a rejection of parole, if it does not mean that a retributive tariff has not yet been satisfied, must entail a judgment that deterrence or reeducation has not yet "taken" and that further danger is to be expected. The parole system is thus intensely predictive and in recent decades parole boards have been in the habit of turning frankly to statistical tables to assist them in making such predictions.

It is too early to tell whether the present climate of rejection of the parole system is well advised. Indeterminate sentences joined with the possibility of parole had the apparent good sense of refusing to make conclusive judgments at the time of judicial sentencing and relying rather on the seemingly more accurate procedure of periodic review while a prison term was being served. In the laboratory of the prison, it was thought, the assessment and prediction could be made with infinitely greater accuracy after observation and study. However, the predictions of parole boards are made in the light of an artificial history of purely institutional conduct and without the adversary due-process joinder of issue that we associate with proceedings that lead to deprivation of liberty. A revulsion against the parole system was inevitable but it ought not necessarily to be coupled with a rejection of the underlying proposition that an assessment of future dangerousness is a relevant consideration in sentencing.

III

For a considerable time, future dangerousness has been recognized as a decisive or at least relevant consideration in several kinds of statutory provisions to do with sentencing.

Some state statutes have provisions relating to mentally abnormal sexual offenders (traditionally referred to as sexual psychopath laws) that require a very lengthy or indeterminate sentence after conviction of a sexual offense coupled with a finding of mental abnormality and future dangerousness. A few jurisdictions have taken up the broader drafting of the Model Penal Code and provide generally for the imposition of lengthy sentences on mentally abnormal dangerous offenders. These statutes rest on the predicate of a finding of mental abnormality but the federal version is broader and discards this foundation. The federal statute (18 U.S.C. § 3575), enacted in 1970, provides for enhanced sentences for offenders who are found in a separate proceeding to be both "special" and "dangerous." A *special offender* under this statute is one who has two or more previous convictions for offenses punishable with imprisonment for more than one year and who has actually been imprisoned before. The offender must also be *dangerous,* which depends on a finding that "a period of confinement longer than that provided for [the felony for which he has been convicted] is required for the protection of the public from further criminal conduct by the defendant". The standard of proof for this supplementary hearing, which is held by a judge without a jury, is a preponderance of the evidence; the same statute provides generally that no limitation is to be placed on the information concerning the background, character and conduct of a person that the federal court may receive and consider for the purpose of imposing an appropriate sentence. If the finding is made, the statute authorizes a sentence up to 25 years.

This federal statute is exceptional in eliminating the need for any finding of mental abnormality while requiring an explicit finding of future dangerousness. Much more common are traditional state recidivist statutes that do not expressly pose the question of future dangerousness but provide for greatly increased sentences for habitual criminals. But the absence of such an express reference in these statutes should hardly induce doubts about the justification perceived for them. The legislative history of many of these provisions, combined with the sentencing observations often made by judges when they are invoked, clearly reveal the blend of justifications that are conflated in the notion of incorrigibility. This is the practical expression par excellence of the suggestion we have made earlier that desert and incapacitation are virtually inseparable notions in the business of sentencing. A history of repeated offenses is taken to characterize the individual as more deeply deserving of punishment and at the same time to identify him as particularly menacing for the future. Society needs to be protected from dangerous persons who in turn have no moral claim to escape lengthy detention since they have failed to profit from earlier opportunities to learn a lesson. We could give this a desert theory turn by saying that a person deserves to be confined not only because he has done wrong but because by his wrongdoing he has willfully caused us apprehension about the future. Menaces and threats may be met with punishment and there is no worse menace than the exhibition of a propensity to continue with dangerous criminal acts after previous convictions and sentences. Desert and incapacitation are thus mutually supportive concepts.

But the array of sentence enhancing statutes listed here has in practice not been very much used. There are several reasons for this. The habitual criminal statutes have traditionally been drafted so broadly that they are applicable to cases involving comparatively innocuous previous offenses, certainly a range of offenses unconnected with violence though not necessarily unconnected with dangerousness in some attenuated sense of that concept. There is a natural reluctance to apply statutes with so sprawling a scope that always trail the risk of constitutional attack on the ground that their application might constitute cruel and unusual punishment. Thus, whereas habitual criminal statutes have been an important chip in the process of plea bargaining, they have been actually applied in a small minority of the cases where they might have been invoked. This fragmentary and very occasional pattern of application itself raises questions about selective prosecution and about the efficacy of the statutes as a rational way of pursuing any legitimate sentencing aims.

If a statute is not simply a general recidivist one but (like the federal provision and the sexual psychopath laws) depends on an explicit finding of dangerousness that cannot be satisfied simply by pointing to previous convictions, then other influences combine to make prosecutors loath to employ these provisions except on rare occasions. The procedures raise a cloud of dubious and unresolved questions about due process and aspects of the law of evidence, which are taken up in the next section. Rather than run into these thorny issues, prosecutors may prefer to pass by the opportunity to rely on the special provisions. But these troublesome issues linger as concealed wounds that will impair the health of the system if they are not exposed and confronted. It seems likely that franker treatment will in the future be afforded them for two reasons.

First, the reappearance of capital punishment procedures as a prominent feature of our criminal justice system is already forcing such an appraisal. Several capital statutes contain provisions for a separate sentencing hearing in which a finding of dangerousness is one aggravating feature on which the capital sentence may rest. Second, the recent theoretical emphasis on incapacitation either as a prime justification for any sentence of imprisonment or as a good reason for enhancing sentences has brought to the surface the subterranean, semiacknowledged practice of relying on such estimates of future conduct as a prime factor in all sentencing practice. The intense drama of the capital sentence case combined with the general consciousness raising about the connection between sentencing and estimates of future danger ensure a deeper consideration of the issues involved from a variety of standpoints—the perspective of moral philosophy, the medical and social science learning about the possibility of reasonably accurate prediction, and, finally, the relevant constitutional and legal principles.

A major and complex issue that pervades this field is the drawing of distinctions between the proof of guilt and the sentencing stage of a criminal proceeding. There is no lack of agreement that all the accoutrements of due process of law, including proof beyond a reasonable doubt, the opportunity to confront witnesses against one, as well as less purely constitutional doctrines such as the prohibition on hearsay, apply to the proof of guilt stage. Sentencing, however, has traditionally been regarded as a proceeding of a wholly different nature. Here, the search has been for a complete profile of the defendant; the life he has led, the things he has done and, in the widest sense, the kind of person he is are all proper subjects of inquiry. Information is sought and worked up by probation officers, and the judge may order a medical and/or psychiatric examination of the defendant to assist him in reaching a disposition. Hearsay allegations may be made in the presentence report, some of them favorable to the defendant and some damaging. Perhaps it will be said that he is a good husband and father or perhaps that he neglects his family and associates with known members of organized crime groups. The defense may present its own submissions but it cannot counter in the classic way that it might employ at a confrontational trial, for the sources of allegations in the presentence report are not necessarily produced for cross examination.

Are such informal procedures tolerable? Is the distinction between the trial stage and the sentencing stage so demonstrably radical that the interests defended by due process principles and the rules of evidence no longer need protection? The decided cases give obscure and uneasy responses to this difficult set of questions.

IV

The definitions of many crimes contain elements that may be called aggravating circumstances. We may have a general offense of robbery consisting of stealing from the person with violence or threats of force and we may then have a higher degree of robbery distinguished by the additional circumstance of carrying a gun in the commission of the offense and punishable with a higher maximum sentence. Suppose these definitions were shuffled by having only one offense of robbery but adding an auxiliary provision that after a robbery conviction a court should hold an inquiry into whether the defendant was carrying a gun when the offense was committed and, on such a finding, might or must increase the sentence. Suppose further that this provision went on to say that at the gun hearing the burden of proof on the prosecution was only a preponderance of evidence, that a jury could be dispensed with and that the usual rules of evidence were suspended so that, for example, hearsay could be introduced. There can be no doubt that this transparent device would be howled down indignantly as a blatant and sinister formalism, aiming at the creation of a serious criminal offense while dispensing with the requirements of the Constitution.

In its decision in *Specht v Patterson* (1967),* the Supreme Court of the United States seemed to make this instinctive response. The Colorado statute reviewed in that case provided that, following a conviction for certain sexual offenses, there should be a hearing to determine whether the defendant "constitutes a threat of bodily harm to members of the public or is an habitual offender and mentally ill." The statute required a complete psychiatric examination of the defendant with a written report. An affirmative finding after such a hearing led to an indeterminate sentence of from 1 day to life, a maximum sharply more severe than that prescribed for many of the underlying sexual offenses taken alone. In striking down this procedure as unconstitutional on due-process grounds, the Supreme Court held that the statute amounted to the creation of an aggravated degree of the offense on the basis of a finding of additional facts (dangerousness), and that such findings could only rest on the adversary procedures that due process demands to ensure accuracy and fair participation for the defendant. This would necessitate representation by counsel, the right to compulsory process to offer evidence and the right to confront witnesses for the state by cross-examination. The Court did not say that trial of the issue by jury was constitutionally required, nor that the burden of proof must be beyond a reasonable doubt though at that date it had not been held that these rights were due process components applicable to the states. It did quote approvingly from a Pennsylvania case that had stated that in such a hearing the full panoply of due-process protection must be afforded.

Justice Douglas's pronouncement in *Specht* that the statutory procedure involved amounted to "the making of a new charge leading to criminal punishment"† might seem to bode ill for free-ranging inquiries into dangerousness at the sentencing phase. But the distinction between a circumstance that amounts to a new factual element, aggravating the degree of the offense, and a circumstance that is merely relevant to sentence was not pursued rigorously in *Specht*. The Court in *Specht*, for example, looked for support to its earlier decision in *Graham v West Virginia* (1912)‡ which concerned the propriety of a state procedure for determining whether the defendant had been previously convicted for

*386 U.S. 605.
†*Id.* at 610.
‡224 U.S. 616.

purposes of increasing the sentence. But Mr. Justice Hughes, in *Graham*, stressed that the habitual criminal statute did not create a fresh offense nor a higher degree of the offense committed, but "goes to the punishment only."* If Hughes's point was that the specified condition (being a recidivist) had nothing to do with the way in which the instant offense was committed then the same would be true of *Specht*, for a determination of dangerousness is not necessarily connected with any particular mode of committing the offense for which the defendant has been convicted. Of course, to query whether such statutory provisions can reasonably be regarded as creating fresh offenses does not solve the due-process problem, for we could abandon that point and simply fall back on the position that, however we classify it, the statute does provide for an increased period of detention and therefore triggers due-process requirements for that reason alone. After all, some due-process elements are necessary for civil commitment in the absence of any allegation of crime. The problem in criminal cases is rather whether the due process already extended in the proceedings leading to a finding of guilt suffices or whether fresh due process must be provided for the sentencing stage.

In this regard, *Specht* is difficult to weld into a harmonious principle with other leading cases from the Court in the area of sentencing. Even before *Specht*, uncertainty had already been introduced by two earlier decisions. In *Townsend v Burke* (1948)† the Court found a due-process violation where a trial court had taken into consideration false information concerning previous convictions at a sentencing proceeding where the defendant had no counsel. But shortly afterwards in *Williams v New York* (1949),‡ a capital case, the Court refused to find that due process required any special procedures to be followed at sentencing. The jury in *Williams* had recommended life imprisonment but the judge overrode this and imposed the death sentence, relying on information in the presentence report alleging that the defendant had committed many other crimes (of which he had not been convicted) and that he possessed a "morbid sexuality." The defendant was given no opportunity to challenge this information. Writing for the Supreme Court, Mr. Justice Black upheld the death sentence and stressed the importance of allowing a free flow of information to the judge at the sentencing stage to further the aim of appropriately individualizing punishment. The overriding importance of this rehabilitative goal (an ironic point in a capital case) rendered a due-process insistence on trial standards of presenta-

---

*Id. at 624, quoting *McDonald v. Massachusetts*, 180 U.S. 311, at 312 (1901).
†334 U.S. 736.
‡337 U.S. 241.

tion of evidence inappropriate. In *Gardner v Florida* (1977),* another capital case, the Court took a different view from *Williams* and, although *Williams* was distinguished on the facts, it would seem to be virtually overruled for death penalty cases. The Court rested *Gardner* chiefly on the special nature of the death sentence though at one point in his opinion Mr. Justice Stevens stated that "it is now clear that the sentencing process, as well as the trial itself, must satisfy the requirements of the Due Process Clause."† The force of *Williams* as a precedent may therefore be somewhat weakened though it is presumably still applicable in noncapital cases.

Decisions in this area seem, indeed, to run in pairs where each case, if not quite irreconcilable with its companion, can be squared with it only by strenuous exertion. So in *United States v Tucker* (1972),‡ the Court disapproved the practice of relying in sentencing on previous convictions where the defendant had not been represented by counsel in the earlier case. *Tucker* can be taken to show respect for the importance of accuracy in the information that a court looks to in sentencing since the prime vice of the absence of counsel at a criminal trial is the unreliability of any ensuing conviction. Alternatively, *Tucker* may be read simply as an instance of a kind of exclusionary principle—that no use should be made in subsequent judicial proceedings of an earlier proceeding that is vitiated by a practice now condemned as unconstitutional.

But *Tucker,* in turn, has to be set alongside *United States v Grayson* (1978)§ where the trial judge had enhanced the sentence on the avowed ground that the jury's guilty verdict demonstrated that the defendant must have been consistently lying and fabricating when he testified in his own defense. This could be construed as imposing an extra bit of time for perjury, an offense for which the defendant had never been indicted and never convicted in any formal proceeding. (The jury's verdict of guilty perhaps logically entails the proposition that they did not believe the defendant when he testified, but it does not logically entail the proposition that the defendant was lying; certainly, had the government indicted him for perjury, they could not have obtained a guilty verdict simply by pointing to the transcript of the first trial.) The majority of the Supreme Court, however, contrived to find the procedure in *Grayson* unexceptionable by stressing the importance in sentencing of the likelihood of the defendant's being rehabilitated and declaring that the impression formed by the judge of the defendant's conduct when he testified was an invaluable index of this prospect. The opinion of the

*430 U.S. 349.
†*Id.* at 358.
‡404 U.S. 443.
§438 U.S. 41.

Court in *Grayson* refers frequently in an approving manner to *Williams* and thus appears to rehabilitate that decision in the noncapital area.

Grayson epitomizes as well as any other case the peculiar intractability of the sentencing process in the light of familiar constitutional principles. It also exemplifies the tight fusion of justifying principles for punishment that we have noted earlier. If the defendant is thought to have persistently perjured himself at his trial, does he deserve a greater sentence because (a) this overly exuberant attempt to evade his just punishment stains his character even deeper than commission of the crime itself, or (b) because this conduct amounts to a bad forecast for the likelihood of his repentance or renunciation of criminal habits? Perhaps for both reasons, though, in its opinions, the majority of the Supreme Court stressed the latter and by so doing at least obliquely validated the propriety of enhanced sentences based on a prediction of future behavior. This may not be quite the same as a recognition of incapacitation as a supreme justification since the stress is on the need for more time to rehabilitate the defendant rather than the protection of society. But why is rehabilitation important? Certainly it may be in part because we have a social obligation to help people by purging them of their criminal impulse, but it would be naive not to recognize at least the coexistence of a purpose to protect other citizens from them. *Grayson* is therefore hard to understand in any way except as in some measure validating informal assessments of future dangerousness by a trial judge as a proper part of the sentencing process.

But why is it permissible for such an evaluation to be made informally without any adversarial joinder when the *Specht* case repudiated a more formal version of the same calculation under the Colorado sex offender statute? Does everything simply turn on the point that in *Specht* the Court was dealing with the express imposition of an enhanced sentence by a statute where there was a finding of a statutorily specified condition (albeit one as vague at the edges as dangerousness)? Is the *Grayson* situation effectively removed from the weight of the principles defended in *Specht* simply because the sentence imposed was still within the range of the maximum laid down for the original offense and there was no question of any special enhancement prescribed by statute for any specified circumstance or condition?

The paradox here is that the more the state articulates special sentencing considerations in separate proceedings with a demand for specific findings and a definite sentence enhancement the more it may fall under constitutional scrutiny. But where special statutory criteria and separate proceedings are wholly absent and findings (predictions) as to the future are simply collapsed into general sentencing discretion, the less control will be exerted by the Supreme Court. States wishing to avoid federal intervention will not be slow to learn this lesson.

Indeed, separate formal proceedings after a finding of guilty and going expressly to the issue of dangerousness are, as we have seen, rare. The habitual criminal statutes are not properly counted here since they do not depend on an explicit additional finding of dangerousness. But when such a formal special hearing is held under statutory authority, then the requirements of *Specht* will have to be observed. These requirements may be more stringent where the procedure is before a jury than where it is before a judge sitting alone because, as we shall see below, the possibility of prejudice is thought to be much greater where a question is sent to a jury. But if the language of *Specht* is taken to heart and such proceedings are perceived as the creation of an aggravated degree of the offense depending on an additional finding of fact, then a powerful argument could be advanced that the defendant may not constitutionally be deprived of a jury to adjudicate the supplementary question.

In such a proceeding before a jury, it would be necessary (in the absence of defense waiver) for any witness (psychiatrist or otherwise) to testify orally as to the defendant's dangerousness and to be subject to cross examination. As the capital punishment cases will show, prior questions might arise as to the circumstances of any examination of the defendant conducted by a psychiatrist who testifies for the prosecution. Was the defendant adequately advised by counsel? Did he realize that the results of the examination might be used against him? If not, then violations of his constitutional right to counsel and privilege against self-incrimination may have occurred. The burden of proof is another due process element that may cause difficulty. If future dangerousness is an aggravating element that may take a case into the realm of the death penalty or some other enhanced penalty, then how can it be acceptable to show it only by a preponderance of evidence? But once we say that proof beyond a reasonable doubt is required, how could this standard ever be satisfied? With the present state of knowledge about the accuracy of predictions of dangerousness, it is almost unimaginable that any professional could testify that he can predict future behavior with such confidence. There is, indeed, a general logical difficulty about demanding proof beyond a reasonable doubt of future events. The law is accustomed to asking for this degree of proof as to whether something happened or not, even as to whether someone did something with a certain intent or not, but to ask for such a response to the question of whether something will happen in the future is to move into a different category of discourse. The lurking implication of this line of analysis is that future dangerousness perhaps cannot be entertained at all as a legitimate aggravating circumstance.

But if we travel this far along the road, we shall meet the hardest problem. Does the logic of the discussion up to this point also compel us to direct judges to purge their minds of every consideration of future dangerousness in the everyday business of sentencing where there is no question of any statutory specification of sentence-enhancing conditions? Such a proposal would surely run against stubborn obstacles. One would be the practical difficulty of monitoring a judge's sentencing deliberations. If a judge does not call for reports or a hearing on a defendant's possible future dangerousness, how shall we know that the court did or did not take that factor into account? A judge is not obliged to make a full statement of the factors that led him to select a particular sentence. Even if a judge were prohibited from receiving any express estimates as to future dangerousness, still in his review of the circumstances of the crime, perhaps in the demeanor of the defendant at the trial, certainly in the defendant's past record and life history (for surely we could not want to bar knowledge of these) information is available that makes it seem vain to expect the suppression of all assessments of the defendant's danger to the community.

But attempts to make the sentencing process both more open and more controlled are not necessarily doomed to failure. At least they might bring about some desirable improvements over the present situation. An experiment in reform might be devised along the following lines. Before passing sentence, a court would be required to present to the prosecution and the defense a "proposed sentence statement" that would contain both a statement of the sentence the court tentatively proposes to impose and a statement of reasons justifying this sentence. Within a prescribed period, either side could object to the proposed sentence, respond with rebutting information on any factual matter, request a hearing where any factual matters were in dispute, and argue as to the propriety of the sentence. After this exchange, and any hearing that might be necessary, the court would pass its final sentence. This, however, would be subject to full review on appeal, as is currently the practice in England where the Criminal Division of the Court of Appeal frequently changes sentences and usually accompanies its action with a short opinion stating the principles and facts that led it to take such action.

A procedure of this kind might do a good deal towards ventilating the sentencing process. In itself, such a reform would be neutral as to reliance by the court on estimates of future dangerousness, though it would at the least place an obligation on the judge to state openly that he is looking to such a factor and would then give the defense an opportunity to make a response. We might seek to go further and provide that courts might not take future dangerousness into account at all in sentencing. Coupled with the procedure suggested here that would ensure that courts would make no reference to this factor in their proposed sentencing statements; conscientious judges would also make every effort to expel such reflections from their minds. Whether such ostracism is desirable we consider at the end of this discussion.

V

Even if an inquiry into future dangerousness is clothed in the formal dress of a due process hearing, it can still be contended that its basic nature is unredeemable and that it must be expelled altogether as an impermissible subject of inquiry. We have already seen the seeds of this position in the point raised above about the difficulty of imagining future dangerousness as established beyond a reasonable doubt. This argument will now be expanded into its connections with general principles and rules of the law of evidence, some of which have constitutional connections.

To be admissible, evidence must be relevant. We must distinguish here between issues and evidence. Most people would think the *issue* of future dangerousness is properly relevant to the question of an appropriate sentence (though some, as we have seen would disagree on moral grounds and might seek to translate their disagreement into a constitutional argument), but the question now arising is what *evidence* is relevant to the issue of future dangerousness? We know the general forms that proferred evidence is bound to take. It may consist solely of proof of the defendant's past criminal record and his apparent failure to behave acceptably in spite of earlier convictions and sentences. It may consist of reports of the results of clinical examinations and testing by psychiatrists or allied professionals. And it may also include projections based on actuarial tables. But is any of this relevant?

This may at first appear a strange question because, if this kind of evidence is not relevant to the issue, then what could be relevant? But under the most appropriate concept of relevance the answer may well be that nothing is relevant. McCormick in his text on the law of evidence states that "the most acceptable test of relevancy is the question, does the evidence offered render the desired inference more probable than it would be without the evidence?"* This kind of question is constantly presenting itself to courts. For example, evidence of a defendant's flight is generally taken to be relevant, as an indirect admission of guilt, to the general issue of whether he committed a crime. But there will be many difficult marginal cases where the question is whether evidence tendered can properly be considered as evidence of flight at all. Suppose it is shown that a defendant charged with committing a murder in New York

*McCormick, EVIDENCE 437 (2d ed. 1972).

City on January 1 took a plane to Miami on January 2 and stayed there for 1 month. Does this amount to evidence of flight? Questions like this are usually not susceptible to probability checks against statistical tables. They have to be determined in the light of established principles which in turn are expressions of judicial distillation of the general experience of the community in such matters.

There are two important differences between the "flight as proof of guilt" question and the issue of predicting future dangerousness. First, if we disallow the evidence of the trip to Miami as an indirect admission of guilt we shall in most cases have other evidence of the defendant's involvement in the crime. He is not likely to be charged with the murder for no other reason than that he went to Miami. But in the prediction of future dangerousness cases, the question is not just that of disallowing one kind of evidence as insufficiently probative to be relevant. The contention is the radical one that, in the present state of science and social science, there is no imaginable evidence that could be taken to make it "more probable" that a person will be dangerous at some distant future time. If this contention is accepted, then it would not just expel a certain kind of evidence but would expel the whole issue as an illegitimate one, for if there is no admissible evidence that could ever be adduced to prove a fact then that fact cannot be raised as an issue in the trial of a case. If the question whether a person is going to be (or is more likely than not to be) dangerous in the future is like the question of whether a ball in a roulette game will lodge in a black or red slot on the next turn of the wheel, then it has no place in any legal disposition, much less one on which prison time or the imposition of the death sentence may turn.

The second difference between predictions of dangerousness and evidence of flight as showing the commission of crime is that the first is more susceptible than the second to verification. Because it is an area where medicine and the law converge the question has in fact been subjected to considerable examination with an accumulating body of literature, culminating recently in the invaluable survey by Professor John Monahan, *The Clinical Prediction of Future Behavior*. In a summary of part of his conclusions, Professor Monahan comments:

> Outcome studies of clinical predictions with adult populations . . . lead to the conclusion that psychiatrists and psychologists are accurate in no more than one out of three predictions of violent behavior over a several year period among institutionalized populations that had both committed violence in the past and were mentally ill.*

*Monahan, THE CLINICAL PREDICTION OF VIOLENT BEHAVIOR 60 (1981).

Professor Monahan acknowledges a superior ability in psychiatrists to predict violence in the near future on the part of disturbed patients or inmates; but this is not very relevant to the sentencing context where the defendant, even in the absence of a prediction of future dangerousness, will typically receive a prison sentence of some years, so that the prediction we seek relates to his likely conduct a number of years in the future. (He may of course be violent to wardens or other inmates in prison but sending him to prison for a longer term is not well designed to prevent that.) It seems overwhelmingly clear that in the present state of knowledge no method of prediction can get close to 50% accuracy when dealing with this question. If this is so, the argument about relevancy of evidence climbs to a due-process stature for it ought surely to be held a violation of due process to sentence a person to an increased term of imprisonment on the basis of evidence that is not only irrelevant to his guilt for the underlying crime but also irrelevant to his prospects for future behavior and rehabilitation. In the litigation, this argument has been for the most part raised in the capital punishment cases, but it seems equally appropriate in cases where there are special statutory procedures for enhanced sentences and also in the great range of everyday cases where estimates of dangerousness may be taken into account in fixing a sentence within the maximum for a charged offense.

Several states have capital sentencing statutes that require juries, in a penalty hearing, to make specific findings before the death penalty may be imposed. For example, the Texas statute requires the jury to decide "whether there is a probability that the defendant would commit criminal acts of violence that would constitute a continued threat to society." In other states, such as California, though the relevant statute does not require a special finding on the question of dangerousness, courts have nevertheless been in the habit of permitting such testimony on the ground that it was generally relevant to a determination of the appropriateness of the death penalty.

The Supreme Court's first encounter with this question came in *Jurek v Texas* (1976),* where the Court declined to invalidate the Texas statute but did not enter on any full discussion of the propriety of using psychiatric predictions of dangerousness as a standard for imposing the death penalty. (In *Jurek*, the testimony was not that of medical experts.) The Court again looked tangentially at the question some years later in *Estelle v Smith* (1981).† The holding in *Smith* was that a psychiatric report on the defendant's future dangerousness had been wrongly admitted in

*428 U.S. 262.
†451 U.S. 454.

the penalty phase of the trial because he had not been afforded an opportunity to consult with counsel before the examination and had never waived his privilege against self-incrimination. This holding does not of course generally invalidate the use of psychiatric predictive testimony or reports provided proper procedures, neglected in *Smith,* have been followed. Indeed, the Court commented that its decisions in the area "in no sense disapprov[e] the use of psychiatric testimony bearing on the issue of future dangerousness."*

The question came squarely before the California Supreme Court in *People v Murtishaw* (1981).† California does not include future dangerousness among the specified findings that are a necessary predicate for the imposition of the death sentence, but in *Murtishaw* the trial court had permitted testimony on this question by a psychopharmacologist during the penalty phase. This testimony was to the effect that the defendant

> will continue to be a violent, assaultive and combative individual . . . in a prison . . . because of his latent rage and hostility and violence. . . . He could show the same types of homicidal tendencies that he has shown in the past, with no ability to morally or physically constrain himself.‡

The jury passed a sentence of death on Murtishaw.

The California Supreme Court annulled the death sentence because of what it held to be the impropriety of admitting psychiatric predictions of violence. The Court pointed out that the statute did not require a finding of dangerousness and the trial court had therefore exercised a discretion in admitting the testimony at all. This discretion was improper in view of (a) the weight of studies suggesting that such predictions had a very high rate of unreliability and (b) the extraordinary caution that a court should employ when dealing with a capital sentence. The court rejected the argument frequently made that the reliability of evidence does not affect its admissibility but goes only to its weight, which can be challenged by cross examination and argued by counsel to the jury or court. In a capital case, the potential for prejudice was, in the view of the Supreme Court of California, so great that the evidence must be excluded altogether.

The California Court's decision would not necessarily apply to cases where the capital sentence was not involved, especially if a statute actually required a finding of future dangerousness. The opinion rests largely on the extraordinary nature of the death penalty and on the unnecessary intrusion of the evidence where the statute did not ex-

---

**Id.* at 473.
†29 Cal. 3d 733, 631 P. 2d 446.
‡29 Cal. 3d at 767, 631 P. 2d at 466.

pressly raise the issue of future dangerousness. Even in a capital case, the court indicated the possibility of two exceptions where psychiatric testimony on this question would be sufficiently reliable to be admissible. These would be where the psychiatrist who reported had had a long term professional relationship with the defendant and, second, where the defendant has "a long-continued pattern of criminal violence such that any knowledgable psychiatrist could anticipate future violence."*

Although the case presents the clearest condemnation of expert predictions of future dangerousness offered by a leading court, the *Murtishaw* opinions still seem not fully developed. If the vice of psychiatric prediction is its inherent unreliability then how can that be saved by the presence of a statute that expressly demands a finding of future dangerousness? Such a demand does not elevate the reliability of the prediction. And how can it be saved by moving out of the field of capital punishment into the context of enhanced prison terms? As argued earlier, a category of evidence that does not pass a threshold test of making a fact in issue more probable than not is simply irrelevant and therefore inadmissible, and this will be so whether the disposition that turns on it is electrocution or paying a fine of $100. The due-process implications of its own analysis were thus left undeveloped in *Murtishaw*. In addition, the two exceptions allowed by the Court seem dubious. A long professional relationship between a psychiatrist and the defendant may perhaps strengthen the chance of accurate predictions of violence in the short term, but there is no reason to suppose that it significantly improves the quality of predictions for the distant future. As for the second exception, which conceded expertise to psychiatrists generally when there has been a "long-continued pattern of criminal violence," the most appropriate comment might be that we hardly need psychiatrists to count previous convictions. Clerks and computers do this just as well and if it is the history of past violence that is the decisive factor, when psychiatrists are no more peculiarly qualified by virtue of their special training than anyone else. The exceptions thus seem to be anaemic compromises that evade the rigorous conclusions demanded by the court's initial premise that the literature studying predictions of long-term future violence does not demonstrate a degree of accuracy sufficient to constitute the basis for enhanced punishment.

The Supreme Court of the United States was again called upon to pass on a challenge to psychiatric testimony introduced to predict future dangerousness in the sentencing phase of a capital case in *Barefoot v Estelle* (1983).† In this case, once more involving the Texas statute, the

*29 Cal. 3d at 774, 631 P. 2d at 470.
†77 L.Ed. 2d 1090.

jury had passed a death sentence at the penalty phase after hearing the testimony of 2 psychiatrists who had not examined the defendant personally but who gave answers to hypothetical questions. The petitioner argued on appeal that psychiatrists generally are incompetent to predict with any acceptable degree of reliability that an individual will commit other crimes in the future and pose a danger to the community. The majority of the Supreme Court responded to this argument by suggesting that it amounted to an invitation to the Court "to disinvent the wheel." By this piece of hyperbole, the Court was apparently referring to the fact that there was some authority that psychiatric predictions were admissible at special sentencing hearings and that the practice of looking to future dangerousness was so well settled in other connections, such as the granting of bail and parole and making civil commitments, that its displacement would be highly disruptive.

As far as capital cases are concerned, the Court's remarks clearly exaggerate the weight of authority. Whereas *Jurek* supported the Court's position, there was also respectable authority to the contrary (as in *Murtishaw*), and for the Court to have taken the contrary position in *Barefoot* would hardly have been a cataclysm in the field of capital sentencing. One senses that the Court was not so much worried about the special question of psychiatric testimony in capital cases but was rather concerned about the general implications of arguments to do with the propriety of making any kind of question turn on evidence about predictions of future dangerousness. If psychiatric testimony were disallowed in a capital case, how could any kind of testimony on this question be allowed in any kind of case? This was perhaps the large issue that the Court could not bring itself to confront at this point and it is the ultimate issue that must be faced in this discussion.

In *Barefoot* itself, the Court embarked on what may seem to be a rather lame defense of the admissibility of psychiatric testimony. Referring to Professor Monahan's study and acknowledging the embarrassing fact that the *amicus* brief of the American Psychiatric Association agreed with the position of the petitioner, the Court nevertheless observed that the petitioner and the Association did not contend that psychiatrists are always wrong in their predictions, but only that they are wrong most of the time. But this, the Court argued, can be brought out by a defendant on cross examination and by adducing his own evidence on the question.

There is, of course, formal logic in the Court's position that the proposition that a psychiatrist is likely to be wrong on a certain question most of the time does not mean that he will be wrong in any given case, but that hardly appears to be the most persuasive consideration. Before we weigh a piece of expert testimony, it is necessary to establish that the subject is a fitting one for the reception of expert evidence at all and that there is a class of people who may fairly be called experts. This was the gravamen of the issue raised by the petitioner and the court's defensive response that psychiatrists after all are likely to be right some of the time (just as someone playing roulette will be right some of the time) hardly seems a sufficient answer. This question can best be explored further by some consideration of doctrines relating to scientific evidence and the testimony of reports of experts.

VI

The law of evidence has developed doctrines relevant to the problems arising from the proof of future dangerousness. These doctrines deal with the questions of what must be shown to render evidence admissible as "scientific" and what circumstances must be present to admit the opinion evidence of an expert. Because most people are impressed by science and experts, such evidence, once admitted, will tend to be very weighty unless it is convincingly controverted by other experts.

The question of whether evidence is scientific has usually arisen with respect to testing procedures that are offered in support of a conclusion relevant to a fact in issue. So ballistic tests and fingerprint tests had to struggle for acceptance while a certain amount of controversy is still engendered by some breath-testing procedures for blood alcohol content. The polygraph or lie detector test procedure continues to be rejected by the great majority of courts. The chief criterion with respect to such procedures was stated in the foundation case of *Frye v United States* (1923),* where the defendant in a criminal case had sought to introduce evidence of a favorable outcome in a lie detector test. The court recognized that in their infancy scientific principles have to struggle to cross a line between "the experimental and the demonstrable stages." Before a court may admit a conclusion deriving from a new procedure, the principle or technique must, in the view of the *Frye* court, "have gained general acceptance in the particular field to which it belongs."† This *Frye* doctrine is not free from obscurity, as there may be arguments about what exactly must have gained acceptance and exactly among whom, but the thrust of the decision has been widely adopted by other courts.

As the *Frye* test implies, the questions of whether a procedure is scientific and whether a question is accessible to scientific analysis are ones of time and place. McCormick in his treatise on evidence quotes a

---

*293 F. 1013 (D.C. Circuit).
†*Id.* at 1014.

court in 1923 as saying "the statement that one can know that a certain bullet was fired out of a .32 caliber revolver when there are hundreds and perhaps thousands rifled in precisely the same manner and of precisely the same character is preposterous."* Improved optical instruments have overturned that judgment just as the great advances of medicine have rendered acceptable expert evidence on the causes of illness or disease that might have been wholly speculative a few decades ago. We have to work with what we know or think we know at a particular time. The "humors" theory of the etiology of disease appears as fanciful today as a microbe theory might have appeared in medieval times. Predictions of future dangerousness may become quite precise in the future but the question is what value and weight they have today. Given the circumstance that the American Psychiatric Association has repeatedly addressed *amicus* briefs to courts with the message that psychiatrists have no reliable technique for predicting future violence, it is apparent that the *Frye* principle could be used as a vehicle for excluding such evidence.

Rules on the admissibility of scientific evidence overlap well-known principles of the law of evidence respecting the testimony of experts. If a matter is fully accessible to the knowledge and experience of the general run of people, then no special explanations or interpretations are needed. A jury may draw its own conclusions from evidence of the underlying facts. But some matters, though well accepted as being within the realm of technological process or scientific analysis, are of so specialized or complicated a nature that no one should come to a judgment on them without hearing the evidence of specially qualified persons. The details of the most modern methods of producing steel, the nature of the generally accepted best methods of treating certain diseases, the workings of a commodity market would be a few of countless examples. Here, the practice is to introduce testimony by a witness qualified as an expert. The general view is that expert evidence is not to be too tightly confined but may be admitted not only in cases where the ordinary person could have no well-based knowledge or understanding of a subject but also in cases where, although ordinary people might have some general knowledge or experience, there is a special class of persons who have a deeper knowledge that can enrich or expand the understanding of the ordinary person. Predicting future dangerousness might be thought to fall into the latter category if, indeed, it can rise at all to the level of scientific or even relevant evidence.

We have seen that part of the problem here is that the question involves future events but this is not necessarily an insuperable obstacle,

---

*McCormick, EVIDENCE 489 (2d ed. 1972), n. 28 citing *People v Berkman*, 307 Ill. 492, 139 N.E. 91 (1923).

because many instances of predicting the future might properly be regarded as having a scientific basis and might be the subject of expert testimony. The prediction that persons suffering from an identifiable stage of a certain disease, with certain specific accompanying symptoms, will die within twelve months might be made with a very low percentage of false positives. Perhaps there is a certain ambiguity in the term *scientific* in this context. One sense might refer to the accuracy of predictions and might deny the title to any technique that produced less than a very high percentage of true positives. But another sense might concentrate more on methodology and might be willing to call a technique scientific, and recognize its exponents as experts, even if its practice resulted in a considerable number of false positives as long as it complied with a set of criteria for identifying scientific method. Long-range weather forecasting may be a good example. Such forecasters are certainly scientific in the ways in which they have constructed and endeavored to refine their methodology, but their science is still primitive in that we could not base important decisions on their prognostications with great confidence. However, if we have to take decisions that will be vitally affected by future weather we would be foolish not to follow the advice of professional meteorologists, assuming that their advice is by and large better than results obtained by tossing a coin.

Compare this kind of advice with the advice we might receive from the self-proclaimed chiliastic expert who assures us that the world will end on a day and hour certain in the not too distant future. Here, the very title of expert rings hollow because we do not believe there is anything knowable to be expert about. It is not that knowledge about the date of the end of the world is of no interest to us. Most of us might change our behavior substantially if we heeded the warning that the end would come soon. The point is that we simply do not believe that anyone else can know this. Predictions of future dangerousness perhaps fall somewhere between long-range weather forecasts and prophesies of apocalypse. They are like weather forecasts in their earnest pursuit of scientific method and their rudimentary construction of scientific techniques, but more like prophecies in that their accuracy level is very low.

To what extent we make use of them ought to depend overridingly on who is asking the question of whom, in what context, and for what reasons. Suppose I am compelled to take a long journey through the desert, away for days from any other people except one companion; and suppose that I must choose as my companion either x or y, neither of whom inspires me with great confidence, though I am inclined to think x the more reliable. But a psychiatrist who knows them both well tells me that x is a good deal more likely than y to collapse emotionally under the strain of a desert journey. Handbooks on this kind of prediction tell me that psychiatrists tend to be correct in such predictions 54% of the time. It may be a close question whether I am more persuaded by the psychiatrist's slender qualification as an expert or by my own intuition, but I would be foolish in such a situation not to ponder the psychiatrist's forecast carefully. And this is principally because I have no choice but to make a choice. I cannot banish the question because I must travel either with x or with y.

But the proper response in the criminal justice system does not have to be the same because it is at least logically possible to expel the question altogether. Although we have suggested earlier that it is difficult not to think about future dangerousness in the process of sentencing, still an attempt could be made to suppress the consideration. And certainly it is not necessary for a statute to pose the question specifically to juries as a precondition for an enhanced sentence and even for the death penalty. The most objectionable aspects converge in such procedures. The question is asked by the state in the context of a criminal proceeding with a view to enhancing punishment. Under many statutes, it is asked of a jury. The very posing of the question in a statute has a tendency to persuade a jury that it is susceptible of a convincing response. And when psychiatric testimony is admitted by the court as that of experts, the endorsement is doubled. A natural lay respect for doctors may be reinforced by their introduction as witnesses for the state, certified by the court as eminently qualified to respond to a question whose legitimacy is in turn certified by its appearance in a statute. To persuade juries in these circumstances that the evidence of the state's psychiatrist is to be taken lightly and that, indeed, no response to the question posed ought to be viewed with any confidence may be a daunting task for the defense. The context and aim of the proceeding and the entrustment of the question to the jury combine to create a potential for the most acute prejudice—in the case of the death penalty, what might be called extreme prejudice.

Rules about the exclusion and admissibility of evidence in the common law system were devised for the most part with the institution of the jury in mind. Traditionally, application of the rules of evidence has been relaxed when a question is to be decided by the court without the participation of a jury. In some states, the death penalty question is for the judge, whereas the ordinary sentencing procedure, lacking any special hearing on dangerousness, is naturally usually a matter for the judge alone. This raises the question of whether in this general sentencing context there may not be a better case for permitting consideration of future dangerousness and even specific psychiatric testimony going to that issue. Whatever the best answer to that question, it seems that, given the unreliability of the evidence, it is wrong in principle to allow the question to be made a condition for enhanced punishment when the matter must be decided by a jury. But unreliability is not the only difficulty here and the other problems, as we shall now see, affect even hearings before a judge without a jury.

VII

The recent gathering stream of studies on the reliability of predictions of dangerousness has demonstrated that the most useful underlying procedures are those which rest in an actuarial way on broad data bases. Professor Monahan has commented:

> The most important single piece of information one can have in prediction [sic] violence is the base rate for violent behavior in the population with which one is dealing. The base rate is simply the proportion of people in the population who will commit a violent act in a given time period.*

Even so, Monahan summarizes research studies as indicating that "psychiatrists and psychologists are accurate in no more than one out of three predictions of violent behavior over a several year period among institutionalized populations that had both committed violence in the past and were diagnosed as mentally ill."† Statistical methods relying on other demographic data may improve accuracy but they are plagued by moral and constitutional questions arising out of the fact that apart from past violent behavior (which itself usually includes behavior as a juvenile) the most important variables as those of sex, race, employment, and alcohol or other drug abuse. Can we properly take these factors into account in a legal context even assuming that their use could lift the accuracy of predictions to a more acceptable level?

Certainly, any plans for preventive detention (preceding a finding of guilt) that rested on such factors would be constitutionally very vulnerable. If, for example, in determinations of dangerousness relating to the granting or denial of bail we were to rely on factors such as the defendant's race, or sex, the equal protection clause of the Fourteenth Amendment would be implicated. The State may not use the suspect classifications of race or sex as a basis for imposing any disadvantage unless it can demonstrate a compelling interest. Even if protecting citizens from the threat of violence could be regarded as a compelling interest in some general sense, it would be rendered much less than compelling in the context of the disposition of an individual defendant by the very low credibility that could be attached to the small degree of

---

*Monahan, THE CLINICAL PREDICTION OF VIOLENT BEHAVIOR 39 (1981).
†*Id.* at 60.

increased accuracy conferred on the prediction by the use of the suspect categories. Do these arguments lose any of their force in the context of a special hearing as to the dangerousness of a convicted offender, whether it be for the enhancement of a prison term or for deciding whether to impose the death penalty, or in the general process of sentencing?

It is possible to attempt to distinguish the situations. The argument might run as follows. It is an absolute principle of the morality of our system that punishment can only rest on the finding of guilt for doing a forbidden act. But the convicted offender is already identified as a member of that class. For him, the question is no longer whether he is properly punishable at all but only what is the proper punishment. Suppose his history of violence as a juvenile together with present unemployment statistically increase the chance that he will be violent in the near future. It is true that our system's principles demand that we treat every offender as an individual human being, but what does it mean to treat someone as an individual? Is his past violence not a part of his individual personality and is his present unemployment not a part of what makes him individual? Perhaps he is not to blame for his present unemployment and in some sense not to be blamed afresh for what he did wrongly in the past, but the question that we have to consider (the most appropriate sentence) should not be thought of as just a question of weighing present blame. It may also take into account how long a term of detention is appropriate in the interests of society for a person who has independently been indentified as seriously blameworthy. Any potential for excessive harshness could be checked by restraints and stops. We could limit the permissible amount of enhancement of sentence and we could exclude the death penalty altogether for independent reasons to do with the extreme nature of the sentence.

This line of argument has some plausibility but cannot prevail without important modifications. Its fatal defect is its inability to defend against the charge that it justifies detention or the prolongation of detention by circumstances over which offenders have no control and for which they are therefore in no way responsible. This is patently so with sex and race and is probably usually so with employment, in spite of recent suggestions that a deliberate choice to pursue crime as a way of life may sometimes be responsible for unemployment. Looking to such factors to assess future dangerousness for purposes of fixing a criminal penalty will inevitably be seen as punishing people because they are young, unemployed, black males. Explanations that it really amounts to incapacitation and not punishment are not likely to mollify when what is imposed is exactly the kind of disposition traditionally regarded as the most unpleasant outcome of a criminal proceeding.

This conclusion does not altogether deny the propriety of taking dangerousness into account in sentencing, but it does require that the only indicia of dangerousness to which a court may look are those over which the defendant had control, for which he can be held responsible in the classic understanding of that concept in the criminal justice system. We must be faithful to the system's deepest level of principle. This restricts us to taking into account only what people have done and not what they are or, to put it better, it confines the concept of what people are to a review of the things they have responsibly done. In essence, this means that the defendant's previous record of dangerous behavior will be the only proper material to be consulted.

The most difficult case here will be the commission of previous offenses while a juvenile. The theory of our juvenile proceedings does not deny that juveniles are in some measure responsible but regards them as having a special potential for reclamation and perhaps as in some way having a diluted responsibility. These strands have combined to develop rules that bar the introduction of juvenile offenses as evidence for most purposes in subsequent proceedings against the defendant as an adult. And yet the commission of violent acts as a juvenile may be one of the most helpful predictors of future dangerousness. Perhaps the most reasonable response would be a version of a limitation period by which juvenile offenses could be counted for some years in determining the disposition for a fresh offense but would eventually (perhaps after 5 years) be a prohibited consideration in fixing a sentence.

The proposal advanced here is by no means a reversion to a full desert theory. Estimates of future dangerousness will be permitted in the sentencing process and are justified on mixed grounds that comprise the demonstrated inadequacy of past deterrents, a need for a longer period in which to rehabilitate the offender or change his disposition, and the social defense principle of protecting the public through extended incapacitation. Although a deserved punishment is the foundation on which all else must be built, the length of the sentence need not be justified in "pure" desert concepts. But in each case the disposition will turn upon an evaluation of the defendant's criminal individuality and special dangerousness as exhibited in criminal acts for which he was responsible. This is fully consonant with basic values of the criminal justice system and with the traditional mixed approach to sentencing.

There remains the problem of reliability. Evaluations of future dangerousness based solely on a past criminal record or a history of past violent acts are likely to be even less reliable than those arrived at by the infusion of additional data of the demographic kind that we have suggested must be excluded. It is not, therefore, even more unjustifiable to rely upon such fragile forecasts? But let us assume that a history of past violence does establish *some* increased risk of future dangerousness as compared with offenders who do not have this record. Predictions of future violence for offenders with a past record will still include a high number of false positives, but the number will be lower when the past history is considered than when it is not. When this history is factored into our estimate, we shall still be wrong a lot of the time but without it we would be wrong most of the time. Does this constitute a sufficient warrant to make use of the record as a consideration in sentencing?

There is a respectable argument that it does confer that right. The defendant is now convicted again for a violent or otherwise dangerous crime. This conduct on his part may fairly be taken to operate as a forfeit of the right that others enjoy that we should not pay attention to anything less than overwhelming predictions of future dangerousness. Part of the routine social price to be paid for the repetition of bad acts is that people will not take a chance on one in the future, even if they judge the chance to be quite small. This is the principle that operates here. We do not need to call for the degree of proof we should demand in a civil commitment situation or even in a quarantine case where no fault is to be laid at the door of the respondent. Repeated criminal violence for which an offender is responsible deservedly incurs the risk of society's responding in a self-protective manner by adverting to the risk of repetition in its disposition of the offender, even if this risk cannot be established beyond a reasonable doubt nor even by a preponderance of the evidence. It is, however, necessary that the record be relevant to a finding that the defendant is more likely to be violent in the future than other offenders who do not share his past history.

VIII

If the lines of the above proposal were followed, considerable difficulty would remain in building a fair and orderly practice of sentencing. As we have seen, there are presently two rather different situations in which questions of future dangerousness can arise. One is the structured hearing for purposes of possible penalty enhancement, as in some death penalty statutes and in the general federal statute relating to special, dangerous offenders. Here existing procedures afford large elements of due process, including a hearing in an adversary style, but there are still important distinctions between this hearing and the trial phase because proof by a preponderance is accepted and, under the federal statute, the hearing is before a court without a jury. All the federal courts of appeal that have considered attacks on the federal statutes have upheld its constitutionality and have taken the view that it does not create an aggravated offense but is rather only a sentencing inquiry and, indeed, affords rather more due process than sentencing inquiries generally do. The earlier discussion should demonstrate that this conclusion is not easy to accept. The federal statute provides for a specific enhancement of the penalty above the maximum for the underlying offense. And this depends not simply on a prior record but on a separate, additional finding of dangerousness. But the argument of the federal appellate courts to the effect that judges have always unofficially and informally considered dangerousness in ordinary sentencing deliberations, without any burden of proof requirement, is a challenging one and forces us to confront the question asked earlier as to whether a procedure should be condemned merely because it expresses a statutory specification of dangerousness as a precondition for an enhanced sentence. Does drawing the line at this point become a mere formalism, and, if so, is the right answer an attempt to introduce stricter due-process controls into the general process of sentencing?

The drawing of the line can be defended. When there is a special sentence enhancement based on special findings arrived at in a penalty hearing, the state has initiated a procedure aiming at a recorded judgment that the offender falls into a special category that brands him as worse than other offenders by reason of some special antisocial character. The principle residing in the *Specht* decision of the Supreme Court, discussed earlier, rightly points to the necessity to apply full due-process guarantees in such a situation. But with ordinary sentencing, we do not have such an escalation of the nature of the judgment. The jury verdict relates to a single range of badness and gravity within which judges have been assigned the task of making the subtler judgment of the precisely appropriate sanction. It is, of course, possible that legislatures could evade this distinction by simply providing very high maximum sentences so that courts could "enhance" for perceived dangerousness beyond what might be regarded as the desert maximum for the offense itself. But we have to begin by assuming that legislatures are acting honestly and, if they are not, we may fall back on other principles such as that prohibiting cruel and unusual punishment.

When a jury convicts a defendant, it finds that he committed the offense beyond a reasonable doubt, but it does not find beyond a reasonable doubt whether he did it atrociously or moderately or with mitigating circumstances. To some extent, these distinctions may inhere in the division of offenses into degrees, but they are never expressed in full exactitude, and there is always room for assessing how bad an instance of a particular category of crime an individual offender's act amounts to. This is, of course, what judicial discretion in the sentencing process is designed to address itself to. But the old tradition that this judicial response need not receive a reasoned expression and is generally not subject to any review in an atrocious one. If dangerousness based on a past record is a matter that courts may generally take into consideration in sentencing, fairness imposes certain demands. As we have suggested, a court should state in a presentencing statement the facts relating to dangerousness that the court finds relevant. In so far as these relate to past criminal convictions, there should be no difficulty with their verification, though the defendant may wish to file a statement explaining or mitigating the significance of earlier convictions. Insofar as the court's statement refers to events in the past life of the defendant alleged by the prosecution in its presentencing statement but not supported by previous convictions, the defendant may contest the prosecutor's version and should be entitled in that case to a hearing and the court should ignore allegations that are not established convincingly. Some of these requirements are already pretty well incorporated into sentencing law and practice, and they represent a welcome infusion of due-process notions into the sentencing phase.

After factual matters have been investigated in this way, the sentencing court should be entitled to take into account any established past actions by the defendant that tend to increase the risk of his future dangerousness, provided that the past record includes at least one previous conviction for the kind of offense that indicates dangerousness of the relevant kind. But the court should not look to any demographically based projections nor to psychiatric reports. The first are to be excluded insofar as they do not relate to acts done by the accused and the second in part for the same reason and, insofar as they are based on the defendant's past record, because psychiatrists have no more expertise to predict on this basis than anyone else. The court's sentence supported by a final statement of reasons should be subject to review by an appellate court.

If this procedure commends itself, then special sentence-enhancing statutes based on a finding of dangerousness should be regarded as unwise and in the best view unconstitutional, even though the courts have not yet been ready to come to this conclusion. Such statutes specify a future risk that must be proved by a preponderance of evidence but, as we have seen, in the present state of knowledge and technique proof in this measure cannot be made. The heightened risk that is the most that can be shown falls far short of proof to this degree and therefore ought not to serve as the basis of a statutory judgment that an offender merits a higher degree of punishment than that prescribed for the underlying offense for which he has been convicted. The analogies of bail and civil commitment proferred by some courts to justify such statutes are quite unconvincing, because these situations involve prediction of the short-term future, where there is greater reliability. Also they do not entail judgments of guilt or punishment and so do not trigger the same constitutional demand for the highest degree of proof.

By contrast in the ordinary sentencing situation (as opposed to special statutory enhancement), though judicial discretion can be partly controlled, it would probably be impossible to expel considerations of future dangerousness altogether. If the attempt were made, courts could reach the same results by viewing the defendant's past record as indicating the need for sharper deterrence, or a longer period for rehabilitation or even as evincing a worse character calling for greater retribution. It is better to accept the inevitability of such consideration and to endeavor to make it open and subject to some principled control and appellate review.

IX

If these conclusions and proposals are defensible, they virtually rule out any role for the psychiatrist or allied professional in this aspect of the sentencing process. Psychiatrists confront the prospect of dangerousness in persons whom they examine or who are their patients in a number of contexts. There is, for example, the question of whether a psychiatrist has a duty to bring a patient's dangerousness to anyone's notice if he believes the patient to be a threat to a specific potential victim or to society generally. At any rate, with respect to the threat to a specific potential victim, some courts have begun to recognize a duty in this respect. But to acknowledge such a duty (a conclusion itself fraught with controversy) does not invalidate the arguments against a psychiatrist's offering such predictive testimony in the sentencing phase of a criminal proceeding. The interest of protecting another person's life may in some cases be taken to outweigh the values of confidentiality and privacy in the doctor–patient relationship. Warning is all that is contemplated and some appreciable apprehension of danger may be enough to justify this or even impose a duty to warn. But much more is required for a prediction to be counted as a proper foundation for incarceration.

Psychiatrists can properly be seen as having in general terms a public duty to offer their expertise to institutions of government for the protection of society, but such a duty has clear limitations. It would be improper for psychiatrists to refuse to take part in the inquiry that may take place in a criminal trial into the responsibility of the defendant when a defense of insanity is raised. Although medicine may not deal in concepts of responsibility, the law must do so and it is an accepted part of our social morality that mental or emotional illness of a certain kind or intensity may refute responsibility. Psychiatrists can properly be asked to give us a description of the kind of illness or condition a defendant was suffering from so that we may use that profile in answering questions about his responsibility.

Psychiatrists may also properly be asked to give us the benefit of their clinical skills in predicting whether a person is likely to be dangerous to himself or others in the immediate future so that some kind of temporary detention may be ordered, for it does seem to be the case that psychiatrists are better than lay persons at such estimates. But a quite different responsibility is assumed by those who speak as to sentencing especially when they know that what they say can scarcely fail to be highly influential. Here, the justification for proferring an opinion must be a special expertise that enables the witness to comment with a high degree of confidence. When that is absent, the proper course of action is silence. If the law itself has not yet recognized this, psychiatrists can teach the courts a useful lesson by not participating in sentencing hearings.

III

Aspects of Psychiatry and the Civil Law

5

Psychiatry and Civil Law

JONAS R. RAPPEPORT

PSYCHIATRY AND CIVIL LAW

When one thinks of forensic psychiatry, which Seymour Pollack has defined as "the application of psychiatry to legal issues for legal ends, legal purposes,"[1] the immediate image is of the insanity plea and the psychiatrist's role with criminal law. We hear much less of psychiatric involvement with civil law. Reflecting this, there is little in the psychiatric literature about civil law issues. (I know of only three books,[2,3,4] two monographs,[5,6] and a few articles[7] on the subject.) Because, as far as the law is concerned, all that is not criminal is essentially civil, the subject matter covers a vast area. In an oversimplified sense, criminal law maintains public order and essentially deals with crimes against the state; civil law protects individual rights and attempts to resolve disputes between individuals (or between an individual and the State).

Forensic psychiatrists involved with civil law may be called in on cases ranging from child custody determinations through wills/testamentary capacity and including, but not limited to, determinations regarding personal injury, malpractice, worker's compensation, and Social Security disability. This discussion will focus on worker's compensation, Social Security disability, private insurance disability claims, and personal-injury-related psychiatric impairment.

In preparing this article, I looked through the index of the latest three-volume edition of the Kaplan et al. "Comprehensive Textbook of Psychiatry."[8] *Social Security* was not listed; "disability" sent me to the

JONAS R. RAPPEPORT • Medical Service of the Circuit Court, Room 503, Courthouse West, Baltimore, Maryland 21202.

glossary. There was no listing for *impairment*. Under "occupation," I could find only "stress" and was referred to the section on "other conditions not attributable to a mental disorder." Does this sparsity of writings reflect psychiatry's lack of knowledge in these areas; or is there actually little psychiatric impairment related to these issues; or is this lack of information the result of the law's failure to appreciate psychiatric impairment in determining disability?

Recovery without Physical Injury

Lawmakers appear to be leery about looking at the emotional factors involved in the areas of civil law I am discussing. Although decisions have varied, the general attitude has been if there is no actual physical injury, the patient may not recover damages. There are, however, cases allowing for recovery without physical injury that go back as early as 1882, when a British telegraph office worker was allowed compensation for emotional disturbance without physical injury following his being frightened when a locomotive smashed through one wall of the office in which he was working. He received payment for temporary disability due to "fright"; however, in 1896, a woman who allegedly had a miscarriage as a result of fear over the actions of a mismanaged team of horses was denied redress. The court said, "If emotional caused ills were compensable, injury may be easily feigned without detection and damages may rest on mere conjecture and speculation—a wide field would be opened for fictious or speculative claims."[9] It is clear that the court was saying that, if we allowed recovery without actual physical injury, we would be opening a Pandora's Box for claims in an area that cannot easily be verified.

Another legal reason for a restriction on psychological claims following injury rests on the doctrine of foreseeability, or duty, which is one of the foundations of Tort (injury) Law. In essence, this rule states that the defendant owes a duty to avoid injury to the plaintiff only as far as the natural and probable consequences of his acts dictate. Thus, the defendant should not be held liable for the plaintiff's individualized reaction to an occurrence. However, when physical injury occurs, such as a head injury to a man with a paper-thin skull, the defendant is held responsible on the legal theory that he takes the victim as he finds him. Why is the plaintiff's emotional vulnerability treated differently? A thin skull is not easily feigned but neither is an hysterical neurosis. In recent years, there have been inroads on the law's resistance, some of them somewhat ludicrous, as in the case of the woman sitting in the front row of a circus who suffered severe psychic trauma after one of the horses defecated on her. In this case, the court allowed an award for her emotional symptoms based on the actual contact between the horse and her.[10]

In other cases, the courts have allowed for psychic trauma on the basis of the *"zone of danger"* concept; that is, where the plaintiff's proximity to danger resulted in emotional trauma from the fear of possible injury. Other recent cases have allowed recovery where the plaintiff was clearly exposed to obvious severe emotional stress when standing outside of, but near, the zone of danger and helplessly observing severe physical trauma to a loved one.[11]

Evaluating Impairment

It is important to separate the medical concept of impairment from the legal concept of disability. Impairment is a medical term; disability is a legal term. In the words of R. Buckland Thomas:

> Psychiatric impairment is defined in terms of the degree of loss of total functional capacity that is directly related to a definite psychiatric illness . . . Disability, although related to impairment, is a different concept. Its meaning implies disadvantage, restriction or—probably more frequently—the inability to pursue an occupation because of physical or mental impairment . . . the determination of disability is considered to be legal or administrative as opposed to a medical determination of impairment.[12]

It is imperative that we keep this differentiation in mind. In criminal law, the forensic psychiatrist renders an opinion as to a person's psychic impairment, which affects competency or responsibility, but the law determines whether or not that person is in fact legally competent or responsible, that is, suffers such a disability. In civil law, the forensic psychiatrist renders an opinion as to the degree of psychic impairment and how it affects his daily or work performance and the law then ascribes the degree or percent of disability.

Some distinctions between general psychiatry and forensic psychiatry may be important in evaluating impairment. Forensic psychiatrists must not forget that they have been consulted not for therapeutic reasons but to help the patient deal with a third party. There is a great likelihood that the patient will not be as truthful as he or she would be in other circumstances. The law recognizes that an accident victim who consults a physician for treatment is likely to be truthful about how the accident occurred so that he or she can be treated properly. The same patient consulting a physician for an examination long after the accident for the purpose of obtaining expert testimony in a lawsuit may not be as truthful. (I have written, elsewhere, about the differences between general and forensic psychiatry.)[13] In this circumstance, psychiatrists must shift their attitude completely; not only may they not believe everything the patient says, but they must suspect malingering as opposed to denial, suppression, or distorted perception. They must obtain information from any source that will help. It must be constantly kept in mind that the information furnished by patients or their attorneys may be distorted; psychiatrists must be cautious about basing their opinion solely on that information. Too often, when confronted with other contradictory information, psychiatrists have stated that they are not detectives; they have based their opinion merely upon what the patient told them.

In the treatment situation, the therapists defend such an attitude by stating that they do not want to "pass judgment" on their patients. Many would question the validity of this stance, but I will not argue the point here, because my focus is on the forensic setting. I do not believe that a report based only on what the patient and his or her attorney have said represents a "scientific" or "medical" report unless there is a *caveat* indicating the limited sources of information. Are not single-source forensic reports really adversarial discussions rather than medical reports? I raise this question here because I believe it bears on the evaluation of impairment. Of course, time and money limitations may interdict more thorough evaluations; however, we do need to keep this issue in mind. (Single-source opinions based on unvarified facts without clear-cut symptoms, etc., are not scientific and may not warrant the status of expert opinions.)

Now let us look at the actual process of assessing impairment for civil law purposes. Richard Rosner[14] described the sequence of steps a physician should take after being requested to testify on behalf of a patient suing an employer. The physician should ask the patient to have his or her attorney call and then attempt to find out the specific medical/legal issue involved. (Each of the four types of on-the-job injury compensation that I discuss later—tort liability, worker's compensation, Social Security disability, and compensation under a part of a disability insurance plan—entails different rules of law and legally defined criteria, and each may require different medical data.) Next, the doctor should ask the patient's attorney to explain the legally defined criteria of relevance to the specific medical/legal issue. Each of the 50 states has its own constitution, legal statutes, and body of case law (i.e., previously adjudicated lawsuits). In addition, the federal courts have their legal statutes and case law. It is important to find out how a given jurisdiction defines the tort liability for a medical impairment due to on-the-job injury.

Rosner noted that psychiatrists must list both their "hard" and "soft" findings; that is, their interpretation of the verifiable facts, limitations, other medical reports and clear-cut objective symptoms, and soft or subjective complaints, and how these produce impairment and then how they relate to the definition of disability. The psychiatric examination must focus on clinical data that are relevant to the legally defined criteria for the specific issue. Elsewhere, Rosner[15] cautioned that

> much psychiatric-clinical data is extraneous and distracting in a psychiatric-legal setting. . . . To determine what is relevant, one must have a knowledge of the legal issue (step one) and a knowledge of the applicable criteria that determine the meaning of the legal issue (step two).

The fourth step Rosner[15] described is articulating the *causal* connection between the findings and the legally defined criteria. He emphasized the absolute necessity of explaining the *logical* connection between the clinical material and the expert opinion. This is merely the verbalization of the reasoning process that has already occurred in a good psychiatric-legal evaluation. It involves a report on how the pertinent findings of the psychiatric examination directly respond to the legally mandated criteria. In this context, it must be remembered that causation has totally different meanings in medicine and in law. What the law is interested in is not the scientific cause but the proximate cause.

The concept of psychic injury or impairment is often blurred by our own negative and positive feelings about suffering. On the one hand, suffering can evoke resistance, denial, negativism, hostility, and suspicions of malingering; on the other hand, we identify with the ill and downtrodden. Emmanuel Tanay noted that our resistance to observing the consequences of psychic trauma stems from the human need to feel invulnerable. We need to believe that a normal individual can recover from an overwhelming experience after a period of time without lasting damage to the psyche.[16]

We work hard and complain little; this whining, depressed, "impaired worker" may not arouse our sympathy. Is this malingering, a presentation of past psychopathology, or the result of other life issues unrelated to the trauma in question? Parlour,[17] who considers himself a defense psychiatrist, cited data from a number of studies which document the use of physical injury and subsequent disability payments as a solution to ongoing psychological problems. He noted that a study by Selzer and Vinokur demonstrated a significant relationship between life change and current subjective stress, on the one hand, and traffic accidents, on the other. In short:

> It may become more difficult to assert that psychiatric disabilities are job related. The evidence is persuasive that most affective disorders, schizophrenic disorders, and many anxiety disorders have substantial hereditary components. It may thus be argued that the disability would have occurred anyway.[17]

A further area of confusion is the variability of reactions to comparable events. What is psychologically stressful to one person will not seem to affect another. Raskin spoke of "affect and tolerance," the ability to deal with feeling aroused by the incident.[18] Modlin spoke of ego impairments that prevent the integration of, and adaptation to, the stress.[19] The forensic psychiatrist faces the difficult task of determining the degree of impairment and then presenting this to the court in such a way that it can determine the degree of disability. I believe that it is exceedingly difficult to clarify many of the issues involved in a completely satisfactory way. There are those who claim that attorneys tell their clients to exaggerate their symptomatology and not "get well" until the case has been settled. Edward Colbach[20] wrote of the "mental-mental" muddle in Oregon, the state with the highest cost of worker's compensation insurance in 1978. In 10 years, there was a 49% increase in claims found to be disabling, especially those of the mental-mental type; that is, "some sort of mental stress has resulted in a mental problem."[20] Now public policy decisions must be made. Did Pandora's Box open too wide?

Worker's Compensation

The establishment of worker's compensation represented a legal attempt to assist the worker in obtaining compensation for injuries that occur in the line of duty through no one's fault. The original premise was that the worker would give up the hope of a large award and the risk that he might lose the case for a lesser award determined in a more liberal fashion. In the same way, the industrialist or manufacturer would give up hope of prevailing and instead buy insurance against workers' disabilities and submit conflicts to a special administrative court. Recovery for pain and suffering was eliminated. As a social policy decision, worker's compensation has been broadened so that the causal connection may be minimal. (Remember cause and etiology are not the same.) If a factory worker has a heart attack while working, it may be assumed that the heart attack was the result of his employment (i.e., his employment was the proximate cause of the heart attack). Yet, the truth may be that if the worker had been subject to any stress—or no stress—the coronary arteries would have occluded at that time. Because the attack occurred in the work situation, it may be compensable. In fact, even if it occurred outside of the work situation, but could be related to some particular stress that occurred in the work situation, it might be compensable. In some ways, worker's compensation is a form of social insurance.

The emotional effects of workplace stress, however, have not been so readily accepted, harking back to the Pandora's Box concept of the court in 1896. A landmark case that helped pierce this mental illness barrier (*Carter v General Motors*) involved a young man working on an assembly line who could not keep up with the work and was pressed to do more and more by his supervisors; he eventually developed an overt paranoid schizophrenic psychosis, was hospitalized, and subsequently received worker's compensation. Many believe that this 1961 case was the door-opener for the admission of psychic trauma into this area of civil law.[21]

A 1976 case (*Swiss Colony, Inc. v the Dept of Industry, Labor and Human Relations*)[22] involved a woman who had worked for Swiss Colony, a mail-order cheese company located in Monroe, Wisconsin, since 1955. She became the purchasing agent for the fast-growing company in 1961. This job subjected her to numerous stresses and strains. In the Spring of 1971, she began to feel rattled and disorganized and less able to withstand the mounting pressures of her job. In November 1971, she consulted a physician and, on November 7, was admitted to St. Clare Hospital in Monroe suffering from weight loss, insomnia, exhaustion, and depression. After staying in the hospital, on November 18, she was released but she was readmitted on November 29 in a psychotic state diagnosed as schizophrenia. She was again released on January 10, 1972 but did not return to work until October of that year. She then returned to work half time in a position of reduced responsibility and pressure. On January 2, 1973, she began to work full time in this reduced position. She entered the claim that she had become disabled by mental illness caused by the stresses and strains of her employment and that this illness constituted an accidental injury arising out of her employment. The lower court agreed. On appeal, the question was asked, "Was the claimant subject to stresses and strains which were out of the ordinary from the day-to-day stresses and strains which all employees must experience and, if so, did these out-of-the-ordinary stresses cause the claimant's mental disability?" The Court of Appeals answered both questions affirmatively and said:

> There is no question that . . . the claimant was subject to stresses and strains which were out of the ordinary from the day-to-day stresses and strains which all employees must experience. It is true that, as both psychiatrists and the psychologist testified, mental health specialists believe that all schizophrenics have a genetic predisposition to this condition, although an examination of the claimant's family history revealed no mental problems of this type. The condition of schizophrenia does not exist until it is created by life stresses, and in this case it did not exist at all until the claimant's gradual decline and breakdown in the Fall of 1971. This is not a case where there is a history or evidence of prior mental or mental-physical disabilities later aggravated by work stresses. There is extensive credible evidence in this case that the cause of the claimant's mental disability was the usual work stress which she was subject to in 1971. The claimant's admitting psychiatrist . . . testified that this work stress was the major contributing factor to the claimant's mental dis-

ability (and) . . . that, if this unusual work stress had not been present, the claimant would not have experienced her mental breakdown. The claimant had had marital difficulties, especially in 1968–1969, but her psychiatrist discounted these prior difficulties as a minor stressful situation in 1971. He testified that the claimant would not have suffered her disability because of her marital problems alone, and that she would have experienced a break-down regardless of her marital situation. . . . Finally, it is undisputed that the actual precipitating factor of the claimant's initial breakdown in October 29, 1971, was a work-related incident. Accordingly, there was sufficient medical proof in this case to substantiate the claim of a 25 percent permanent partial mental disability.[22]

In the 1981 Oregon case, *James v SAIF (State Accident Insurance Fund)*[23], the claimant clearly had preexisting psychiatric illness. In explaining the difference between an occupational disease and an accident, the court said that

accidents are sudden and unexpected. An occupational disease, on the other hand, is recognized as an inherent hazard of continued exposure to conditions of a particular employment and comes on gradually. It would appear that Ms. James's neurosis would constitute an occupational disease and not an accident. Therefore, to be compensable, it must be caused by circumstances to which an employee is not ordinarily subjected or exposed except during a period of regular employment.[20]

After examining Ms. James's history, the court pointed out that she was apparently highly sensitive to any criticism, both on and off the job, and had become quite upset a few months before she left work after a school principal was critical of her in an incident involving her child. In this case, the court thought that there was a fact question as to whether the claimant's condition was caused by circumstances "to which an employee is not ordinarily subject or exposed to other than during a period of regular actual employment."[20]

Parlour has delineated special problems in managing psychiatric aspects of workmen's compensation cases. He believes the legal system encourages claims of psychiatric impairment in various ways, including the common attribution of personal misery to the work experiences.

Despite these inherent disadvantages, skilled defense psychiatrists can frequently mobilize the healthful motivation of plaintiffs by helping them improve their maladaptive life-styles, thus minimizing disability claims. In other cases, defense psychiatrists can develop credible documentation that plaintiffs' residual disabilities should not be completely attributed to job exposures.[24]

Parlour proposed that the American Psychiatric Association "form a Task Force on worker's compensation to facilitate education and communications in this field, and to consult with interested outside groups, notably legislatures, bar associations, insurance carriers, businessmen, and labor unions."[24]

An important obstacle to the resolution of the worker's compensation problems I have been discussing is the lack of motivation on the part of insurance companies and plaintiffs' attorneys to deal with this problem in other than an economic (raise rates) and legal (case law) fashion. Neither appears interested in encouraging medical research. Should the situation get out of hand, I suspect we can depend on court decisions such as that in the *James* case to reduce findings of disability.

Before leaving this subject, it is important to mention what is probably the largest area of worker's compensation, disability for veterans, which to my knowledge has received *no* attention in the literature. Dan Sprehe, in a 1980 presentation, commented on this.[25] Tens of thousands of veterans receive disability benefits, some for psychological or physical injuries that seem only remotely related veterans' military service. Does this represent a social policy decision placed on the staff of caduceus?

Social Security Disability

In 1981, the Reagan Administration made changes in the standard for social security disability that resulted in 500,000 mentally ill individuals being taken off of the social security disability rolls. Obviously, this had a tremendous social impact, as well as a devastating personal impact, on those patients and their families. Public pressure and the efforts of the APA caused a reversal of this policy, and we have seen significant changes. Nevertheless, this unfortunate episode highlights how vulnerable legal decisions about disability are to changes in the rules. The impairments never changed, the disability did.

The Social Security Administration has attempted to describe objective standards for assessment of psychiatric impairment. Nussbaum has written extensively on this topic.[26] He has attempted to organize a factor analysis related to symptoms that produce impairment and to quantify these symptoms. This new approach, although clearly not without its problems, is helpful in dealing with the difficult issue of gleaning the necessary information from doctors' reports. Forensic psychiatrists daily confront the difficult task of objectifying the subjective complaints of those they evaluate. That is what makes the assessment of psychiatric impairment so difficult.

Private Insurance Disability Claims

I refer here to claims filed by individuals who own private disability insurance policies. To my knowledge, this category applies exclusively to individuals who are self-employed. In my experience, such claims have been made by self-employed professionals who have had periods of psychiatric hospitalization and whose insurers have wanted an up-to-date (posthospitalization) evaluation. I wonder if any disability claims have been made on the basis of a psychological condition that never required hospitalization, such as a phobia or obessive-compulsive neurosis that might disable an individual to the extent that he or she could not go to work. For example, a cardiac neurosis after a coronary might prevent work. I suspect such claims are extremely rare because, generally, individuals with this type of disability insurance are high-level executives or other professionals who tend not to be so incapacitated by a mental illness that does not require psychiatric hospitalization.

Further, it has been my impression that, in private insurance disability cases, for reasons that are not clear to me, the insurer does not press hard to disallow a claim and may even attempt to make a lump-sum settlement when the prognosis for recovery is poor, as in severe cases of paranoid schizophrenia. I can imagine other situations that might require psychiatric evaluation; for example, a disability claim where there is a question concerning the individual's ability to do the type of work required by the insurance company or any work for which he is trained. Disability policies of this type are written in many different ways; some allow disability if the individual is unable to do his or her usual occupation, while others allow disability only if the individual is unable to do any type of work. How does one determine whether a person is so impaired that he or she is unable to do any type of gainful work? I know of nothing in the literature that speaks to any of these problems.

Psychiatric Impairment after Traumatic Personal Injury

Here, we find a rich field for claims and counterclaims. Psychiatric impairment resulting from a fright, a possible fright, or the so-called *functional overlay* from a physical injury. (This latter term is frequently used loosely to describe any symptoms related to a physical injury that cannot be accounted for by physical findings.) Bromberg noted that functional overlay is not a recognized psychiatric diagnosis. He differentiated functional overlay from organic conditions and from malingering.

> Functional overlay is not malingering; the former is based on preconscious and unconscious mechanisms, the latter is consciously induced. In considering psychiatric reactions to pain and disability, a gradient of simulation, malingering, symptom exaggeration, over-evaluation, functional overlay and hysteria is useful. The dynamics of overlay are a combination of anxiety from body-image distortion and depression from decreased efficiency of the body, as well as the resulting psychosocial disruption in a patient's life."[27]

An example of the fright, or disaster-produced trauma, is seen in the Buffalo Creek Disaster in which the coal company dam ruptured, unleasing over 130 million gallons of water upon the 16 small communities of the valley below. Over 125 people died, leaving 4,000 survivors.[28] This led to a $13.5 million settlement from the Pittston Company.

> Serious psychological impairment has been found in more than 600 adult and child survivors of the 1972 Bufalo Creek disaster in West Virginia, and there is strong indication that the effects of the survivors' psychological trauma are becoming entrenched.[29]

The reaction in response to the Three Mile Island nuclear accident was quite different.[30] A study of the effects of this accident on 151 patients from the Three Mile Island area and 64 from a comparison site sought to isolate the risk factors for those who were most distressed by it. The results showed that those most at risk for trauma (a) lacked a supportive network and (b) continued to view their situation as dangerous for up to 1 year later. The study concluded that "disaster does not significantly increase the abnormalities of psychiatric patients."[30] However, in the year following a disaster, the presence of both risk factors should trigger the clinicians' concern as to whether members of this subcohort sense impending doom and alienation from fellow human beings. The need for clinicians specifically to inquire about these variables and not assume that they will become evident through treatment is supported by data indicating service-use patterns for high and low distress groups were identical in the year following the incident.[30] This latter statement clearly points to some clinical responsibility on the part of the community mental health center and therapist. Does a clinical responsibility develop for the forensic evaluator? Should it be emphasized in the latter's report?

Modlin was one of the first to describe a post accident anxiety syndrome,[19] which was eventually called traumatic neurosis. Today, the concept of the traumatic neurosis may have been lost in the DSM-III category "Post Traumatic Stress Disorder".[31] The initial requirement is exposure to a

> psychologically traumatic event that is generally outside the range of usual human experience. The characteristic symptoms involve reexperiencing the traumatic event; numbing of responsiveness to, or reduced involvement with, the external world; and a variety of autonomic, dysphoric, or cognitive symptoms.[31]

Thus, such common traumas as simple bereavement, business loss, and marital conflict are not included in this category. The stressor may be a natural or man-made disaster and may include a physical component (e.g., rape, assault, torture), in some cases causing direct damage to the central nervous system (e.g., malnutrition, head trauma). The authors of DSM-III noted that "the disorder is apparently more severe and longer lasting when the stressor is of human design."[31]

The DSM-III definition of the stressor covers a multitude of situations and, unfortunately, still leaves us with a subjective foundation. As psychiatrists, we can understand the concept of the overwhelmed ego, the invasion of body space, etc. Can the law understand this? Can we quantify this issue sufficiently to give the law a clearer understanding? Is the law afraid of the Pandora's Box concept with reference to traumatic neurosis? Many of the problems arising here are quite similar to those related to worker's compensation; in fact, in many cases, they are exactly the same. Like other types of disability claims, those involving traumatic personal injury come up against issues of preexisting condition, secondary gain, and functional overlay.

The law is skeptical, as we should be. Did we never see such cases until we gave them a name? Were the symptoms of World War I "shell shock," World War II "combat fatigue," and the "post Vietnam veterans' syndrome" any different? Does the Vietnam outreach project "produce" cases of the stress disorder? Does that program attempt to blame too much character-based behavior on the Vietnam experience? Is psychiatry being "used" in order to justify a social policy; if so, is this good for psychiatry and, more importantly, is it good for the impaired? (In other contexts, Robitscher[32] and Halleck[33] have written about these issues.)

Although the attempts of DSM-III to delineate psychiatric syndromes are meritorius, the "Post Traumatic Stress Disorder" presents a symptomatic picture that can be very subjective. How carefully do we question the patient–plaintiff during an examination requested by his/her lawyer's? Do we search for exaggeration of symptoms? Do we attempt to obtain verification of symptoms from the spouse, relatives, fellow employees? I'm not sure we do, even when we examine for the defense or for a neutral party. Parlour suggested that we work as carefully in civil forensic examinations as we would in criminal forensic ones, utilizing all of the ancillary sources of information available.[17] I do not want to belabor this point; however, if we are to be recognized as legitimate, we must recognize that patients can easily learn which "symptoms" to present to us. We must be thorough and complete.

Other forms of psychiatric impairment occur following either physical or emotional trauma. I refer to the DSM-III category of "Somatoform Disorders," which includes" Conversion Disorder," "Psychogenic Pain Disorder," and "Hypochrondriases."[31] They are subject to the same questions and doubts, and can be prey to the same kind of subjective evidence I have just discussed. Often we must evaluate impairment in gray areas where there seems to be pathology but we are hard put to verify it, clarify it, and relate it to total personality development. We are also faced with the issue of determinism versus causation that arises in civil law, a cause as well of problems in the form of determinism versus free will in our interface with criminal law. Obviously, there are no easy answers. The law must make decisions now and calls on us to assist in any way we can. We must do our best, always seeking to extend the limits of our knowledge.

CONCLUSION

Forensic psychiatrists involved in civil disability cases can and must try to do more. In assessing psychiatric impairment, we must think about and try to implement more research, gather more data, look deeper, and verify more. We must try to develop techniques for treatment and, more important, to test some of the questions that have been raised by defendants and their counsel. Do these patients recover miraculously after a satisfactory settlement of their claims? Are many of the types of impairments I have discussed exaggerated and based on little more than subjective symptoms? Many believe these last two statements are the exception rather than the rule, but we do not really know. In this connection, one wonders why the 1971 *Guides to the Evaluation of Permanent Impairment*[34] has not been converted to DSM-III, and why the insurance companies that frequently criticize us do little to support research. There is no doubt that there is some impairment in many who have suffered injuries, whether of the physical-mental, mental-mental, or any other type. The challenge to forensic psychiatry is to do our best to fully evaluate these patients and present our findings as objectively as possible.

REFERENCES

[1]Pollack, S: Forensic psychiatry, a specialty. *Bull Amer Acad Psychiatry Law*, 2:1–6, 1974.

[2]Leedy, J (ed.): *Compensation in Psychiatric Disability and Rehabilitation.* Springfield, IL, Charles C Thomas, 1971.

[3]Keiser, L: *The Traumatic Neurosis.* Philadelphia, J. P. Lippincott, 1968.

[4]Trimble, MR: *Post Traumatic Neuroses From Railway Spine to the Whiplash.* New York, John Wiley & Sons, 1981.

[5]*Group for the Advancement of Psychiatry (Committee on Psychiatry in Industry): What price compensation?* Vol. IX, N. 99, June 1977.

[6]Williams, T (ed.): *Post-traumatic stress disorders of the Vietnam Veteran.* Cincinnati, OH, Disabled American Veterans, 1980.

[7]Post-traumatic stress disorders. *Behavior Sciences & the Law*, Vol. I, N. 3, Summer 1983.

[8]Kaplan, HI, Freedman, AM, and Sadock, BJ: *Comprehensive Textbook of Psychiatry/III, ed 3.* Baltimore, Williams & Wilkins, 1980.

[9]Morris, C: Emotional disturbances and personal injury cases. *Med Trial Tech Q (Annual),* 157–162, 1961 Also cited in Rappeport, J: Traumatic neurosis, in G. Balis, *et al.* (eds.) *Psychiatric Foundations of Medicine (Vol III).* Reading, MA, Butterworth, 1977.

[10]*Christy Bros Circus v Turnage*, 38 Ga. App. 581, 144 S.E. 680 (1928).

[11]D'Ambra v US, 354 F. Supp 810 (D.R.I. 1973).

[12]Thomas, RB: Psychiatric impairment and disability. *The Psychiatric Forum*, Vol. 23, Spring 1973, pp. 22–24.

[13]Rappeport, JR: Differences between forensic and general psychiatry. *Am J Psychiatry, 139*: 3, March 1982, pp. 331–334.

[14]Rosner, R: Medical disability compensation: a practicum. *New York Univ Medical Q, 34*(1):3–6, Summer 1978.

[15]Rosner, R (ed): Critical Issues in American Psychiatry and the Law. Springfield, IL, Charles C Thomas, 1982.

[16]Tanay, E: Psychic trauma and the law. *Wayne Law Review* 15:3, Summer 1969, p. 1033.

[17]Parlour, R and Jones L: Theories of psychiatric defense in workmen's compensation cases. *Bull Amer Acad Psychiatry and Law*, Vol. VIII, N. 4, 1980, pp. 445–455.

[18]Raskin, H: A view of traumatic neurosis. *Bull Amer Acad Psychiatry and Law 1*:2, April 1973, pp. 124–141.

[19]Modlin, H: The post accident anxiety syndrome: Psychosocial aspects. *Am J of Psychiatry 123*:8, Feb. 1967, pp. 1008–1012.

[20]Colbach, E: The mental-mental muddle and work comp in Oregon. *Bull Amer Acad Psychiatry and Law*, Vol. 10, N. 3, 1982, pp. 165–169.

[21]Carter v General Motors Co., Mich. 577 106 N.W. 2d 105 (1961).

[22]Swiss Colony v U.S. Department of Industry, Labor and Human Relations, 240 N.W. 2d 128 (Wisconsin, 1976).

[23]James v State Accident Insurance Fund, 290 Or. App.343, 624 P.2d 565 (1981).

[24]Parlour, R: The psychiatric defense of worker's compensation cases: A proposal. *"Newsletter" of Amer Acad Psychiatry and Law*, Vol. 8 N. 3, Dec. 1983, pp. 32–33.

[25]Sprehe, D: Worker's Compensation—What happens after the ratings? *International Journal of Law and Psychiatry, 7,*165–178.

[26]Nussbaum, K: Objective assessment of degree of psychiatric impairment: Is it possible? *The Johns Hopkins Med J*, July 1973, Vol.133, N. 1, pp. 30–37.

[27]Bromberg, W: Functional overlay: An illegitimate diagnosis? (Forensic Medicine), *West J Med*, 130:561–565, June 1979.

[28]Stern, G: *The Buffalo Creek Disaster, The Story of the Survivors' Unprecedented Lawsuit.* New York, Random House, 1976.

[29]2 *Clinical Psychiatry News*, Oct. 1974, p. 1.

[30]Bromet, E, Schulbert, H, and Dunn, L: Reactions of psychiatric patients to the Three Mile Island nuclear accident. *Arch Gen Psychiatry 39*:725–730, June 1982.

[31]*Diagnostic and Statistical Manual of Mental Disorders III.* Am Psychiatric Assn,Wash,DC,1980.

[32]Robitscher, JD: *The Powers of Psychiatry.* Boston, Houghton Mifflin, 1980.

[33]Halleck, SL: *The Politics of Therapy.* New York, Science House, 1971.

[34]*Guides to the Evaluation of Permanent Impairment.* Am Med Assn, Chicago, American Medical Assn, 1971. Since this article was written, a second edition using DSM-III has been published: Chapter 12, pp. 215–221.

6

Last Will and Testament: Forensic Psychiatry's Last Frontier?

The Psychiatrist's Role in Will Contests

ROBERT LLOYD GOLDSTEIN

The will! The testament!
Shakespeare, *Julius Caesar*

A *will* is a legal instrument that is executed in accordance with certain formalities, by which a person directs the disposition of his property to take effect following his death. The principal distinction between a will and other types of conveyances (i.e., transfers of title to property) is that a will takes effect only on the death of the maker of the will. In order to protect all persons involved, the law surrounds the making of a will with certain specified formalities, which may vary from state to state depending on local statutory schemes. Each state has its own laws dealing with the right* to make testamentary disposition of one's property (although a number of states have adopted the Uniform Probate Code,† which

---

*The right to bequeath one's property has never been regarded as one of the so-called "natural rights" of man. Testamentary disposition is rather a "privilege" which springs from the law and is completely subject, therefore, to legislative control.

†The American Bar Association approved a Uniform Probate Code (UPC) in 1969 which has been adopted by several states.

ROBERT LLOYD GOLDSTEIN • Department of Psychiatry, The College of Physicians and Surgeons, Columbia University, New York, New York 10032.

simplifies the requirements and procedures). The person who makes a will is the *testator* (*testatrix* in the case of a woman). A *will contest* is a probate proceeding (*probate* means literally *prove*; a *probate proceeding* seeks to prove the will of the deceased).

The four main requirements for the formation of a valid will are

1. the testator must have had *testamentary intent* (*Animus Testandi*) at the time he executed the will (i.e., he must have subjectively intended the particular words to be his will);*
2. the testator must have had *testamentary capacity* at the time of execution of his will (to be discussed in detail);
3. execution of the will must be free of fraud, duress, undue influence or mistake (undue influence to be discussed in detail); and
4. the will must have been duly executed in compliance with applicable statutory requirements.†

A psychiatrist may be called upon to testify at a probate proceeding if a will is challenged (usually by an expectant heir whose hopes were disappointed). Less than 3% of all wills probated in the course of a year are contested and less than 15% of those that are contested are overturned.‡ Psychiatric opinion is generally sought to evaluate *testamentary capacity*. Occasionally, the psychiatrist is asked to address the issue of *undue influence*.§

Testamentary Capacity

The question of testamentary capacity usually must be determined on a *postmortem* basis.‖ The testator is dead by the time a will contest arises, which confronts the psychiatrist with the uncertain task of reconstructing a past situation (as he must also do, for example, in the evaluation of an *insanity defense* in a criminal proceeding) in order to reach a conclusion as to whether or not the testator possessed the requisite capacity at the time the will was executed. However, in contrast to the *insanity defense* situation (which already poses clinical and scientific diffi-

---

Lister v Smith, 164 Eng. Rep. 1282 (A duly executed will is presumed to have been executed with the requisite intent).

†Every will, other than a holographic will (one which lacks formal attestation and execution) or a nuncupative will (an oral will) must be executed in accordance with certain formalities prescribed by statute. The common law of wills is founded on the original Statute of Wills (1540 A.D.).

‡Slovenko, R: *Psychiatry and Law*. Boston, Little, Brown, 1973, p. 336.

§Perr, IN: Wills, Testamentary Capacity and Undue Influence. *Bull Amer Acad Psychiatry & Law*, 9:15–22, 1981.

‖Slovenko, *Psychiatry and Law*, 1973, p. 336.

culties of sufficient magnitude to disenchant many observers of the psycho-legal partnership*), in will contests, the psychiatrist does not even have the opportunity to examine the individual, albeit after the fact. The testator is not available for evaluation. The psychiatrist must glean his data from witnesses who can describe the testator's state of mind and behavior at the time the will was made (witnesses whose powers of observation and disinterest in the outcome of the proceeding are suspect), hospital and nursing home records and other scattered fragments of factual or circumstantial evidence that may be produced. Conclusions arrived at on such a basis must necessarily be regarded as far less reliable than most other conclusions called for in forensic psychiatry. It has been suggested that, after all is said and done, a finding of testamentary incapacity or undue influence by a court has little to do with the convincing scientific proof offered by the expert psychiatric witness. Rather, these issues may constitute an artificial basis or pretext that enables the court to set aside a will it judges to be unfair or unnatural.[†]

Before he hazards an opinion in an area where uncertainty and speculation are everpresent pitfalls, the psychiatrist is obliged to understand the legal framework of testamentary capacity (which is a completely different concept than mental capacity for any other purpose, e.g., capacity to stand trial). Testamentary capacity is a subjective matter, comprised of four elements:[‡]

1. The testator must have actual knowledge of the nature of his undertaking, that is, he must know that he is making his will.
2. The testator must have the capacity to understand the nature, extent, and condition of his property.
3. The testator must have the capacity to understand the relationship between himself and those persons who ought to be in his mind at the time he makes his will: the *natural objects of his bounty.*
4. The testator must have the capacity to interrelate the foregoing factors to form an orderly scheme of disposition.[§]

These standards suggest that capacity must be judged by all the circumstances of the case, taking into consideration the particular testa-

---

*Halpern, AL, Rachlin, S, Portnow, SL: New York's Insanity Defense Reform Act of 1980: A Forensic Psychiatric Perspective. *Albany Law Rev., 45*:661–677, 1981.

†Slovenko, *Psychiatry and Law,* 1973, pp. 342–344.

‡*Gilmer v Brown,* 186 Va. 630; *Estate of Bullock,* 140 *Cal. App.* 2d 944.

§This requirement is analogous to the standard set forth in *Dusky v United States,* 362 U.S. 403 (1960) (To be competent to stand trial, a defendant must have a *rational* as well as a *factual* understanding of the proceedings).

tor, his personal circumstances and the particular will under scrutiny. The requirement of testamentary capacity, therefore, is quite variable, depending among other things on the complexity of the estate involved and the scheme of disposition as well as on the psychological functioning of the testator.* Wills are made by all types of individuals, in every stage of life and condition of health. One is not prevented from making a valid will merely by virtue of being old, uneducated, sick, or lacking in business experience. The psychiatrist must understand that the "sound mind and memory"† that many statutes require as a standard for testamentary capacity is not a mind without fault nor a memory without flaw. Less mental capacity is required to execute a will than any other legal instrument.‡ Courts have rejected the notion that an excellent memory or a high degree of intelligence is required to make a will.§

A testator must understand that he is making a will and thereby disposing of his property under its terms. He need not have a lawyer's understanding of the legal terms of the will, but merely a layman's appreciation of its plan and effect. He must be aware of the nature, extent, and condition of his property and to be able to call it to mind in a general way. This does not mean that he must be able to state from memory everything that he owns and its precise value.∥ He must be able to recall the persons who are the natural objects of his bounty (his relatives, dependents and associates). There is, however, no requirement that he mention them in his will or leave them a bequest. He may cut them off without a penny and still possess testamentary capacity, provided that he was able to recall who they were and what their relationship to him was at the time the will was executed.#

As an expert in psychopathology and its many manifestations and effects, the psychiatrist may be called on to evaluate the impact of the following disorders on testamentary capacity.

---

*Holloway: Testamentary Capacity. N.Y.L.J. 12/2/68, 12/3/68, p. 1, col. 4.

†Some jurisdictions speak of "sound mind and memory" as a standard for capacity. The Georgia statute is particularly colorful, requiring the testator to possess a "decided and rational desire as to the disposition of his property. His desire must be decided, as distinguished from the wavering, vacillating fancies of a distempered intellect. It must be rational, as distinguished from the ravings of a madman, the silly pratings of an idiot, the childish whims of imbecility, or the excited vagaries of a drunkard." *Ga. Code Ann.*, tit. 113, § 202.

‡Matter of Coddington, 281 App Div 143, 118 NYS2d 525, affd 307 NY 181, 120 NE2d 777.

§Matter of Strong, 179 App Div 539, 547, 166 NYS 862.

∥Davidson, HA: *Forensic Psychiatry.* New York, Ronald Press, 1965, pp 124–125. Davidson says that the testator does not have to know "to the square inch the exact acreage of his land nor . . . the serial numbers of his government bonds."

#Davidson, *Forensic Psychiatry,* pp. 124–125.

Psychosis.   Perfect sanity is not required to make a will. Even the existence of a psychotic illness at the time an individual makes his will does not perforce invalidate it. This is analogous to the proposition that all schizophrenics are not thereby incompetent to stand trial* (or the proposition that all involuntarily committed patients are not incompetent to refuse treatment[†]). Even an adjudication of insanity or incompetency for other purposes does not conclusively establish that an individual lacks testamentary capacity (although it may raise a presumption of testamentary incapacity). It must be proven that the psychosis impaired one or more of the essential elements required for testamentary capacity. Therefore, an individual who has been committed to a psychiatric hospital or who has been found not guilty by reason of insanity may still be competent to make a will.[‡]

On the other hand, the presence of *insane delusions* (a legal term of art)[§] that have an effect on the testator's disposition of his property may suffice to set aside a will. Delusions of marital infidelity, of the illegitimacy of one's children, of great wealth or of poverty may serve to invalidate a will.[‖] But not every false belief can be categorized as a delusion. Wills do not depend for their validity on the testator's having reasoned logically or on his freedom from eccentricities or prejudices. "One has the right to make an unjust will, an unreasonable will, or even a cruel will."[#] Shortcomings such as a prejudiced, narrow, or bigoted viewpoint do not destroy testamentary capacity. Indeed, even the presence of a delusion does not necessarily lead to a finding of incapacity. Delusional ideation and testamentary capacity may coexist![**] A testator is incapacitated only when the delusional thinking directly affects the specific factors required for making a will. Persons suffering from encapsulated delusions may be otherwise perfectly competent to manage their own

---

*Goldstein, RL: The Fitness Factory. Part I: The Psychiatrist's Role in Determining Competency. *Am J Psychiatry, 130*:1144–1147, 1973.

[†]Brooks, A: The Constitutional Right to Refuse Antipsychotic Medications. *Bull Amer Acad Psychiatry & Law, 8*:179–221, 1980.

[‡]Wadsworth v Sharpsteen, 8 NY 388, 393.

[§]An insane delusion exists when a person persistently, against all evidence and probability, believes supposed facts which have no existence except in his imagination. The belief must be utterly preposterous and unfounded.

[‖]In re Kahn's Will, 5 NYS 556.

[#]In re Willits' Estate, 175 Calif. 173, 165 Pac. 537 (1970).

[**]To set aside a will on the ground of insane delusions, it must appear that the will was formulated in reliance on the irrational belief. Generally, supernatural or fanatical religious beliefs (e.g., beliefs in witchcraft or spiritualism) do not in themselves lead to a finding of testamentary incapacity. However, a will would be invalid in a case where "the testator was laboring under a delusion that the spirits of the dead were directing him in all his business" and instructing him as to how he should dispose of his property. *Middleditch v Williams*, 45 N.J. Equity 726.

affairs and conduct themselves in accordance with the demands of society.*

Organic Brain Syndromes. The most common condition within this classification that affects testamentary capacity is dementia (senile or presenile type). Memory lapses, disorientation, confusion, delusional ideation, and other impairments may result from advancing degeneration of brain tissue. It should be noted, however, that advanced age alone is no basis for a finding of incapacity.† "The infirmity, listlessness, untidiness or irascibility of old age raise no inference of incapacity."‡ It is always a question of degree. The uncertain progressive nature of the dementias and their varying effect on different individuals require that the psychiatrist return once again to the basic criteria for testamentary capacity and apply them as his yardstick in a particular case.

Toxic or infectious conditions, congenital disorders, and injuries may also lead to testamentary incapacity. This group would include substance abuse, iatrogenic intoxication (e.g., medications administered to alleviate suffering in terminally ill patients), uremia, encephalitis, syphilis, epilepsy, brain injuries, and so on. Manifestations may be primarily organic in nature (acute or chronic), primarily psychotic, or mixed.§

Incapacity cannot be presumed merely on the basis that the testator was an alcoholic or a drug addict or even that he was intoxicated at the time a will was made.‖ The relevant inquiry is did the testator meet the specific tests for testamentary capacity? Testators who were afflicted by physical ailments at the time of the execution of their wills (e.g., cancer, malnutrition, paralysis and many other "deathbed" maladies have been reported) are not deprived of their capacity to make a will unless it can be demonstrated that the infirmity prevented them from grasping one or more of the specific factors essential for will-making.#

Mental Deficiency. The testator's mental deficiency may be probative of testamentary incapacity only if it impairs his ability to satisfy the specific criteria outlined above. The cases discussing mental deficiency indicate that comparatively little intelligence is required for will-mak-

---

*Swanson, DW, Bohnert, PJ, Smith, JA: *The Paranoid.* Boston, Little, Brown, 1970, pp. 72–75.

†Warren's Heaton: *Surrogates' Courts* (6th Ed) § 186–C, ¶9(c) (lists the decisions by age of the testator).

‡Matter of Beneway, 272 App Div 463, 71 NYS2d 361.

§Slovenko, *Psychiatry and Law*, 1973, p. 340.

‖Matter of Heaton, 224 NY 22, 120 NE 83.

#No presumption of invalidity arises from the fact that, when he executed his will, the testator was on his deathbed. Matter of Seagrist, 1 App Div 615, 37 NYS 496, affd 153 NY 682, 42 NE 1107. For a discussion of the validity of a will executed during a "lucid interval," see Davids: *New York Law of Wills* §§30–33.

ing.* As noted above, less mental faculty is required to execute a will than any other legal instrument. This view arises, in part, from the fact that, for example, a contract requires some degree of adversary negotiations, whereas a will does not (however, this is something of an oversimplification, because wills, and contracts, may differ greatly in complexity).†

Undue Influence

As with testamentary capacity, the question of undue influence usually must be determined *postmortem*. An influence which destroys the testator's free agency is an undue influence. It must be established that the influence of another person was such that the other's will or intention was substituted for that of the testator.‡ A lesser degree of impairment of the testator is required to establish undue influence than to establish testamentary incapacity. The following four factors are indicia of undue influence:

1. The testator was susceptible to undue influence (e.g., he was in a weakened state, mentally and/or physically, and thereby vulnerable to domination by others).
2. There was an opportunity present for undue influence to be exerted (e.g., the testator was isolated from the outside world by the beneficiary, who may have been a child or friend).
3. Personal gain can be inferred as a motive for the exercise of undue influence.
4. The will was *unnatural*, for example, children were excluded or the beneficiary received much more than would ordinarily be expected.§

According to Perr, a court should consider not only the physical or mental condition of the testator but also all of the surrounding circumstances, including the role and actions of those who allegedly exerted undue influence on him. He outlines a number of factors to consider, such as the dependent and impaired condition of the testator, significant evidence of impaired mental functioning (although falling short of testamentary incapacity), and control of the testator's environment by the beneficiary to the point of seclusion from the outside world.‖

Questions of undue influence may arise in the context of a fiduciary

*In re Carpenter, 145 NYS 365, 373.
†Davids: *New York Law of Wills* §22.
‡Davidson, *Forensic Psychiatry*, New York, Ronald Press, 1965, p. 129.
§Perr, Wills: Testamentary Capacity and Undue Influence, 1981.
‖Perr, Wills: Testamentary Capacity and Undue Influence, 1981.

or confidential relationship that existed between testator and beneficiary (e.g., doctor–patient, attorney–client, priest–penitent). For example, the power of the transference that arises in psychiatric treatment (and in other contexts as well) may serve to invalidate a bequest by a patient to his psychiatrist or to a clinic or hospital, if undue influence is found.*

Ethical Considerations

At this point, one may be left with the impression that the psychiatrist's task in evaluating testamentary capacity is but a further example of what a recent author had in mind when selecting the title *The Impossible Profession*.† It may indeed be impossible in most cases to draw a reasoned clinical opinion from the available data, and psychiatric conclusions in this area are often speculative and unsatisfying. To compound this unsettling state of affairs, such evaluations have also been subject to attack on ethical grounds. Once again, psychiatrists are vilified as the agents of a monolithic state, trampling on and thwarting the rights and last wishes of the poor deceased for the distribution of his property, if his desires conflict with society's expectations and demands.

Slovenko points out that the validity of a will may often depend on the extent to which it affords protection to the interests of the family:

> There is a deep-seated aversion to the power of arbitrarily diverting the natural course of the devolution of property. Generally speaking, the interests of society in family maintenance are greater than its interests in the protection of the freedom of testation. In order for that preference to be given priority, it is necessary for a will contestant to allege, in effect, that the testator was crazy. Will contests based upon a testator's supposed lack of testamentary capacity are simply 'litigatory trappings which the contestants assume'.‡

Furthermore, as noted above, the evaluation of testamentary capacity generally does not allow for direct examination of the testator. This is an outright violation of the Canons of Medical Ethics, which unequivocally declare that it is unethical for a psychiatrist to offer a professional opinion about an individual, unless he has conducted a personal examination of that individual.§

*Slovenko, *Psychiatry and Law*, 1973, p. 341.

†Malcolm, J: *Psychoanalysis: The Impossible Profession*. New York, Knopf, 1981. The author quotes an analyst, Adam Limentani, who states "As psychoanalysts, we are only too aware that our profession is not only impossible but also extremely difficult." Apparently, this is no less true for forensic psychiatrists!

‡Slovenko, *Psychiatry and Law*, 1973, pp. 343–344.

§Principles of Medical Ethics, With Annotations Especially Applicable to Psychiatry § 7(3)(1981)("[I]t is unethical for a psychiatrist to offer a professional opinion unless he/she has conducted an examination").

   As if we as a profession have not suffered enough casualties in "The Great War between law and psychiatry",* the area of the evaluation of testamentary capacity promises to be a field day for the anti-psychiatry establishment. Not only are we accused of oppressing the mentally ill while they are alive and still capable of experiencing the day-in-and-day-out distress that we allegedly inflict on them under the aegis of the "Therapeutic State,"† but now we are vulnerable to charges of committing a sort of psychiatric sacrilege by thwarting the competent wishes of the deceased and by labelling him mentally ill *after the fact*. Not even death, it seems, can liberate the psychiatric patient from our clutches!

Case Illustrations

SYLVESTER F.

   After his retirement, Sylvester F., a high school principal for 20 years, became increasingly isolated and lonely. He lost touch with his old friends (many of whom had moved out of state) and stopped seeing his family. A bachelor, who had always been thrifty and hardworking, Sylvester had saved and invested his money over the years, accumulating a small personal fortune in excess of $750,000. He became friendly with a group of neighborhood people who owned a family grocery store. He moved out of his home and rented a room in the home of his new friends, the Baileys. Mrs. Bailey cleaned his room, prepared his meals, and ran errands for him. Sylvester was already in his late seventies. As time went on, Mrs. Bailey began to assist Sylvester with his finances. He relied on her to go over his bankbooks and other holdings, make deposits and withdrawals for him, and so on. He arranged for her to have power of attorney and to sign his checks. A number of unusual financial transactions took place over the years: Large sums were expended to purchase gifts for the Baileys, including two new automobiles. Certain tuition and medical expenses were subsidized by Sylvester as well. At one point, Sylvester loaned Mrs. Bailey $25,000 to buy a small cafe, which she had always wanted to do. When the purchase fell through, he told her "to forget it and keep the money," because he did not really need it. Sylvester kept a drawer in his room stuffed with hundred dollar bills. The Baileys had his permission to go to the drawer and take money "whenever they needed anything." No accounting was kept of any of these transactions and Sylvester showed no interest in the disposition of his funds. On his 80th birthday, Sylvester went to the Baileys' family lawyer to draw up his will. He excluded his 3 surviving sisters (all in their sixties and seventies and financially well off) and left everything to the Baileys.
   Shortly thereafter, Sylvester fell and fractured his hip. While in the

---

*To the best of my knowledge, Dr. Alan A. Stone was the first to use this phrase.
†Schur, EM: *Labeling Deviant Behavior*. New York, Harper & Row, 1971.

hospital, it was noted that he was confused and often lost track of what he was saying. A psychiatric consultant reached a diagnosis of Primary Degenerative Dementia. He noted the presence of confusion, memory loss, loss of critical faculties, impaired judgment, child-like dependency, indifference to managing his own affairs, inappropriate expansiveness and recklessness in a previously prudent and cautious individual, and heightened suggestibility.

The hospital administration was concerned about Sylvester's possible incompetence and notified his family. Sylvester remonstrated with the hospital, his sisters, and their attorneys. He protested that he enjoyed taking care of the Baileys, that it made him feel important, and that he did not care if they (the Baileys) handled his money, because he was "very old anyway" and did not need much for himself.

Before any legal action could be taken to appoint a conservator for Sylvester, in order to protect his assets, he died suddenly in his sleep and his family promptly sought to overturn his will. After a protracted court battle, the will was overturned in favor of Sylvester's family. The court based its decision on elements of both testamentary incapacity and undue influence, referring to the incontrovertible evidence of progressive cognitive decline, personality changes manifested by his extravagant and reckless handling of his funds, his deteriorating judgment, and his childlike dependency on the Baileys. The court noted that his friends had attempted to seclude him from the outside world and to encourage his total dependency on them. The record supported a conclusion that they had flagrantly exploited his vulnerability, even to the point of having their own lawyer prepare his will. The decision also made reference to the "unusual situation" in this case, that a psychiatric assessment of the testator, performed before he died (and around the time he executed his will), had been available. In the words of the decision "probative evidence of this sort was of inestimable assistance to the court." The extensive documentation of his psychiatric impairment, based on live examinations, in the context of all the surrounding circumstances, resolved many of the uncertainties which often plague courts in such cases.*

MARY S.

After her husband's death, Mary S. became increasingly depressed and was repeatedly hospitalized in psychiatric facilities. Her diagnosis was

---

*The lawyer for the Baileys argued that far from exploiting Sylvester, the Baileys had cared for him during his last years and had earned his trust and his love. "It had given Sylvester pleasure to be generous to them and his will was an expression of his true heartfelt wishes." He argued further that to overturn the will in favor of "relatives in name only," who had shown little interest in Sylvester while he was still alive, was the equivalent of robbing Sylvester of his last wishes for the disposition of his wealth. Was this decision another example of Professor Slovenko's thesis that psychiatric illness is used as a pretext to overturn wills which do not conform to society's usual expectations? (See note p. 114 and accompanying text.)

Involutional Melancholia and several courses of E.C.T. were administered. After a chronic and deteriorating clinical course, she died of natural causes, after spending almost 10 years in a state psychiatric institution. Only after her death did it come to light that she had prepared a will during a period of acute illness. Shortly after a brief psychiatric hospitalization (during which she had received E.C.T.), she had spent a few days with her son and his family. During this short visit, her son took her to his lawyer and a will was executed. The terms of the will were favorable to the son and his wife, to the virtual exclusion of Mary's two daughters. During the ensuing will contest, psychiatric experts were called by the daughters. In their opinion, Mary's mental status around the time of the will's execution called into question her testamentary capacity. The hospital records had described her as "confused, disoriented, preoccupied with somatic and delusional ideation and possibly suicidal." Other hospital record entries were equivocal. There was also evidence that she had written checks around the same time to pay her bills. It was uncertain whether she had done so on her own initiative or had merely written them while being directed to do so by her son. Her son contended that she had had a "lucid interval" when she made her will. The lawyer who drew up the will also testified that she had appeared competent at that time and that he had noticed no abnormalities. She had never been adjudicated incompetent to manage her funds and had entered all the psychiatric hospitals on a voluntary basis. After a heated trial, the will was overturned. The verdict has been appealed. In this case also, psychiatric evaluations were carried out during life and around the time the will was made, allowing the factfinder to reach a more informed decision.

SUMMARY

The legal framework for the making of a valid will was outlined and the psychiatrist's role in a will contest was discussed. Testamentary Capacity and Undue Influence were reviewed in some detail, with a focus on the interrelationships between psychiatric issues and the surrounding legal framework. The psychiatrist must have a clear understanding of the relevant legal issues in order to make an intelligent contribution. The imposing clinical and ethical difficulties in this area may understandably dissuade most psychiatrists from undertaking these specialized forensic evaluations. These clinical and ethical issues were discussed and two case illustrations were provided.

7

The Plaintiff's Case
in Psychiatric Malpractice

ROBERT L. SADOFF

INTRODUCTORY COMMENTS

Prior to discussing the plaintiff's case in psychiatric malpractice, it would be helpful to present general concepts of malpractice and specifically malpractice issues that arise for psychiatrists. *Malpractice* is a concept that develops from a claim of negligence on the part of a professional who has a specific duty to another person who is damaged in some way by the professional's negligence. In medicine, the physician has a particular duty to his patient. If the physician is negligent, or derelict in his duty, and the patient is damaged as a direct result of that negligence, the necessary four elements are present for a malpractice suit. I have elsewhere referred to these four elements as the four *D's*.[1] In psychiatric malpractice cases, the psychiatrist also has a specific duty to his patient that must not be breached or a malpractice suit may arise if damage occurs.

There are several areas in psychiatric paractice in which a malpractice suit may arise. There have also been shown recently to be minor modifications in the four Ds, especially when the psychiatrist has been held liable for the violent behavior of his patient and the damage occurred to a third party, not to the patient. The traditional areas of malpractice in psychiatry include suicide, improper use of medication, breach of confidentiality, treatment without proper informed consent, and failure to properly restrain a self-destructive patient. Newer issues

ROBERT L. SADOFF • Center for Studies in Social-Legal Psychiatry, School of Medicine, University of Pennsylvania, Philadelphia, Pennsylvania 19104.

that have recently arisen in malpractice suits in psychiatry include the following: failure to warn a third party of the violence of the psychiatric patient, failure to properly restrain a patient who presents a risk of harm to others, and mishandling of the transference in psychotherapy that results in improper relationships between psychiatrist and patient.

In all of these cases, the issue to be determined is the standard of care required for proper treatment. The standard of care is national and not local at this time. Means of communication and transportation are such that the expectation of the psychiatrist in a rural setting would be to obtain proper consultation from the university settings or urban areas in the event of an unusual or challenging case. It is no longer appropriate to consider that the standard of care is higher in the teaching hospitals than it is in the outlying districts where there may be only one psychiatrist in a 100 mile radius. His means of practice may vary or be different from those of psychiatrists in a crowded urban section, but the standard or quality of care is expected to be the same. The standard of care is one that is accepted by the majority of psychiatrists and represents the average treatment available, not necessarily optimal treatment or very specialized treatment espoused by a few psychiatrists. The standard of care is not what the expert witness would have done under the same circumstances, but it is the practice that would have occurred by the average general psychiatrist at the particular time of the incident in question with the information available prospectively, and not retrospectively. That is to say, if a patient has successfully suicided, the argument may not be made that the treating psychiatrist naturally was in error because his treatment was not sufficient to keep his patient alive. There may have been no way of predicting that this particular patient under the circumstances of his treatment would have killed himself. The treating psychiatrist may have instituted every treatment regimen that appeared to be proper at that time with the information that was available to him through the patient, the family, or previous treatment sources. However, there are guidelines that may have been breached by the treating doctor that did directly lead to the suicide of his patient.

The law speaks of proximate cause as the direct relationship between the breach of duty and the damage to the patient or others. In psychiatry, we consider a direct relationship or link between factors, but proximate cause may also include indirect relationships. Examples of such indirect relationships are included in the more recent cases in which the psychiatrist is asked to predict whether his patient is going to harm someone else or be violent if he is released from the hospital or if he is not properly hospitalized. Often such predictions are not within the expertise of the psychiatrist except if the violence is imminent. An example follows.

The author was approached by a plaintiff's attorney to evaluate the records of an individual who had been hospitalized 5 years previously at a particular hospital in a state other than the one in which the author worked. The patient had been released and had subsequently been hospitalized at three other hospitals during the succeeding 5 years. This patient had then attacked a stranger in the street resulting in her death. The victim's husband sued the hospital at which the patient had been initially admitted 5 years before with the claim that had the hospital kept the patient, this tragedy would not have occurred. As a potential plaintiff's expert, I evaluated the data and concluded that I could not be of help to the plaintiff because too much time had elapsed between the initial hospitalization and the ultimate violent behavior. Also, there were three other hospitalizations between the first hospital and the violent behavior that needed to be accounted for. I did not see how a direct or indirect link could be made between the treatment given by the hospital in question and the violence that occurred 5 years later. The plaintiff's attorney argued that he was not so concerned about the intervening hospitalizations, but had the first hospital properly treated, restrained, or kept the patient for a longer period of time, his illness would have been either "cured" or his condition better stabilized so that he would not have several years later committed the violent act against his client's wife.

I raise the example noted above for several reasons:

1. To point out the indirect link that many plaintiffs' attorneys may confront potential experts with in assessing psychiatric malpractice.

2. To note the distance between the alleged act of malpractice and the potential expert witness. Often plaintiffs' attorneys can not find a psychiatrist in a particular locality to testify against a colleague and must travel many miles to find a psychiatrist who is not familiar with the defendants in a particular case.

3. To alert the potential expert witnesses that all cases that come their way need not be accepted. It is quite appropriate for a psychiatrist, consulted by plaintiffs' attorneys (or defense attorneys for that matter), to reject the offer of serving as an expert witness. Unless the expert is committed to the appropriateness of the case, he cannot properly help the case.

Each of these points will be considered in greater detail in this presentation.

THE ROLE OF THE FORENSIC PSYCHIATRIST IN PSYCHIATRIC MALPRACTICE CASES

The psychiatrist may be approached by either the plaintiff's attorney or the defendant's attorney in assessing and evaluating a medical malpractice case. In general medical malpractice cases, the psychiatrist may be called by either side's attorney to assess damages only. It would not be proper for a psychiatrist to testify about negligence of an orthopedic surgeon or an internist or a radiologist. He can, however, testify about damages to the patient as a result of the trauma experienced within the alleged medical malpractice event. Patients who are harmed iatrogenically often have psychiatric symptoms which are directly related to the trauma experienced. These symptoms must be assessed and determined to either be related to or separate from the alleged medical malpractice. The patient must also be evaluated for the possibility of malingering which is defined as conscious deception. Malingering is not a psychiatric diagnosis. It is a euphamism for *faking* or *lying*. The patient knows that he or she is deceiving the physician by giving the symptoms that do not exist. Some patients are well educated or well trained to present bizarre symptoms in order to fool the psychiatrist and claim a large award. The psychiatrist must be in a position to assess the degree of deception if present and to distinguish malingering from bona fide psychiatric diagnoses or symptoms such as conversion symptoms, dissociative phenomena or psychosomatic illness.

In psychiatric malpractice cases, the expert witness will be required to assess not only the damage to the patient but also the deviation from the standard of care by the treating psychiatrist that led to the damage to the patient. Damage may be physical, emotional, or economic. Some treatment in psychiatry may damage a patient physically such as inappropriate use of medication which could lead to kidney damage, brain damage, or other systemic difficulties. Economic damage may occur with breach of confidentiality that might lead to loss of job or income. By far the most common damage to be assessed by plaintiff's expert is psychological damage or emotional illness claimed to result from the breach of duty by the defendant psychiatrist.

There are a number of practical considerations with respect to accepting the assignment as plaintiff's expert in a psychiatric malpractice case. When a plaintiff's attorney calls and requests consultation in a psychiatric malpractice case, the potential expert should ascertain immediately who the defendant's psychiatrist is and whether he has any affiliation with that psychiatrist or the hospital that is being sued. Any direct or indirect relationship that exists should immediately be given to the plaintiff's attorney to determine whether there exists a potential conflict of interest. It would not be appropriate for a psychiatrist to become involved in a case against a good friend, an individual with whom he works, or against a hospital at which the potential expert has an affiliation. If such a conflict occurs, the psychiatrist may refer the plaintiff's attorney to a number of other forensic psychiatrists who would not have such a conflict. Perhaps the defendant hospital or psychiatrist is fairly well known in the area, and the plaintiff's attorney must turn to resources in other states. There is a directory of forensic psychiatrists published by the American Academy of Psychiatry and the Law to which the plaintiff's attorney may be referred for alternate consultants.

Following a preliminary assessment that there is no conflict of interest, the plaintiff's attorney should then mail the potential expert the medical records, a statement of the complaint against the defendant's psychiatrist, and any other relevant material that would be important for the initial assessment of liability. Only after careful review of all materials that are available at that time should the potential expert indicate by telephone whether or not he would be willing to serve as a consultant in this case. If, after review of the records, the psychiatrist determines that he cannot be of help, he should let the plaintiff's attorney know as soon as possible. It is preferable to call the attorney than to put this opinion in writing, because the plaintiff's attorney may be required to turn all reports he has received over to the defendant's attorney through a process of discovery. It is always best to adhere to the wishes of the attorney who is directing the strategy for his case.

If the potential expert can agree to serve as consultant based on his review of the materials provided, he should then call the plaintiff's attorney and ask whether a written report is required. The psychiatrist should again follow the directions of the attorney in giving him either a brief report or a lengthy detailed report outlining the reasons for the psychiatrist's ultimate conclusions. Some attorneys require a long detailed report and others would wish only a one page summary of the opinions of the potential expert witness. Following the initial evaluation, further information will be provided to the potential expert witness. He will receive the interrogatories by both plaintiff and defendant and the answers to same. He should receive transcripts of depositions of the principal parties to this legal action. He must collect the review all relevant information or data in order to present as credible an opinion as possible. It is also possible that some of the information he receives will weaken his opinion and other information will strengthen it. He should be clear to point out to the plaintiff's attorney what information is helpful and where the weakness of his opinion exists and is vulnerable to cross-examination.

Throughout the early stages of the collection of information, the forensic psychiatrist acts as a consultant to the attorney that calls him. In this case, he is consultant to the plaintiff's attorney and as such has the option of interviewing the plaintiffs and/or family members. He may not have the option of interviewing the defendant psychiatrist. There are many reasons why such an interview would not be allowed: The plaintiff's attorney may not want any direct confrontation between his expert and the defendant. He may be concerned that the plaintiff's expert would begin to identify with his colleague and accept the defendant's rationale for his treatment of the patient. He also may be concerned that defendant's attorney may claim undue influence if there arises a disagreement in the interview between the defendant's psychiatrist and the plaintiff's expert. It may appear to the plaintiff's expert that collecting all information including data "from the other side" would be scientific and valuable in a proper assessment. However, we are dealing here with an adversary system and not a scientific one. What appears to be helpful and proper in a medical environment may not be appropriate in a legal adversarial case. It is always best to check with the attorney who is directing the case before proceeding in uncharted or potentially conflicting areas. The expert is the consultant to the attorney and should be guided by the attorney's decisions in these particular matters.

The psychiatrist may be required to give a deposition regarding his findings and his opinions. A *deposition* is a discovery technique by the defendant's attorney in order for him to ascertain clearly what the plaintiff's expert will testify in court. He does not want to be surprised when the case is before the jury or the judge. He needs time to prepare his questions and his cross-examination. In order to do this, he must know on what factors the plaintiff's expert bases his opinion and his conclusions. The psychiatrist must have a predeposition conference with the plaintiff's attorney in order to prepare his deposition testimony. There is usually no direct and cross-examination at such depositions as there is in court, but there is primarily the cross-examination by the defendant's attorney, usually in the privacy of the psychiatrist's office both with the attorneys and the court reporter present. The deposition is taken under oath and the psychiatrist must have the records available in order to document his conclusions and opinions from the records. He may or may not have prepared a written report at the time of the deposition, but all of his records and notes are discoverable at that time. That means the defendant's attorney will take his chart or records and review any notes or correspondence the psychiatrist has had in the preparation of his opinion. It is important for the psychiatrist to obtain a transcript of his deposition in preparation for the trial because it is certain that the defendant's attorney will have a copy of that transcript available during cross-examination at the time of trial.

Following the deposition, the case may go to trial. Many of these cases do settle before trial or on the doorstep of the courthouse at the time of trial. Nevertheless, the plaintiff's expert must be prepared to testify in the event the case does not settle. He must have a pretrial conference with the plaintiff's attorney to discuss all questions that will be asked on direct testimony. He must prepare his presentation to the jury in a skillful manner so that his communications are clear, precise, and based on the material in the records. He must be aware of all information gathered by the plaintiff's attorney that might tend to detract from his opinion or to support his opinion. He must also have available the transcripts of depositions of the defendant's expert witnesses to be familiar with the defense case and the theory on which they will base the defense of the alleged malpractice action. In the pretrial conference, he will also give information to the plaintiff's attorney on potential weakness in his testimony and vulnerability on cross-examination. Having become familiar with the defense theory of the case, he will also provide the plaintiff's attorney relevant questions for cross-examination of defendant's expert. In all pretrial conferences, consultations, or preparations of reports, the plaintiff's expert serves as a consultant to the plaintiff's attorney in helping him prepare the case from a psychiatric standpoint. Once the psychiatrist takes the witness stand at the trial, he serves only the fact finder, that is, the judge or the jury, and assumes the role of teacher rather than adversary or consultant to the plaintiff. His objectivity and neutrality add to his credibility. The fact finder will be faced with opposite opinions and must determine which side to believe, that is, which side is more credible.

The Malpractice Trial

Having been duly prepared, the plaintiff's expert is called as the principal witness in psychiatric malpractice cases. The responsibility for proving the elements of liability and damage rests mainly on his shoulders. The burden of proof in psychiatric malpractice cases lies with the plaintiff to show that there was negligence and that that negligence directly led to damage to the patient. Thus, the plaintiff's expert must present his information to the jury in a clear, comprehensible manner that will be understood by them despite the need for use of technical or psychiatric words. All such words should be clearly defined by the expert and explained when necessary. The expert may always clarify his responses or his answers so the jury is not confused. He should be prepared to discuss standards of care and how the defendant deviated from such standards. He must be prepared to discuss the diagnosis of the patient and the proper treatment.

On cross-examination, the plaintiff's expert is likely to be asked a number of potentially embarrassing questions designed to unnerve him or confuse him. Such questions include the manner in which he became involved in this particular case. Does he testify exclusively for plaintiffs against his colleagues in psychiatry? Was he called through a medical malpractice service which is devoted to plaintiffs' cases exclusively? He may be asked how often he testifies for defense or plaintiff and how frequently he testifies in court. There will be an attempt to label him as a *hired gun* who frequently testifies against his colleagues. He will be asked how much he is being paid for his opinion. The response, of course, is that he is paid for his time and his expertise and not for his opinion. He must be prepared to acknowledge what his fees are and how they have been paid. Any and every legitimate attempt to discredit his credibility will be offered prior to the substantive testimony about the merits of the case and the validity of his opinion. In some cases, he may be put on trial just for testifying against a colleague.

On cross-examination, he may be asked if the defendant psychiatrist was "wrong" in what he did or whether the defense psychiatrist whose opinion differs from his was "wrong" in his assessment of the information and the material. To the former question, he may respond that the defendant psychiatrist deviated from the standard of care. Whether this is right or wrong may be a moral question, but it is not the relevant question for the lawsuit. If the judge allows such a question, the plaintiff's expert must respond according to his opinion and his conscience. To the second question regarding the opinion of his adversary, the defense expert, he may respond that the opinions may differ but that does not necessarily mean that his adversary is wrong. It does not become a matter of right or wrong. It is a matter of opinion about the deviation from the standard of care. It may be that each psychiatrist has a different opinion about what constitutes the standard of care with respect to that particular treatment issue.

Practical Considerations

Prior to accepting the assignment as consultant to the plaintiff in a psychiatric malpractice case, the psychiatrist should properly assess all ramifications of the case and determine whether or not he requires further specialized consultants. For example, the case may center around misuse of medication. If the forensic psychiatrist is not an expert in the use of that particular medication or is not as familiar with psychopharmacological principles as another colleague, he may wish to consult with other psychiatrists who are more familiar with the use of that particular medication or drug. He may wish to have a suicidologist in cases of suicide. He may wish to consult with a forensic psychologist or a neuropsychologist in order to properly assess damages to the plaintiff. In cases involving children, he most certainly would want to consult with a child psychiatrist and may want to have a team of experts rather than a single expert in that particular case. It is important for the forensic psychiatrist, in whatever kind of case, that he stay within the areas of his own expertise. Especially in psychiatric malpractice cases, however, is this important and essential. He will be stretched to the limit of his expertise on cross-examination and tested with respect to his degree of confidence and his experience in working in particular fields of psychiatry. Thus, it becomes even more important for him to establish the boundaries of his expertise and consult with colleagues who will complement his expertise and extend the boundaries of the case beyond his own experience.

With respect to fees, there are a number of practical issues regarding plaintiff's experts. Initially, it should be established that the plaintiff's attorneys work on a contingency basis rather than on a retainer fee as they might in criminal cases. This is done for a number of reasons including the fact that most plaintiffs do not have sufficient funds to provide retainer fees and should not be precluded from suing because they cannot afford the expenses. It is unethical for the psychiatrist to work on a contingency fee arrangement. That is, he may not ask for a percentage of the case if his side wins. Similarly, he should not be assured by plaintiff's attorney that his fees will be paid out of the settlement or the award at trial. Suppose there is no award? If there is no settlement, there is no money to pay psychiatric fees. Thus, it is important in plaintiff's cases, not only in malpractice, but in all tort cases when working for the plaintiff, to accept a retainer fee in advance. I do this for two reasons: Initially, I want to guarantee my fee, and secondly, I want to be certain that my testimony is not contingent on whether or not I am paid. When requested by a plaintiff's attorney to evaluate materials in order to determine whether or not I will serve as an expert witness, I will ask for a retainer fee with the materials so that if I am unable to help, I will still be paid for my services and for my time. There are a number of attorneys who cannot afford to, or will not, pay experts who cannot be of help to them. Similarly, all work that is done must be paid in advance. Any deposition time must be paid prior to the deposition. There may be a delay in the deposition, or one of the attorneys may not show up, or one side may not have called the court reporter, and the deposition may not proceed. What is the psychiatrist to do with the time that he has reserved for such a deposition, and for which he has perhaps rescheduled a number of patients? It is important to ascertain who pays for the discovery deposition in that particular jurisdiction. It varies depending on the state and the agreements between and among counsel. It is certainly important for the plaintiff's expert to be paid for his time in court prior to his testimony. He will most certainly be asked whether he has been paid, and how much. Having indicated one's fee in court and relating to the jury that that fee has already been paid, will add to the aura of neutrality and credibility such that there cannot be any implication that the stronger the expert adheres to his opinion the more he will be paid subsequently.

A word about medical malpractice services. There are a number of attorneys who require expert witnesses for medical malpractice cases who are unable to obtain them in their local area. They often turn to national medical legal services that provide expert consultation with respect to medical malpractice cases. Most of these services are legitimate and are run by attorneys who have experience in the field. Their consultants may be renowned experts who agree to evaluate a case but not testify subsequently. In other cases, the expert who evaluates and concludes that he can agree that malpractice occurred also agrees to become the expert witness. There is nothing unethical about working through a medical malpractice service or being on such a "list" of experts. Defense attorneys may attempt to discredit a plaintiff's expert by indicating that he was called through such a service. The most effective rebuttal to that accusation is to indicate that the expert also works for defense attorneys or insurance companies in defending similar claims.

SUMMARY AND CONCLUSIONS

This presentation has attempted to outline a number of the difficulties the plaintiff's expert may encounter in serving that role in psychiatric malpractice cases. It behooves the plaintiff's expert to be as complete, thorough, and comprehensive in his evaluation prior to agreeing to serve as an expert witness against a respected colleague. Having reached his opinion, however, it is also important for the plaintiff's expert to present his information, his conclusions, as clearly and as relevantly as possible in court. He will be attacked on cross-examination for testifying against his colleague. The plaintiff's expert may be reassured that his role is a legitimate and respected one in the sense that we must govern and regulate our own practices through legitimate standards of care or surely somebody else will regulate our practice for us. We must all adhere to the standards that are set and make sure that our colleagues do so as well. We must all ensure the high quality of care by being available to consult with attorneys when malpractice does occur in psychiatry, and utilize our experiences to teach our colleagues what is appropriate, what is acceptable, and most importantly, what is harmful to the patient. Despite all the rhetoric and the strategy and courtroom tactics that may occur in a heated psychiatric malpractice case, the important consideration is the well-being of the patient. We must all work toward improving our services rendered to the patient by continually improving our standards of care and providing the highest quality of treatment whenever possible.

REFERENCES

[1]Sadoff, RL: *Forensic Psychiatry: A Practical Guide for Lawyers and Psychiatrists*, Charles C Thomas, Springfield, IL, 1975, p.205.

8

The Defense of a Psychiatrist Charged with Malpractice

ALAN J. TUCKMAN

Who, in the rainbow, can show the line where the violet tint ends and the orange tint begins. Distinctly we see the difference of the colors, but when exactly does the one first blendingly enter into the other?

Herman Melville, *Billy Budd*

AN OVERVIEW

To function as a forensic psychiatrist, evaluating individuals engaged in legal matters, and then testifying in their behalf, is an arduous but challenging task. Many learned treatises and conferences have been devoted to the basics, the ethics, and the nuances of this difficult and complex specialty. Yet, after a number of years, as with any task performed repeatedly, one becomes comfortable and proficient in it. Although there exists the constant challenge of the new case and the planned-for appearance in the courtroom, the "expert" in forensic psychiatry is trained to pursue his/her task along time-honored pathways.

To add to this responsibility, the evaluation and testimony in the defense of a fellow psychiatrist charged with malpractice complicates that role enormously. Alan Stone, at the Annual Convention of the American Academy of Psychiatry and Law, in New York City, in 1982, called forensic psychiatry a "moral minefield." If that be the description

ALAN J. TUCKMAN • Department of Psychiatry, School of Medicine, New York University, New York, New York 10016.

of forensic psychiatry, generally, then adding to it malpractice defense is like adding nuclear weapons to that minefield, with unexpected issues arising from unanticipated directions, suddenly exploding on the scene. For example, we may have developed a full awareness of our own reactions to criminal and civil clients seen over the years, but, how prepared are we to deal with emotional reactions stimulated by a client so much like ourselves, threatening our own reputations.

In addition, another complicating factor is the unique nature of psychiatric malpractice, in which the sympathies of the jury will more likely not be neutral but will rest with the plaintiff–patient due to the currently tarnished image of the physician in our society. The psychiatrist, testifying for the defendant-psychiatrist, will have a more difficult task, requiring greater believability to overcome the frequently held belief that "doctors protect their own."

Although some of our colleagues, such as Karl Menninger, believe that psychiatrists do not belong in the courtroom in most types of cases[1], none can dispute that it is mandatory for us to be there in psychiatric malpractice.

This chapter will be devoted to guidelines, as well as pitfalls, along the path from first contact to final testimony in psychiatric malpractice defense. It is not designed to advise psychiatrists on how to avoid malpractice, which is covered elsewhere, nor is it a guide to legal strategies during the course of the proceedings. That task is properly the function of the defendant's attorney. Instead, its focus, as well as its philosophy, is on the function of the forensic psychiatrist in a defense role in this increasingly broadening area of law.

It should be noted, interestingly, that whereas there are many articles and books devoted to psychiatric malpractice, none have been written to help a colleague defend himself/herself when confronted with a malpractice action. Yet, the number of malpractice cases against psychiatrists is definitely increasing. Although some writers believe that these suits are "a positive development, overall, as it may produce a more unified profession, instead of over 200 modes of psychotherapy,"[2] we are quite aware that each suit lost by a psychiatrist must also be considered a black mark against the whole profession.

It is evident, though, that the nature of psychotherapy produces a very low risk of liability, not because malpractice is less common among psychotherapists, but because there are formidable obstacles to developing a malpractice suit. It may be impossible to prove that a therapist deviated from customary professional practice when there are widely varying modes of treatment and the relationship between the emotional injury and the alleged breach of duty may be too distant to recognize.

As Joel Klein, APA Counsel, stated,[2] "Verbal psychotherapy will continue to be impervious to most damage suits. Psychiatric malpractice either involves a 'big hurt,' which can be readily proven, or a 'big bill,' in which a patient sues as a tactic to get out of a large debt owed to a psychiatrist." On the other side, as Schetky and Cavanaugh noted,[3] "Practicing good medicine provides no immunity from a malpractice suit. You don't have to be worth a million to be sued for a million."

PERSONAL ISSUES

Forensic psychiatrists, although needed to participate in these cases, often do not recognize the unique nature of this type of work. Counter-transference reactions relating to the age, marital status, problem presented and other issues are all potential areas for conflict and clouding of the therapist's objective distance. But none are as potentially threatening as that produced by working with a fellow psychiatrist, which may even produce a reluctance to do this type of work. Every physician knows the mixed feelings of relief and anxiety when hearing of a colleague accused of a misdeed in their practice. Many will think, "Thank goodness, it's not me; but it certainly could have been me. No one is immune and none of us is pure enough to escape." Thus, an early impulse will be to distance oneself from the accused. Everyone is susceptible to the feeling of not wanting to be identified with that person for fear that they will be contaminated by the problem and the stigma will rub off if they are too sympathetic. Or, we might want to distance ourselves because of the assault to our own sense of omnipotence, feeling, "if he/she is imperfect or susceptible, I could be too." All too frequently, possibly as a method of "identifying with the aggressor," one becomes overly judgmental and punitive and withdraws, not wishing to help at all, or finds fault out of proportion to the harm allegedly done, and allies oneself with the accusers.

Added to this emotional reaction to the accused, are the exaggerations of normal reactions to the judicial system itself. Schetky and Colbach noted[4] that "the Courtroom is a minefield for the psychiatrist, where counter-transference threats to one's selfhood are much more omnipresent than in the private consulting room." The unique nature of our client, the psychiatrist–defendant, may bring these feelings to the surface more powerfully than in other settings.

Rada[5] pointed out that "countertransference extends to our feelings about the legal system, legal profession and specific participants in the legal process including clients and colleagues and includes issues of sibling rivalry." And how easy it is to take those previously described negative feelings toward colleagues and displace them onto the legal system, find fault with it, and respectably bow out of helping a colleague in need.

On the other side, to be considered when entering a psychiatric malpractice case, are the protective feelings for a fellow psychiatrist in trouble. The "rescue fantasy," identification with the underdog and anti-authoritarian feelings[6] are all intrinsic components of our basic personalities as psychiatrists and may surface to blind us to real issues and problems with these cases.

I am reminded of a colleague, the director of a mental health program, who some years ago was under extreme pressure from staff, community board and legislature, in the early formative days of community mental health programs. He was accused, by a former patient, of drinking with the patient in his office, and acting "unprofessionally," thus affecting negatively the outcome of the therapy and decisions in the patient's life, regarding her own alcohol problem. My protective, nurturing feelings for this psychiatrist at the vanguard of the public mental health movement led me to attempt to muster support for him and actively work with his attorney to prepare an adequate defense. It was not until shortly before the trial that I was faced with material, not heretofore available, pointing to the psychiatrist actually having a disguised drinking problem. Only then was I able to confront him, without my protective feelings "in gear," and get him to admit to the allegations. A reassessment of the case allowed a more limited and realistic defense, producing an out-of-court settlement that included mandatory therapy for the psychiatrist as well as supervision of his work.

Thus, before even joining a case, very powerful feelings and "counter-transference readiness" must be anticipated and dealt with if they do appear to be present.

Another situation to be understood is the great value and power of the psychiatric report, especially in a malpractice case, and the need to exert great care in preparing any material for use by an attorney, even including caution in preliminary remarks to the attorney. The early phase of a lawsuit frequently includes the exchanging of "interrogatories" or written answers to questions posed by the other side. One of these exchanges generally includes the names of the experts and the character of their testimony. It is essential, therefore, to offer no firm commitment to the case, or the position the expert will take, until the evaluations are completed. In addition, the report will be offered to the attorney and may be used in the case, exclusively, to attempt a settlement.

Although Schetky and Colbach[7] pointed out that the forensic psychiatrist "should clearly recognize the diagnostic, predictive and therapeutic limits of psychiatry, maintaining a clear perspective of being only a small cog in a larger and very complicated legal wheel," it is usually the expert's report and subsequent testimony that are the most powerful components of the psychiatric malpractice case. Very few actions get as far as settlement, much less trial, often because of material provided by the defendant–psychiatrist's experts, through their reports.

Slawson, in 1979,[8] described the results of his survey of psychiatrists' experiences with malpractice actions against them, between 1971–1976. Of 105 reported cases, 54% ended with no more than notification of possible claim, 19% were settled before trial for an average cost of $22,400 (interestingly, Slawson's earlier, 1970 study of the years between 1958–1967, noted an average settlement of only $1,034[9]). Only 6% got to trial, with half of those won by the defendant–psychiatrist. Slawson estimates, from his studies, that there is only one chance in 200 of a psychiatrist subjecting his insurance company (much less himself) to a significant loss. Due to the nature of the proof required in these cases, it must be the impact and weight of the expert testimony that influences the outcome to an appreciable degree.

THE EARLY STAGES

A subsequent role for the forensic psychiatrist (complicating his/her life and work even further) has to do with his relationship to the defendant–psychiatrist during the pendency of the malpractice action. This type of client poses another challenge which other types of cases and "regular" clients do not. Rarely will a forensic psychiatrist become "therapeutically involved" with a client during a legal action. Yet, the emotional status of the defendant–psychiatrist and our responsibility to a colleague may require unique handling of that fellow psychiatrist. Because we are seen as experts in psychiatry *and* law (which, in reality, most of us are not), a fellow psychiatrist may approach us directly on being notified by a former patient, or the patient's insurance company, regarding a potential legal action that may be imminent. Our advice is sought about how to proceed with the contact. This early phase is crucial for that psychiatrist and for us as consultants.

The initial feelings of the therapist accused of malpractice, who had been living in a world where the "doctor is the supreme caregiver" and the patient is compliant and helpless, are ones of rage at the patient's ingratitude. This is often followed by intense guilt (frequently unwarranted) and self-doubt. The patient had been expected to assume a child's role, and the physician placed in the position of resolving the patient's problems and receiving gratitude from the patient.[10] Now there is a turnaround in the relationship and the psychiatrist is cast in the role of a parent who has raised and nurtured a child, only to have him rebel, demand his own independence and call the parent to task for his actions. Frequently, as experienced by parents, the psychiatrist feels enraged, helpless, impotent and ambivalent, and this ambivalence may prevent him from taking the necessary action to defend himself in a proper manner.

Discussion with the psychiatrist about these feelings, coupled with *appropriate,* and objective, support can help him at least traverse this highly traumatic initial period more easily. Coupled with this discussion, immediately directing him to contact his insurance company and their attorneys, and to do nothing to endanger his case, whether by contacting the patient, discussing the case with other people (including other psychiatrists), or altering records, will be helpful and can provide emotional support. This support is essential to the defendant–psychiatrist, because, in a very short time, he will feel isolated, different, damaged and estranged from colleagues. He will desperately need the support of at least the forensic psychiatrist and possibly even a therapist, (who he will be reluctant to see, for fear that its exposure will be damaging to his case).

In the same way, the defendant–psychiatrist whose case you enter as an expert may need support throughout the proceedings. Psychiatrists, although human, frequently have difficulty recognizing their own stresses and seeking emotional support from others.

ENTERING THE CASE

The next phase of the process is the evaluation of the appropriateness of the case and the forensic psychiatrist's ability and willingness to participate in it. Several moral issues must be addressed during this period. An important one has to do with how one decides to participate in a case and in what way. It is assumed that most psychiatrists are "ethical" and that there exist only a few "bad apples," those physicians who, consciously and willingly, break the law and the codes of ethics of the profession. Is it proper to help defend only the psychiatrist who we believe is ethical? Or, as some forensic psychiatrists believe, is it not as proper to help an obviously guilty psychiatrist, at least to mitigate or to reduce the severity of the penalty, if found guilty? For example, a psychiatrist is accused of sexual misconduct with a patient and the evidence is clearly sufficient to make his guilt a foregone conclusion. Is it appropriate to help him by showing that there was no emotional damage to the patient and that the patient even improved during the course of the "therapy," thus reducing the potential award to the patient?[11]

Similarly, should the forensic psychiatrist participate in strategy sessions with the attorneys and defendant–psychiatrist or simply function as a psychiatrist, evaluating the data and presenting it to the attorneys for their use. When do we step beyond our expertise as psychiatrists and take on roles more appropriate to attorneys?

These are not easy questions to answer, because we believe in the Anglo-American concept of the accused deserving the best possible defense, no matter how small or limited. Yet, whenever we testify and to whatever we testify, our reputations and images as credible psychiatrists are at stake. We may help win the case, or reduce the award, but at what price to our reputations and future effectiveness?[12]

Objective distance is always necessary and the forensic psychiatrist is first, and always, a consultant. It is not his case to win or lose. This does not mean that we cannot be advocates for our position and that of maligned colleagues. Only the degree and method are at issue.

In beginning the evaluation phase of the case, another questionable practice must be recognized and weighed. Occasionally, an attorney will contact a forensic psychiatrist very late in the course of the case, often with "only 1 or 2 days available" to perform the evaluation, prepare a report, and/or agree to testify in it. Because psychiatric malpractice is one of the more complex types of cases we participate in, it is essential to assess whether it really is appropriate to involve oneself in this manner. No forensic psychiatrist looks very credible when he has to testify that he had only a few days available, and thus, complete and extensive work could not be done and the evaluation or testimony is, therefore, very limited. In addition, we must be ever vigilant that this "last minute" participation was not a tactical maneuver by an attorney hoping to avoid a more in-depth evaluation and assessment by the psychiatrist. Even when the attorney requests an answer to a very limited question, sufficient time must be available to assess the merits of the case and the impact of the forensic psychiatrist's "limited participation" in a globally "bad" case.

UNDERSTANDING THE FRAMEWORK

To participate in psychiatric malpractice cases, significant understanding of the statutes and definitions must be in hand before beginning the actual work, despite the fact that many legal writers point out that

> the substantive rules of law which receive a good deal of attention, are less significant than gathering facts and opinions and presenting them to a jury in a persuasive manner. Most discussions of malpractice pivot around a disputed set of facts and the legitimacy of the expert opinions and credibility of the material disputing the allegations.[13]

But, in order to assess the content of the allegations and compare them with the material gathered, the forensic psychiatrist must have a working definition of psychiatric malpractice and the types of cases encountered.

The most common psychiatric malpractice cases, as defined by Messinger[14], are

1. Failure to properly care for an obvious suicide risk
2. Improper treatment methods
3. Negligent diagnosis
4. Failure to warn of an injury risk (e.g., in ECT)
5. Unnecessary hospitalization
6. Lack of informed consent
7. Inadequate hospital care
8. Sexual improprieties
9. Breach of confidentiality
10. Improper handling of transference
11. Failure to warn of a dangerous patient
12. Undue restraints (in a hospital)
13. Improper commitment procedures
14. Abandonment

There are various guidelines defining psychiatric malpractice[15,16] that generally include

> *negligence* in the *delivery* of professional services, which arises out of a *contract* between the patient and physician. It implies a failure to exercise the *reasonable judgement* and *standard of care* expected of the *ordinary* physician (psychiatrist) practicing in the community. It is a Civil offense or wrong, under tort law, which refers to *harm* done to an individual. . . . Malpractice differs from ordinary tort law by the existence of a doctor–patient *relationship* and by (the requirement of) proof of standard care and its breach, *by expert testimony.* The elements of a malpractice suit include
> 1. Establishing that a *duty existed* between the doctor and patient arising out of the contractual relationship
> 2. Establishing the *standard of care* in the community (or the profession) relative to the issue, as the basis of the suit, and demonstrating a *breach of that standard*
> 3. Demonstrating *injury (or damage)* to the patient
> 4. Proving a *proximate, causal relationship* between the breach of the standard and the specific damages that are alleged to have been done to the patient.[17]

In addition, jurisdictional statutes, professional organization guidelines (e.g., "Principles of Medical Ethic, with annotations especially applicable to Psychiatry," of the American Medical Association and "Rules of the New York State Board of Regents Relating to Definitions of Unprofessional Conduct," for New York residents), and drug company printed materials, when appropriate, must be incorporated into the forensic psychiatrist's thinking, as applicable to the specific case, in order to have a framework to compare alleged deviations with. A very helpful exercise is to develop a two-column checklist comparing each element of the charges with the normally expected behavior, as the material is gathered during the evaluation period.

CLOSING IN

An additional, albeit unofficial and informal, element of the assessment might include the personality of the defendant–psychiatrist. Although there appear to be no published reports pertaining to why specific psychiatrists were sued, some have described variables that may increase or decrease susceptibility to a legal action. Geographical area (urban; California), type of practice (hospital based; use of ECT and drugs) training (adult psychiatry), and sex of the psychiatrist (male) may increase susceptibility.[18] In addition, the personality of the individual psychiatrist may also play a role in promoting a lawsuit by a patient. The psychiatrist who is brusque, indifferent, authoritarian and unwilling to reach out and be available to discuss with the patient his or her concerns about the treatment, may be more prone to a lawsuit. This becomes an important issue, as well, for the forensic psychiatrist's own evaluation. The defendant–psychiatrist you are helping is crucial to the preparation of the case. Poor cooperation, evasiveness or pomposity, must be noted and discussed with the defendant–client. In addition, this personality aberration may become an important component of the defense itself. For example, in a lawsuit charging a psychiatrist with abandonment, the history elicited a story of a patient having seen the psychiatrist for several months and claiming that the psychiatrist dismissed him from treatment without referral to another therapist. The patient made a suicide attempt shortly thereafter, and then proceeded to bring the action against the psychiatrist. In the course of the evaluation, the defendant–psychiatrist claimed that he never discharged the patient but that the patient simply interpreted a particularly confrontive session as one of discharge from treatment. Through corroborating testimony from individuals who knew the psychiatrist, including other patients, the psychiatrist's intensely confronting, brusque and authoritarian personality was described, leaving considerable doubt as to whether the termination of therapy actually was stated by the psychiatrist, or only interpreted in that manner by the patient. The case was dropped and never reached settlement or the courtroom. Yet, it should be noted that throughout the course of the evaluations, the personality of the defendant–psychiatrist continued as an obstacle to the work despite discussions about it. One cannot assume that a psychiatrist will know much more about his particular personality, his methods of relating to patients, or the inappropriateness of his behavior than a lay client.

In proceeding with the evaluation, in-depth meetings should be requested by the forensic psychiatrist of whomever is felt to be germane to the case (defendant, spouse, other collaterals). In some situations, the attorney will be reluctant to allow this, especially if the request by the attorney is for testimony only on general or hypothetical issues, such as the standard of care. It has been found that not having firsthand knowledge of the defendant may be an acceptable practice,[19] but the forensic psychiatrist must question the appropriateness of testifying in a case where he knows nothing of the defendant through personal assessment.

As alluded to previously, it cannot be emphasized enough how much valuable information can be acquired through interviews with family members and, especially, colleagues of the defendant–psychiatrist. Although the attorney may also be using these people as character or factual witnesses, the forensic psychiatrist's evaluation of them may lend significant credibility and corroboration to the material gleaned from the defendant–psychiatrist himself.

In addition, seeing the *plaintiff–patient* for an evaluation, if at all possible, even with their attorney present, can add additional valuable information, at least about the extent or character of the alleged damages and whether the patient had benefitted from the treatment, despite the alleged malpractice.[20] Some psychiatrists and attorneys recommend observing the plaintiff–patient in the courtroom and then testifying to those observations. Serious reservations are held about that practice, because it will, very likely, sound vague and spurious and has been used in the past against the psychiatrist to discredit his entire testimony.[21]

DEVELOPING CONCLUSIONS AND REASONING

As the evaluation proceeds, a picture will start forming of the specific malpractice charged, the attorney's view of the defense, and the defendant–psychiatrist's story. The next step will be to outline the specifics, compare them with the "standard of care," and develop an explanation for any deviation. In a Maryland case[22] entailing an action against a psychiatric hospital and the treating psychiatrists, in the alleged deterioration and death of a patient while in the hospital, a significant issue revolved around the appropriate treatment for schizophrenia in the 1960s. The hospital had treated this chronically ill patient with intensive psychotherapy, alone, and contended that psychotherapy, alone, was an accepted treatment, and that irrespective of the treatment, the natural course of the disease process itself might include remissions, exacerbations, and progressive deterioration over time. Extensive research, in defending this case, included discovering many articles from the psychiatric (and even lay) literature supporting the appropriateness of psychotherapy alone, *in the 1960s*, and to the deteriorating course in some patients, despite any type of treatment.

This last issue is the concept of *causation*, the requirement of a showing of a causal relationship between the psychiatric practice (or alleged malpractice) and the damage charged by the patient. Another common example is one in which a therapist recommends or supports marital separation to a patient; the patient, subsequent to the separation, deteriorates emotionally, and the therapist is blamed for the subsequent deterioration.[23]

In the Maryland case, although there existed no treatise defining the "standard of care" specifically, a body of literature was put together, refuting the contention that medication was required for this patient, and that there existed a "causal relation" between the therapists' actions and the deterioration and death of the patient.

Bringing the reader of the forensic report (and the court) back to the therapist's position, thinking, and judgment at the time of the therapy, in the setting and with the information available at the time, is defined by Campion and Peck as taking a "time machine approach,"[24] a very valuable and effective exercise for the forensic psychiatrist and certainly for the judge or jury.

Some cases may depend on showing that a contractual relationship did not exist between the defendant–psychiatrist and the plaintiff[25] or that reasonable judgement does not entail or require infallibility.[26]

An additional important step might include interviewing psychiatrists to identify the reasonable standard at the time of the alleged malpractice. An interesting example is the use of tricyclic antidepressants in doses greater than those recommended in the *Physician's Desk Reference* or by the manufacturer, and in the use of such drugs as Propranolol for the treatment of the peripheral manifestations of anxiety, which is not a defined use of this drug. In both situations, psychiatrists in the community (and articles from the literature) could be gathered to attest to these common practices. Of course, one might still have to contend with the charge, if made, that the patient did not give adequate "informed consent" prior to the instituting of the treatment.

Further refining of the standard of care would include an assessment of "minimal or reasonable" care, instead of "optimal" care, or that the unique and exceptional nature of the circumstances dictated a deviation from standard care. Wilkinson described a case in which one psychiatrist was not held liable for malpractice when he had terminated professional treatment, yet continued seeing the patient, socially, to avoid a relapse caused by the abrupt (but necessary) end to treatment.[27]

It should be noted that many reputable, ethical psychiatrists in the community take shortcuts in their work but may not admit to it publicly. Menninger stated that the "art of medicine consists in knowing how to make shortcuts and knowing when it is wise and permissible to do so."[28] At least, one could compare the defendant–psychiatrist's actions to these practices, and, perhaps, develop enough material to show evidence of their common, albeit not standard use.

There is generally a wide latitude given to psychiatric practices, as courts are aware that there exist many diverse schools of psychiatric treatment. The psychiatrist will be judged by the "customary practice" in his area and in his school of thought.

Yet, some practices appear to be such "obvious departures that inferences drawn from the facts are within the range of (the layman's) common experience and awareness."[30] But, if the forensic psychiatrist believes that the defendant–psychiatrist acted in good faith, and believed in his mode of treatment, it may be advantageous to speak with other psychiatric experts to attempt to develop backing for this unorthodox approach.

The plaintiff's experts, operating "after the fact," know that the treatment did not work (otherwise, it is not likely that the patient would have brought suit) and can simply point out the departure from "regular or customary" practice. But an argument could still be made that, although the treatment is not usual, it was performed without *foreseeable risk*, in good faith, and was reasonable.[31]

Frequently, the "controlling factor in cases, is whether the psychiatrist could have reasonably anticipated harm to the patient. . . . Perfection and success are not required."[32] Of course, as stated above, the expert must always consider the thinking of the layman, sitting on a jury, and consider what that person would think was unreasonable or even outrageous practice. It is much too easy, in our zeal to believe, and as a result of our liberal and abstract thinking as psychiatrists, to lose sight of what a layman would accept as reasonable or foreseeable. One approach to this potential discrepancy is to have the forensic psychiatrist utilize a group of lay friends, who frequently think more like the general public, as an "unofficial jury" to provide feedback on the believability of a case or its justification. One example was of a psychiatrist who was charged with improper physical (nonsexual) contact with patients. His practice, based on his belief that holding a patient on his lap during a particularly stressful period would provide the security and trust needed to utilize the therapeutic session more adequately, was called into question by one of his patients. This woman, described as hysterical and infantile in her thinking, initiated an action against him for improper practice when she became enmeshed in an eroticized transference and then felt depressed and rejected when he dealt with it exclusively through interpretation. Despite repeated explanations to the unofficial jury that there was no overt sexual contact, they would not accept the psychiatrist's practice as reasonable in the light of so much publicity against physical contact. They were also quite insightful in observing that he should have known that this particular type of patient might very well react inappropriately to this treatment approach.

Another case is of the therapist beating his patient as part of the treatment.[33] Few laymen would not believe this an improper and unreasonable form of treatment, especially if the patient were injured in the course of the sessions. A significant, and probably futile, amount of testimony would have to be offered to overcome this belief.

But, in these cases, an important function of the forensic psychiatrist, after the evaluation, is to advise the attorney and defendant–psychiatrist of the psychiatrically weak and vulnerable areas of the case. This is often a difficult function, as critical care must be taken in not overstating the weak (or strong) points, but attempting to be as neutral and objective as possible. As stated previously, the forensic psychiatrist's opinion will have an enormous impact on many attorneys and may be crucial in influencing them to go to trial on a case or to attempt to settle it. Psychiatrists are certainly considered more knowledgeable in malpractice actions than in criminal or other civil suits, further removed from the mainstream of psychiatry.

In assessing the presence or absence of liability and the extent-of damage, if any, the forensic psychiatrist must spend greater time in deliberating over the material he has gathered before meeting with the attorney, then in other types of cases, since extent of damage is a significant issue when monetary awards are considered.[34]

In addition, it is recommended that the defendant–psychiatrist be present at the meeting with the attorney. If there is any justification to participate in strategy sessions, it would be at this point in the progress of the evaluation process. One other area where the forensic psychiatrist can be helpful in psychiatric malpractice is in evaluating reports and testimony of the plaintiff's psychiatric experts, because psychiatrists may testify to material which is disputable or even totally inaccurate.

Throughout this work, the common tendency for psychiatrists to share "war stories" must be guarded against, both in professional and social settings. Whereas great caution is urged in all case discussions, none are as crucial as those affecting a colleague. Human nature promotes gossiping about the deficiencies of fellow psychiatrists, but the risk of the gossip getting back to the defendant–psychiatrist is great and may have a damaging effect on his self-esteem, promoting greater estrangement and isolation from his peers.

However, there exist few opportunities to be as helpful to a colleague in need as in a psychiatric malpractice action, and to upgrade public awareness in clarifying issues of appropriate disagreement in the field.

REFERENCES

[1]Menninger, K: *The Crime of Punishment,* New York, 1968, p. 139.
[2]Furrow, B: Threats of more malpractice suits may be facing psychiatrists,*Psychiatric News,* July 15, 1983, p. 1.
[3]Schetky, D, Cavanaugh, J: Child psychiatry perspective: Psychiatric malpractice. *J Am Acad Child Psychiatry 21,* 5:521–526, 1982.
[4]Schetky, D, Colbach, E: Countertransference on the witness stand: A flight from self? *Bull Am Acad Psychiatry Law 10,* 2:115–121, 1982.
[5]Rada, RT: The psychiatrist as expert witness, in Hofling C (ed.): Law and *Ethics in the Practice of Psychiatry,* New York, Brunner Mazel, 1981.
[6]Work, H: Career choice in the training of the child Psychiatrist. *J Am Acad Child Psychiatry* 7:442–453, 1968.
[7]Schetky, D, Colbach, E: Countertransference on the witness stand: A flight from self? *Bull Am Acad Psychiatry Law 10,* 2:115–21, 1982.
[8]Slawson, P: Psychiatric malpractice: The California experience. *Am J Psychiatry 136,* 5:650–654, May 1979.
[9]Slawson, P: Psychiatric malpractice: A regional incidence study. *Am J Psychiatry 126,* 9:1302–1305, Mar 1970.
[10]Glass, E: Restructuring informed consent: legal therapy for the doctor–patient relationship. *Yale L. J.* 79:1533–76, July 1970.
[11]Halpern, A: Psychiatric malpractice. Presented at the annual meeting, American Academy of Psychiatry and Law, New York City, Jan. 22, 1983.
[12]Tuckman, A, Schneider M: Society, credibility and forensic psychiatry. *Newsletter Amer Acad Psychiatry Law,* 7, 2, 1982.
[13]Campion, T, Peck, J: Ingredients of a psychiatric malpractice lawsuit. *Psychiatr Q 51,* 3:236–241, Fall 1979.
[14]Messinger, S: Malpractice suits: The psychiatrist's turn. *J Leg Med,* 3:21, 1971.
[15]Slovenkoe, R: Malpractice in psychiatry and related fields. *J Psy Law,* 5–63, Spring, 1981.
[16]Perr, I: Liability of hospital and psychiatrist. *Am J Psychiatry 122:*631, 1965.
[17]Schetky, D, Cavanaugh, J: Child psychiatry perspective: Psychiatric malpractice. *J Am Acad Child Psychiatry,* 21, 5:521–26, 1982.
[18]Schetky, D, Cavanaugh, J: Child psychiatry perspective: psychiatric malpractice. *J Am Acad Child Psychiatry,* 21, 5, 521–26, 1982.
[19]Barefoot v Estelle USSC 82–6080, as described in *Psychiatric News,* Aug. 5, 1983, p. 1.

[20]Halpern, A: Psychiatric malpractice. Presented at the annual meeting American Academy Psychiatry and Law, New York City, Jan 22, 1983.

[21]United States v Hiss 88 F. Supp. 559 (SDNY 1950).

[22]Kappas v Chestnut Lodge, Rockville, Md., 1980.

[23]Wall Street Journal, Nov 6, 1979, p. 1.

[24]Campion, T, Peck, J: Ingredients of a psychiatric malpractice lawsuit. *Psychiatri Q 51*, 3:236–241, Fall 1979.

[25]Last v Franzblau, N. Y., 1980.

[26]Wilkinson, A: Psychiatric malpractice:Identifying areas of liability. *Trial*, p. 73–77, Oct., 1982.

[27]Wilkinson, A: Psychiatric malpractice:Identifying areas of liability. *Trial*, p. 77, Oct., 1982.

[28]Menninger, K: *The Crime of Punishment*, New York, Viking Press, New York, 1968, p. 289.

[29]Perr, I: Liability of hospital and psychiatrist. *Am J Psy* 122:631, 1965.

[30]Olfe v Gordon, 286 NW 2d 573 (Minn.).

[31]Campion, T, Peck, J: Ingredients of a psychiatric malpractice lawsuit. *Psychiatr Q, 51*, 3:236–241, Fall, 1979.

[32]Wilkinson, A: Psychiatric malpractice:Identifying areas of liability. *Trial*, 73–77, Oct., 1982.

[33]Hammer v Rosen 7 App. Div. 2d, 216, 181 NYS 2nd 805 (1959).

[34]Halpern, A: Psychiatric malpractice, presented at annual meeting, American Academy Psychiatry and Law, New York City, Jan 22, 1983.

IV

Adolescent Psychiatry and the Law

9

Adolescent Cognitive and Emotional Development

An Introduction to Adolescent Psychiatry for Forensic Psychiatrists: Clinical Considerations in a Legal Context

BERTRAM SLAFF

It is fundamental to the understanding of adolescents, indeed to the comprehension of all individuals, that the developmental point of view be kept in mind. This may be conceived of as three overlapping circles, one representing physical maturational growth, one expressing cognitive development, one evincing emotional and interpersonal evolution. All of these must be thought of as concurrently dynamic, that is, in a constant state of activity.

Can a child of three lie? Can a child of three steal? Jean Piaget, the great Swiss psychologist and epistemologist, would say no. Children of that age have not yet achieved the capacity for comprehending abstractions such as "truth" or "property rights," a requirement for meaningful lying or stealing. Piaget has studied the vicissitudes of various aspects of learning throughout childhood and adolescence, including such areas as language and thought, judgment and reasoning, the child's conception of physical causality, moral judgment, the child's conception of number, intellectual operations and their development, the early growth of logic in the child, and (with Bärbel Inhelder) the growth of logical thinking from childhood to adolescence.

BERTRAM SLAFF • The Mount Sinai Medical Center, 1100 Madison Avenue, New York, NY 10028.

149

He has described a sensorimotor phase up until about age 2, succeeded by a preoperational or egocentric stage lasting until about age 7.

> Around 7 or 8, the child discovers what we shall call concrete operations (classification, serialization, one-to-one correspondency features, numbers, spatial operations, and the like), which already constitute a kind of logic because of their group structures. But this is a logic of a very limited scope, relating only to objects themselves which can be effectively or mentally manipulated. This logic leads only to restricted systems, corresponding to certain structures of classes, of relationships and numbers, but which do not include the general and formal logic that logicians call the logic of propositions, which in turn makes it possible to reason on assumptions and not merely on objects.
>
> Now, the great novelty that characterizes adolescent thought and that starts around the age of 11 to 12, but does not reach its point of equilibrium until the age of 14 or 15—this novelty consists in detaching the concrete logic from the objects themselves, so that it can function on verbal or symbolic statements without other support. Above all the novelty consists in generalizing this logic and supplementing it with a set of combinations. This set of combinations is not radically new and merely extends, in a way, the classifications and serializations of the level of concrete operations. It is new, however, that these are operations at one state removed, or operations on operations. A set of combinations consists, in fact, in a classification of all the possible classifications, a serialization of serializations (permutations), and so forth.
>
> The great novelty that results consists in the possibility of manipulating ideas in themselves and no longer in merely manipulating objects. In a word, the adolescent is an individual who is capable (and this is where he reaches the level of the adult) of building or understanding ideal or abstract theories and concepts . . . the adolescent is capable of projects for the future . . . , of nonpresent interests, and of a passion for ideas, ideals, or ideologies.[1,2]

Elsewhere, I have enumerated the developmental challenges to the teenager:

> To negotiate the onset of puberty in the face of major changes in body configuration and intensification of sexual drives; to relinquish some of the dependency of childhood; to derive increasing security from his own growing mastery; to tolerate the losing of confidence in his parents and teachers as the repositories of wisdom; to develop his own skeptical and critical powers and to learn more and more how to think in independent terms; to cultivate the growth of his social skills; to learn how to deal with strong emotional states; to begin to be aware of the necessity of thinking ahead and considering goals in a realistic fashion; to deal with sexual strivings and to conceive of love, marriage, and parenthood; and finally, to strive for complete independence. The totality of this development is known as separation and individuation; when it is successfully negotiated, it results in the establishment of an independent adult personality.[3]

Implicit within the developmental frame of reference is the concept of *normative crisis*. This refers to specific events within the normal life cycle which are likely to provoke anxiety. A child's going off to school for the first time is an obvious example of this. It could be noted that this is likely also be be a normative crisis for the mother. Puberty is such a normative crisis. Preparing for sleep-away camp or college may represent such a crisis.

> Dwight, a seventeen-year-old high school senior who wanted to go away to college, was facing the normative crisis of leaving home. He had a childhood history of allergies which had caused much parental and medical concern. During early adolescence his sensitivities had lessened, and he now seemed to be a healthy youth.
>
> In considering colleges to attend, he became concerned by the worrisome thought, "What happens if I get sick?" He was reluctant to tell anyone how terrified he was to be away from his mother.
>
> The family of a close friend invited Dwight to accompany them on a vacation trip. Dwight agonized about what he would do if he became ill. He might throw up, he might sneeze all night, he might suffocate. Determined to keep his anxieties private, he declined the invitation.
>
> However, he really wanted to go on the trip. It seemed a hopeless dilemma. His appetite declined, he slept poorly. Soon his parents realized that he was severely troubled and arranged for a psychiatric consultation.
>
> In the course of the ensuing psychotherapy, it became abundantly clear that Dwight's inner picture of himself was that of a severely allergic youngster, perilously vulnerable to sneezing, choking, and life-threatening attacks of nausea and vomiting.
>
> That he had been essentially well for over five years, that he had matured, and that he could now take adequate care of himself had not been comprehended by the anxious child within.
>
> Dwight was encouraged to open up to the reality of his having outgrown his allergic sensitivities and having become a healthy youth. He was asked to anticipate possible allergic difficulties in the light of his new competence to handle them. He was strongly encouraged to take the proposed trip.
>
> The vacation journey turned out to be successful, though in the final few days Dwight became anxious, thinking his good luck could not continue.
>
> Gradually over the following months Dwight's anxieties faded and his self-confidence grew; he was able to embark on a college career away from home.[3]

As illustrated in the story of Dwight, therapeutic interventions with teenagers should *promote growth*. The goal is to ascertain the presence of roadblocks interfering with growth and to help the individual remove them. It is hoped that the natural tendency for growth will resume. Therapy with such individuals may be of relatively brief duration.

Diagnostic evaluation of a teenager must be a part of a family and environmental study. Some youngsters develop behavioral difficulties in response to unconscious needs on the part of a parent who may, as Adelaide Johnson has noted, have a "superego lacuna."[4] Mixed messages such as, "Don't cheat. But, if you do cheat, at least be smart and don't get caught," clearly express parental ambivalence on the topic.

A parent may subtly incite his child to behave in a particular way by negative suggestion.

Thirteen-year-old Ned stole a substantial sum of money from the church collection in a manner which suggested that unconsciously he expected to be caught. And he was.

Ned's father was a claims investigator for an insurance company, with the responsibility for ferreting out instances of possible fraud. He had nagged his son incessantly about the importance of being strictly honest.[3]

A particular family member, who may be an adolescent, may be elected to serve as the focal point of the family's disharmony. By concentrating the blame on this one individual, the "scapegoat," the other members of the family may be able to avoid confronting their own contributions to the situation.

Fourteen-year-old Debra was the only child of a lawyer– father who lived in Chicago and a painter—mother who kept her own apartment in New York, for professed career reasons. The parents would spend a month or so together in each location; in the course of these periods together, there would routinely be a major battle over Debra's behavior and the parents would then separate again. Debra would stay with one parent or the other, until a toleration point had been reached; she then would be sent back to the other. Her well-off parents had even established her in private schools of comparable status in the two cities, so that, as she was batted about, ping-pong style, school facilities were always available to her.

Both parents had established a "line"; it was Debra's impossible ways that prevented them from being able to stay together. Debra herself had never questioned the validity of this. She believed that she was the serpent who had wrecked the Eden of her parents' lives.[3]

A teenager who is behaving destructively may be acting at the direction of someone else.

A thirteen-year-old youth was described by his parents as severely disturbed. He and his fifteen-year-old brother were angry young people who called both parents "fuzz" and "fascist oppressors." The behavior of the younger boy, Roger, included throwing dishes and threatening to destroy the household. Derek, the older brother, ridiculed the idea of seeing a psychiatrist and refused to consider it. Roger was willing to do so.

In early conversations with the therapist, Roger appeared friendly, lucid, intelligent, and talked with equanimity about what his parents had described as the "state of siege" at home. He laughed, saying his parents had "no sense of humor at all." He admitted that he had thrown dishes several times, when his parents were being "too uptight." Yes, he had threatened to destroy the household, but he really hadn't meant that. "My parents are alarmists; it's not nearly that bad." Speaking for himself and his brother, he admitted, "We tease them a lot."

After some time, the mystery of how Roger could be seen so differently by his parents and by his psychiatrist was opened for discussion. At Roger's appointment one afternoon, Derek, too, showed up, announcing that he wished to report on what was happening at home. He spoke about the persecuting behavior of both parents, occasionally demanding confirmation from Roger, who echoed him without question. He spoke condescendingly about the stupidity of both parents and remarked that it was sometimes necessary for him to get Roger to throw dishes off the table to get through to them.[3]

Diagnostic evaluation of a teenager must include a review of the adaptive successes and failures of the individual throughout development.

Sixteen-year-old Jeremy came to the attention of the student health office at his college after his philosophy instructor expressed concern about him. He was reading far more than anyone else in the class, often seemed preoccupied and withdrawn, and had ideas which seemed to his teacher to be extraordinarily original, possibly highly creative or, on the other hand, bizarre, or both. A careful review of Jeremy's life history revealed that as early as nursery school, he had been noticed as "different." His teacher had reported that he was always sweet and amiable, but seemed to lack some quality of personal responsiveness, as though he didn't really care very much whether or not anyone paid any attention to him. Some years later, he was observed in school to be highly gifted in learning and particularly adept at self-instruction. He was consistently ahead of his class in all his subjects. He cheerfully carried out additional assignments that his devoted teachers prepared for him alone.

At age nine, Jeremy regarded his classmates as childish and told them so. He identified completely with the adult world. Not surprisingly, the other children hated Jeremy and teased him unmercifully. Jeremy seemed not to care very much; by the third grade, he was already teaching himself Italian, botany, and astronomy.

During his childhood Jeremy received much love and support from his parents, who understood and respected his right to be different. If they had fought him on this and pressed him to be more like other children, it is likely that they could have alienated him and that he would then have been even more isolated than he was.

As a young child, Jeremy freely admitted that he was different, saying, in his characteristic way, "That is I."

In the course of the evaluation, his "atypical" behavior at college was felt to be consistent with his earlier character development and was not regarded as cause for concern. It was judged that Jeremy would probably continue to be an atypical person throughout has life, and that he would be likely to continue to gain major gratifications from exercising his intellectual capacities. If at some future time he became upset because of interpersonal difficulties, he might then seek help. Then, too, his "atypicality" would have to be respected.[3]

Curious perceptions or behavior in the present may be rooted in repressed traumatic experiences in the past and may become comprehensible after these connections are made.

A seventeen-year-old boy in psychotherapy developed an insistent and pervasive feeling that his therapist was trying to pull thoughts out of his head.

He knew that people often talk about their "shrinks" attempting to read their minds or pull thoughts out of their heads, but insisted that his concern was literal rather than metaphorical. He also had a feeling that his therapist in some way was going to kill him in the supposed process of helping him. His critical judgment told him that this was "paranoid," and he insisted that he did not really believe this, but nevertheless, he continued to be oppressed by these extremely disturbing preoccupations.

Months later, during a psychotherapeutic session, he began to feel as though his therapist had his hand on his head and was trying to choke him. Panic ensued, accompanied by a terror of being suffocated. A feeling of "It's for your own good" accompanied this anguished reaction.[3]

What had returned to awareness was a long-repressed experience that had occurred at age 2 when he had suddenly developed a respiratory blockage as part of a severe diphtheritic infection of the throat. His parents had rushed their cyanotic child to a physician who lived next door; at once, the physician forcefully removed part of the obstructing membrane from the throat, causing hemorrhaging but permitting the resumption of breathing. This life-saving experience had been perceived from the child's point of view as an assault and a suffocation, with the parents incomprehensibly standing by, saying, "It's for your own good."

With the developmental point of view in mind, we must assume that early childhood events are experienced in ways consistent with the sensorimotor level of development up until about age 2; in an egocentric way, until about 7, and in concrete operational ways until about 11, after which abstract operational thought becomes possible.[1,2] It is hypothesized that derivatives of these maturationally earlier modes of perception continue to be influential later in life. These leave the individual vulnerable to illogical fears, primitively determined assumptions and various conclusions that he may suspect are absurd and yet continue to feel as true.

Erik Erikson has divided the life cycle into "Eight Stages of Man."[5] These include, in sequence: (1) the oral sensory state, in which the issue principally is one of "Trust vs. Basic Mistrust;" (2) the muscular-anal stage, in which the conflict is "Autonomy vs. Shame and Doubt;" (3) the locomotor-genital stage, with "Initiative vs. Guilt;" (4) latency, with "Industry vs. Inferiority;" (5) puberty and adolescence, with "Identity vs. Role Diffusion;" (6) young adulthood, with "Intimacy vs. Isolation;" (7) adulthood, with "Generativity vs. Stagnation;" and (8) maturity, with "Ego Integrity vs. Despair."

Concerning Stage 5, puberty and adolescence, he writes:

With the establishment of a good relationship to the world of skills and tools, and with the advent of sexual maturity, childhood proper comes to an end. Youth begins. But in puberty and adolescence all samenesses and continuities relied on earlier are questioned again, because of a rapidity of body growth which equals that of early childhood and because of the entirely new addition of physical genital maturity. The growing and developing youths, faced with this physiological revolution within them, are now primarily concerned with what they appear to be in the eyes of others as compared with what they feel they are, and with the question of how to connect the roles and skills cultivated earlier with the occupational prototypes of the day. In their search for a new sense of continuity and sameness, adolescents have to refight many of the battles of earlier years, even though to do so they must artificially appoint perfectly well-meaning people to play the roles of enemies; and they are ever ready to install lasting idols and ideals as guardians of a final identity: here puberty rites "confirm" the inner design for life.

The integration now taking place in the form of ego identity is more than the sum of the childhood identifications. It is the accrued experience of the ego's ability to integrate these identifications with the vicissitudes of the libido, with the aptitudes developed out of endowment, and with the opportunities offered in social roles. The sense of ego identity, then, is the accrued confidence that the inner sameness and continuity are matched by the sameness and continuity of one's meaning for others, as evidenced in the tangible promise of a "career."

The danger of this stage is role diffusion. Where this is based on a strong previous doubt as to one's sexual identity, delinquent and outright psychotic incidents are not uncommon. If diagnosed and treated correctly, these incidents do not have the same fatal significance which they have at other ages. It is primarily the inability to settle on an occupational identity which disturbs young people. To keep themselves together they temporarily overidentify, to the point of apparent complete loss of identity, with the heroes of cliques and crowds. This initiates the stage of "falling in love," which is by no means entirely, or even primarily, a sexual matter—except where the mores demand it. To a considerable extent adolescent love is an attempt to arrive at a definition of one's identity by projecting one's diffused ego images on one another and by seeing them thus reflected and gradually clarified. This is why many a youth would rather converse, and settle matters of mutual identification, than embrace.

Puberty rites and confirmations help to integrate and to affirm the new identity.[5]

Establishing a therapeutic relationship with a teenager, particularly the younger adolescent, is often a difficult task. Many young people come to professional attention not because of their own complaints, but because their parents or school authorities or society are troubled about them. It may require considerable skill and patience, to engage a teenager in discussion on terms which are meaningful to him. Flexibility and adaptability on the part of the interviewer are useful attributes.[3]

Many teenagers are emotionally variable. Some have not yet learned how to be verbally expressive about their feelings and do not comprehend the cognitive-emotional link. For these reasons, it is often advisable to interview an individual on a number of different occasions.

In the world of forensic psychiatry, a youth may well wonder,

"Whose side are you on?" An interviewer may be representing the court, either parent in a custody struggle, or either side in various other legal actions. It is most important that the interviewer straightforwardly delineate his role. In most legal determinations, confidentiality can not be assured and this should be clarified with the individual.

It is obvious that the clinician must be firmly grounded in the knowledge of human growth and development in order properly to identify and treat significant deviations from the norms for that development. Many of these deviations will now be explored and additional case vignettes will be provided. These are presented both to illustrate specific conditions and also to convey a sense of the enormous variety of adolescent behaviors. It is hoped that this may give some understanding of how a clinician might recognize health by a process of excluding diagnosable illnesses.

In the interface between psychiatry and the law, there will be many references to DSM-III, *Diagnostic and Statistical Manual of Mental Disorder* (Third Edition),[6] published by the American Psychiatric Association in 1980. DSM-III recommends multiaxial evaluation for each case. Axis I deals predominantly with "Clinical Syndromes;" Axis II deals with "Personality Disorders" and "Specific Developmental Disorders;" Axis III deals with "Physical Disorders and Conditions." The first three axes constitute the official diagnostic assessment. Axis IV deals with "Severity of Psychosocial Stressors;" Axis V deal with the "Highest Level of Adaptive Functioning in the Past Year."

DSM-III includes a section, "Disorders Usually First Evident in Infancy, Childhood, or Adolescence." The disorders described under this heading can be separated into five major groups on the basis of the predominant area of disturbance:

1. Intellectual
   Mental Retardation
2. Behavioral (overt)
   Attention Deficit Disorder
   Conduct Disorder
3. Emotional
   Anxiety Disorders of Childhood or Adolescence
   Other Disorders of Infancy, Childhood, or Adolescence
4. Physical
   Eating Disorders
   Stereotyped Movement Disorders
   Other Disorders with Physical Manifestations
5. Developmental
   Pervasive Developmental Disorders
   Specific Developmental Disorders

Because the *essential* features of Affective Disorders and Schizophrenia are the same in children and adults, there are no special categories corresponding to these disorders in this section of the classification. For example, if a child or adolescent has an illness that meets the criteria for Major Depression, Dysthymic Disorder, or Schizophrenia, these diagnoses should be given, regardless of the age of the individual.[6]

In *Mental Retardation*, "the essential features are (1) significantly subaverage general intellectual functioning, (2) resulting in, or associated with, deficits or impairments in adaptive behavior, (3) with onset before the age of 18."[6] *Mild Mental Retardation* is roughly equivalent to the educational category "educable." This group, with IQs of 50 to 70, represent 80% of the total mental retardation population. *Moderate Mental Retardation*, 12% of this population, with IQs of 35–49, are considered "trainable." The *Severe Mental Retardation* group, 7% of this population, IQs 20–34 and the *Profound Mental Retardation* group, 1% of this population, IQs below 20, complete this survey of the field of mental retardation.

The behavioral disturbances include Attention Deficit Disorder and Conduct Disorder. The essential features of *Attention Deficit Disorder* are signs of developmentally inappropriate inattention and impulsivity. The essential feature of *Conduct Disorder* is a repetitive and persistent pattern of conduct in which either the basic rights of others or major age-appropriate societal norms or rules are violated. The conduct is more serious than the ordinary mischief and pranks of children and adolescents. These are covered more fully by Guggenheim and Garmise in the succeeding chapter, "The Assessment of Psychopathology in Juvenile Delinquency: The Family Court Perspective."

The *Anxiety Disorders of Childhood or Adolescence* include

three disorders in which anxiety is the predominant clinical feature. In the first two categories, Separation Anxiety Disorder and Avoidant Disorders of Childhood or Adolescence, the anxiety is focused on specific situations. In the third category, Overanxious Disorder, the anxiety is generalized to a variety of situations.[6]

Among other disorders is *Oppositional Disorder:*

The essential feature is a pattern of disobedient, negativistic, and provocative opposition to authority figures. . . .

The oppositional attitude is toward family members, particularly the parents, and toward teachers. The most striking feature is the persistence of the oppositional attitude even when it is destructive to the interests and well-being of the . . . adolescent. For example, if there is a rule, it is usually violated; if a suggestion is made, the individual is against it; if asked to do something, the individual refuses or becomes argumentative; if asked to refrain from an act, the . . . adolescent feels obliged to carry it out. The behavior may, in fact, deprive the individual of productive activity and pleasurable relationships.

The continually confronting quality of these individuals is typical of their style and relationships. At times they may appear to be conforming, but in their conformity they still remain provocative toward those around them. Their provocation is often directed toward adults, but may well include other children. If the individual is thwarted, temper tantrums are likely. These . . . adolescents use negativism, stubborness, dawdling, procrastination, and passive resistance to external authority.

Usually the individual does not regard himself or herself as 'oppositional,' but sees the problem as arising from other people, who are making unreasonable demands. The disorder generally causes more distress to those around him or her than to the person himself or herself.[6]

In *Identity Disorder,*

the essential feature is severe subjective distress regarding inability to reconcile aspects of the self into a relatively coherent and acceptable sense of self. There is uncertainty about a variety of issues relating to identity, including long-term goals, career choice, friendship patterns, sexual orientation and behavior, religious identification, moral values and group loyalties.[6]

Nineteen-year-old Warren had dropped out of the prestigious college he was attending, during his second year, because, he said, "I didn't know why I was there." He was an excellent student and a fine athlete. Doing well was what he had always done. He felt that he was programmed to continue this pattern of behavior but had doubts about any genuine commitment to this lifestyle. He felt he had numerous "acquaintances," but not any real friends. He recognized no clues at all regarding career aspirations. In social situations, he constantly monitored his contributions to conversation and worried about how the others would respond to what he had said. He felt himself becoming increasingly oppressed by these preoccupations.

Prominent among the physical disturbances are the Eating Disorders. These include *Anorexia Nervosa,* of which the essential features are "intense fear of becoming obese, disturbance of body image, significant weight loss, refusal to maintain a minimal normal body weight, and amenorrhea (in females). . . . Individuals with this disorder say they 'feel fat' when they are of normal weight or even emaciated."[6]

In *Bulimia,* "the essential features are episodic binge eating accompanied by an awareness that the eating pattern is abnormal, fear of not being able to stop eating voluntarily, and depressed mood and self-deprecating thoughts following the eating binges."[6]

Stereotyped Movement Disorders show an abnormality of gross motor movement. They all involve tics, involuntary rapid movement of a functionally related group of skeletal muscles or the involuntary production of noises or words.

Other disorders with physical manifestations include Stuttering, Functional Enuresis, Functional Encopresis, Sleepwalking Disorder, and Sleep Terror Disorder.

The developmental disturbances include Pervasive Developmental Disorders and Specific Developmental Disorders. About the former:

> The disorders in this subclass are characterized by *distortions* in the development of multiple basic psychological functions that are involved in the development of social skills and language, such as attention, perception, reality testing, and motor movement.
>
> In the past, children with these disorders have been described by many terms: Atypical Children, Symbiotic Psychotic Children, Childhood Schizophrenia, and others. Since these disorders apparently bear little relationship to the psychotic disorders of adult life, the term "psychosis" has not been used here in the name of this group of conditions. The term Pervasive Developmental Disorder has been selected because it describes most accurately the core clinical disturbance: many basic areas of psychological development are affected at the same time and to a severe degree.
>
> Pervasive Developmental Disorders differ from the Specific Developmental Disorders in two basic ways. First, only a specific function is affected in each Specific Developmental Disorder whereas in Pervasive Developmental Disorders multiple functions are always affected. Second, in Specific Developmental Disorders the children behave as if they are passing through an earlier normal developmental stage, because the disturbance is a *delay* in development, whereas children with Pervasive Developmental Disorders display severe qualitative abnormalities that are not normal for any stage of development, because the disturbance is a *distortion* in development.[6]

Among the Specific Developmental Disorders are Developmental Reading Disorder, Developmental Arithmetic Disorder, and Developmental Language Disorder.

DSM-III describes *Schizophrenic Disorders* as follows:

> The essential features of this group of disorders are: the presence of certain psychotic features during the active phase of the illness, characteristic symptoms involving multiple psychological processes, deterioration from a previous level of functioning, onset before age 45, and a duration of at least six months. . . . At some phase of the illness Schizophrenia always involves delusions, hallucinations, or certain disturbances in the form of thought. . . . Onset is usually during adolescence or early adulthood.[6]

Following is a case illustration of an adolescent with a *Schizophrenic Disorder—Paranoid Type:*

> Andrea, a bright, creative, verbal, deeply troubled sixteen-year-old, was to an extraordinary degree similar to Deborah, whose psychotherapy and recovery were described by Hannah Green in *I Never Promised You a Rose Garden.*[7] The presenting behavioral disturbance in both situations was wrist cutting. Andrea, however, was less susceptible to prolonged, severely regressed states.
>
> Andrea reported that she did not have any friends and was highly sensitive as a child. She began to make up names and then invent people to go with them. Increasingly, she believed in the reality of her inventions. At fifteen, she had an intense relationship with a boy which ultimately foundered when she was unable to accede to his sexual advances. "I was living inside then with my made-up people and my made-up things. This depressed me. I wanted to become regular, to be able to talk to people. So I cut my wrists."

Andrea was hospitalized and phenothiazine medication was promptly prescribed. During the early months of her hospital stay, she usually appeared alert and appropriate in her behavior. However, she was susceptible to states of severe withdrawal ("wrapped in cotton"), depression, and apathy, during which she appeared to be seriously ill. Depersonalization, derealization, auditory and visual hallucinations, and paranoid ideation were present to a marked degree.

These episodes of severe disturbance never lasted longer than three to six days. Because of Andrea's propensity for cutting her wrists or for burning herself with cigarettes during these crises, she was of major concern to everyone who cared for her.

Andrea believed that many different figures inhabited her life space. Periodically, she felt displaced. At times, she expressed the wish to jump out of the window (of a fifteenth floor apartment), hoping the impact would "put the pieces back together."

When her suffering was extreme during these states of "daymare," Andrea was sometimes treated with sleep therapy for several days. The plan was to get her to sleep off the "daymare," as one would try to help a person wake up from a nightmare.

It gradually became clear that, probably for over ten years, Andrea had been involved in a paranoid system of thought. She was aware that in some way others posed a threat to this inner world, which she continued to be loath to describe fully. She felt that she was capable of perceiving in a new dimension, and that others were in error in speaking of her private world as "fantasy" or "delusion."

For many months, Andrea believed that her therapist was trying to poison her. Nevertheless, she continued to see him without protest, since she felt she was getting what she deserved, and that he was a relatively kindly poisoner.[3]

DSM-III describes *Affective Disorders:*

The essential feature of this group of disorders is a disturbance of mood, accompanied by a full or partial manic or depressive syndrome, that is not due to any other physical or mental disorder. Mood refers to a prolonged emotion that colors the whole psychic life; it generally involves either depression or elation. The manic and depressive syndromes each consist of characteristic symptoms that tend to occur together.[6]

The essential feature of *Major Affective Disorder—Manic Episode* is "a distinct period when the predominant mood is either elevated, expansive or irritable and when there are associated symptoms of the manic syndrome."[6]

The essential feature of *Major Affective Disorder—Depressed Episode* is "either a dysphoric mood, usually depression, or loss of interest or pleasure in all or almost all usual activities and pastimes."[6]

In adolescent boys negativistic or frankly antisocial behavior may appear. Feelings of wanting to leave home or of not being understood and approved of, restlessness, grouchiness, and aggression are common. Sulkiness, a reluctance to cooperate in family ventures, and withdrawal from social activities, with retreat to one's room, are frequent. School difficulties are likely. There may be inattention to personal appearance and increased emotionality, with particular sensitivity to rejection in love relationships. Substance Abuse may develop.[6]

In *Dysthymic Disorder* (or Depressive Neurosis) "the essential feature is a chronic disturbance of mood involving either depressed mood or loss of interest or pleasure in all, or almost all, usual activities and associated symptoms, but not of sufficient severity and duration to meet the criteria for a major depressive episode (full affective syndrome)."[6]

Seventeen-year-old David was an outstanding student at his large metropolitan high school. He had been elected president of the student body, was captain of the basketball team, and graduated third in his class.

Shortly after learning that he had been awarded an all-expense scholarship to the outstanding college which was his first choice, David underwent a major change in mood. He lost his appetite, slept with difficulty, withdrew socially, questioned his abilities and began to express serious doubts about whether he should accept the scholarship and attend college. It was recognized that he had become depressed, and psychiatric help was sought.

David had for a long time been a "golden lad," generously endowed with health, intelligence, looks, physical and athletic skills, and a relaxed warmth and interest in others.

His parents, fearful that he might become conceited, had for many years reminded him of his good fortune in having inherited superior genes, which permitted him his successes. He was not to claim that he was better than others; he was merely luckier. And, *noblesse oblige*, certainly more would be expected of him because of his good fortune.

At the unconscious level, David experienced his considerable talents as an affliction. His latest success was viewed as an unbearable burden. In their efforts to protect David from becoming too self-assured, his parents had contributed to his developing a severely lowered self-esteem. Future successes seemed to augur further burdens, with the danger of his being expected to perform beyond even his exceptional capacities, and with gratifications apparently not permitted.

In the course of his therapy, David was able to recover from his depression only after he confronted the impasse he had gotten into with his parents. As he studied the meaning of his successes, he perceived that his parents' position was fundamentally unfair to him. He uncovered and allowed himself to experience the rage he felt at them for this and gradually began to permit himself a sense of achievement for what he, not his genes, was accomplishing.

David had only partially internalized his parents' point of view about his successes; his conflicts were partly interior and partly interpersonal. He was in a growth phase in which familiar attitudes frequently undergo major changes; he recovered from his depression fairly rapidly and went on to the college of his choice.[3]

In *Anxiety Disorders*, ". . . anxiety is either the predominant disturbance as in Panic Disorder and Generalized Anxiety Disorder, or anxiety is experienced if the individual attempts to master the symptoms, as in confronting the dreaded object or situation in a Phobic Disorder or resisting the obsessions or compulsions in Obsessive Compulsive Disorder."[6]

Eleven-year-old Marjorie suddenly developed a terror of going to school and absolutely refused to go. She was particularly alarmed about arithmetic, declaring she was stupid and couldn't understand anything at all about what was going on. Further questioning revealed that it was "addition" in arithmetic about which she felt particularly insecure.

What especially confused her parents was that previously Marjorie had been a reasonable bright student (although her grades were not as good as her fourteen year old sister's), and that arithmetic had been one of her better subjects.

She was referred to a therapist who determined that she had developed a school phobia of a nature that contraindicated employing those "first aid" supportive measures that might facilitate a rapid return to school. He recommended that she be withdrawn from school on a medical leave of absence and that she enter psychotherapy.

Marjorie reacted with great relief. She thanked the therapist for rescuing her and with great joy began to work as her father's assistant in the studio where he painted in oils.

The feeling of relief and gratitude ended swiftly when the therapist insisted that the anxieties about school be confronted and discussed. Marjorie then perceived him as an enemy, pushing her to face pain. She felt that she ought to leave psychotherapy, as it was making her feel worse. Nevertheless, she stayed in treatment.

One day Marjorie declared vehemently that she had heard psychiatrists were always looking for a sexual meaning in everything. She wanted it clearly understood that sex had nothing to do with her problem. In fact, she found the whole subject unattractive. Her periods had not started yet, and she was happy about this. She thought from the way her sister talked about them that they were a "messy business." All she wanted to do was to stay a little girl, be at home with her parents, help her father in his studio, and have fun. She denied fearing growing up; rather she declared herself not especially interested in it. She was reacting as though she had the choice of whether or not to permit growing up.

Gradually it became apparent to Marjorie that she was fighting off the acknowledgment of the imminent beginning of her periods. She likened the expectation of having periods to the child's game "Pin the Tail on the Donkey." She elaborated on this by saying it was like having something added to oneself that made one feel different, no longer like oneself.

It was pointed out to her that she had compared the anticipation of her period to having something "added" to her. Suddenly she broke into tears and rushed out of the therapist's office crying, "I hate you!"

Although a period of resistance followed, an important clue had been elicited that contributed to the understanding of her school phobia. Marjorie was terrified of her expected periods, which she feared would be something "added" to her, changing her into something else, not herself. This included fear of the "addition" of breasts. Her defense was to try to go backward, to return to the security remembered from earlier years, to renounce school and learning, to stop time. Nevertheless, implicit in this apparent renunciation of adolescent sexuality was an unconscious return to oedipal sexuality in which, as a little girl, she could spend time assisting her beloved father in his studio, while her older sister was compelled to attend school.

As it became clearer to Marjorie that she was trying to do the impossible, to stop time and growth, she gradually began to prepare to accept the imminent pubertal changes. She agreed to cooperate with home instruction classes for the balance of the term and did return to school when the new term began. The therapeutic goal had been accomplished.[3]

In *Personality Disorders,* DSM-III states:

Personality *traits* are enduring patterns of perceiving, relating to, and thinking about the environment and oneself, and are exhibited in a wide range of important social and personal contexts. It is only when *personality traits* are inflexible and maladaptive and cause either significant impairment in social or occupational functioning or subject distress that they constitute *Personality Disorders.* The manifestations of Personality Disorders are generally recognizable by adolescence or earlier.[6]

Among these are Schizoid Personality Disorder, Avoidant Personality Disorder, Antisocial Personality Disorder, Passive-Aggressive Personality Disorder, and Borderline Personality Disorder.

Finally, in dealing with adolescents one must be sensitive to non-problems, issues that are brought up as psychiatric difficulties which are merely expressions of the uncertainties inherent in the adolescent growth experience.

A fifteen-year-old girl read Radclyffe Hall's *The Well of Loneliness.*[8] She knew that she had had several crushes on woman teachers and wondered if she might be a lesbian. Careful inquiry elicited that this young woman was leading an active social life with young men and that her sexual fantasies were predominantly concerned with men.

It appeared that this girl's concern about homosexual tendencies was more expressive of a literary yearning towards nonconformity than of an actual sexual conflict. It was decided that she needed more time to mature before the presence or absence of a sexual problem could be determined.[3]

SUMMARY

The developmental point of view has been stressed in this presentation on adolescent cognitive and emotional development. This includes physical maturational growth, cognitive development, and emotional and interpersonal evolution. All of these are concurrently dynamic, in a constant state of activity.

Piaget's great contribution to the knowledge of cognitive development has been acknowledged. The substantial body of post-Piagetian criticism is alluded to in the references.[9,10,11,12]

Adolescence, a major growth phase, is presented on the continuum of Erikson's eight stages of the life cycle.

Implicit within the developmental frame of reference is the concept of normative crisis, specific events within the normal life cycle that are likely to provoke anxiety.

It is stressed that therapeutic interventions with teenagers should promote growth. The goal is to ascertain the presence of roadblocks interfering with growth and to help the individual remove them. It is hoped that the natural tendency for growth will resume.

Diagnostic evaluation of a teenager must be part of a family and environmental study. Some youngsters may act out in harmony with a parent's "superego lacuna." They may be responding to a parent's negative suggestion. It is recognized that a particular individual, often a teenager, may be elected to serve as the focal point of a family's disharmony, thus serving as the "scapegoat;" the other members of the family may thus be able to avoid confronting their own contributions to the situation.

Diagnostic evaluation of a youth must include a review of the adaptive successes and failures of the individual throughout development.

Unusual perceptions or behavior in the present may be rooted in repressed traumatic experiences in the past and may become comprehensible after these connections are made.

It is hypothesized that derivatives of maturationally earlier modes of perception continue to be influential later in life. These leave the individual vulnerable to illogical fears, primitively determined assumptions and various conclusions that he may suspect are absurd and yet continue to feel as true.

The difficulties in "engaging" a teenager in meaningful discussion are noted. The frequent variability and nonawareness of the cognitive-emotional link suggest the advisability of interviewing an individual on a number of different occasions.

In the world of forensic psychiatry, an interviewer working with an adolescent must establish clearly whom he is representing. In these situations, usually, confidentiality can not be assured.

In the interface between psychiatry and the law, DSM-III,[6] occupies a major place. An effort has been made to give the flavor of this work and to describe many of the clinical entities which are included.

REFERENCES

[1]Piaget, J: The intellectual development of the adolescent, in Caplan, G, & Lebovici, S (eds.): *Adolescence: Psychosocial Perspectives*, New York, Basic Books, 1969, pp. 22–26.
[2]Flavell, JH: *The Developmental Psychology of Jean Piaget*, Princeton, D. Van Nostrand, 1963.
[3]Slaff, B: Adolescents, in Noshpitz, JD (ed.): *Basic Handbook of Child Psychiatry*, Vol III, New York, Basic Books, 1979, pp. 504–518.

[4]Johnson, AM: Sanctions for superego lacunae of adolescents, in Eissler, KR (ed.): *Searchlights on Delinquency*, New York, International Universities Press, 1949, pp. 225–245.

[5]Erikson, EH: *Childhood and Society*, New York, W.W. Norton & Company, 1950, pp. 227–229.

[6]*Diagnostic and Statistical Manual of Mental Disorders* (Third Edition), Washington, American Psychiatric Association, 1980.

[7]Green, H: *I Never Promised You a Rose Garden*, New York, Holt, Rinehart & Winston, 1964.

[8]Hall, R: *The Well of Loneliness*, London, Covici, 1928.

[9]Gilligan, C: *In a Different Voice*, Cambridge, Harvard University Press, 1982.

[10]Keasey, CB, & Sales, BD: An empirical investigation of young children's awareness and usage of intentionality in criminal situations, in Sales, BD (ed.) *Law and Human Behavior*, Vol I, N. 1, New York, Plenum Press, 1977, pp. 45–61.

[11]Kohlberg, L: *The Philosophy of Moral Development*, San Francisco, Harper & Row, 1981.

[12]Marin, BV, Holmes, DL, Guth, M *et al:* The potential of children as eyewitnesses (A comparison of children and adults on eyewitness tasks), in Sales, BD (ed.) *Law and Human Behavior*, Vol III, N. 4, New York, Plenum Press, 1979, pp. 295–305.

10

The Assessment of Psychopathology in Juvenile Delinquency

The Family Court Perspective

PETER D. GUGGENHEIM AND RICHARD GARMISE

The Mental Health Services of Family Court in New York City functions in a diagnostic/consultative relationship to the court, with an *amicus curiae* status. In cases of juvenile delinquency, a clinical evaluation is requested by the court after a fact-finding (determination of guilt) has been made against a delinquent respondent. The clinic assesses the respondent's mental functioning and recommends to the court appropriate avenues of remediation and rehabilitation, balancing the needs of the juvenile with those of society, all within the context of the "least restrictive" guidelines.

Juvenile delinquency is the outcome of a complex interaction of social, legal, and psychiatric variables, and no single diagnostic classification or theory of aetiology can account for "the delinquent profile." It is well known, for example, that organic factors, as well as major mental disorders, are often prominent in delinquency.[1] From the diagnostic standpoint, most delinquents referred to our clinics are ultimately identified as conduct disorders, although the wider range of impairment is also represented.

PETER D. GUGGENHEIM • Department of Psychiatry, School of Medicine, New York University, New York, New York 10016.   RICHARD GARMISE • Institute of Advanced Psychological Studies, Adelphi University, Garden City, New York 11530.

Our experience focuses on a fairly clearly-defined offender population. Delinquents referred by the court are predominantly male, early adolescent, of minority background and low socioeconomic status, and frequently come from single-parent families. Further, many of the juveniles we see have a history of poor school adjustment, and both gross cognitive impairments and "learning disabilities" are prominent among those referred to us.[2] The intake officers of the court system attempt to refer the less serious delinquencies to a variety of diversion alternatives, rather than proceeding through the legal system, and it is estimated that referrals to the Mental Health Services are ultimately made for no more than 25% to 40% of those youngsters who are eventually adjudicated as delinquents.

This paper highlights some of the unique features in diagnostic work which evolve from our contact with such a clearly defined population, within the context of the Family Court setting. We shall address the structure of the standard clinical interview with delinquents, point out some of the specific problems that the diagnostic process meets in such an environment, and identify the appearance of major psychiatric disorders within the delinquent population.

CLINICAL EXAMINATION

The clinical evaluation of the delinquent begins with extensive preparation before the respondent himself is even seen. The clinician familarizes himself with available background material, which has been gathered and collated by a member of the social services staff. Typically, this material includes the charges filed against the youngster, and a summary of court actions which have led to the judicial finding. There is no invariable correspondence between the nature of the charge or finding, and the mental status of the youngster. Still, the clinician will attend to such detail as can be gleaned from the material (e.g., the time of day or night the youth was apprehended) to begin to formulate relevant areas of investigation. The forensic professional will be aware of the potential discrepancy between the charges and the finding, with the latter oftentimes representing a much reduced version of the former. While one recognizes that the youngster's legal culpability is defined by the finding, the statute governing evidence in a dispositional hearing in a delinquency case indicates that "material and relevant" information is appropriate in the dispositional phase, and one will still inquire in a neutral manner into the circumstances surrounding the actual charges. In a mental health evaluation, we are interested in constructing a full picture of the juvenile's strengths and weaknesses beyond the limitation of the delinquent action, so as to provide an appropriate basis for any needed intervention.

The clinician's preparation may also involve contact with records of previous arrests or PINS petitions, as well as references to other types of court cases (e.g., neglect petitions, custody or visitation suits) with which the respondent's family may have been involved. Because the clinician is making an assessment in part of the chronicity and seriousness of the youngster's behavior, these previous records will be a valuable source of information. Further data may involve contacts with the Department of Probation; this agency investigates relevant family history from a psychosocial point of view, and includes in its reports references to school attendance and other standards of social adjustment. In a certain number of cases, the delinquent will have been seen previously in the clinic, and such material will also be available.

The actual clinical evaluation of the delinquent usually begins in a meeting with parent or guardian. Our service makes it a policy to interview such "collaterals" whenever possible, but in a number of cases the parents are either unavailable or unwilling to appear for interviews. This is in itself important to note, as the court makes clear to the caretaker that part of its own evaluation of the child's resources will reflect the parent's own capacities for cooperation and supervision.

The interview with the collateral has a distinctly different form than the mental health study of the juvenile himself. The parent appears on a voluntary basis. Although the guardian is obviously a focus of court concern, he or she does not fall under the jurisdiction of the court. Thus, the parent's interview tends to concentrate on obtaining a history of the respondent and assessment of the dynamics of the family unit. It is critical to assess the parent's willingness and capacity to supervise the juvenile in a manner that will provide any needed rehabilitative services that may be helpful in minimizing the likelihood of further delinquent actions. One will consider, from this prospective, the veracity and consistency of the parent's narrative, as well as the reactions to the court proceedings and the delinquent actions of the child. Although our clinical practice with these collateral excludes formal mental status as such, one will certainly, when appropriate, investigate the parent's basic psychiatric or medical history as an indication of their potential reliability in providing appropriate supervision.

The interview with the respondent is the heart of the clinical examination. One initiates the session with a brief explanation to the respondent of the purpose of the evaluation, as well as with a reminder that the material discussed will eventually be placed before the court for consideration in the dispositional hearing. Recently, a Court of Appeals decision in New York State has granted counsel the right to be present at clinic evaluations in a different type of court proceeding (termination of parental rights), and applications for observations of the mental health interview by respondent's counsel have subsequently been granted within the Family Court in delinquency matters, on the basis of the Appeal's ruling. Our experience thus far has suggested that the presence of counsel may have a distorting or inhibiting effect on the juvenile's participation; the available literature reflects similar reservations.[3,4] The clinician must observe and attempt to "correct for" such effects, and it is of course of the utmost importance that there be no interaction or actual interference by counsel in the interview session.

The interview proper continues with an exploration or recapitulation of basic biographical information and educational history, including such factors as possible grade failures, special class placement, suspensions, and truancy. Typically, one attempts to engage the respondent in a dialogue about the delinquency itself. The inquiry examines not only the concrete sequence of events, but the frame of mind of the youngster, as well as the social situation in which the delinquency occurred. It is important to assess the motive for the action, insofar as this is accessible. Delinquent activities may be based on desires for financial gain, feelings of anger or revenge, wishes to be recognized as part of a group or subculture, and a variety of other motives. It is particularly helpful to be able to distinguish between delinquencies based on greed and premeditated profit motives and other superficially similar actions which are more impulsive in character.

The respondent is questioned and observed closely as to his reaction to his crime and to his being apprehended. Note is taken of remorse or other manifestations of super-ego functioning. One may well go on to question the youngster about previous arrests; insofar as is possible, one will attempt to investigate these incidents in the same manner. The clinician of course understands that other arrests that have not been the subjects of findings in court are not necessarily indications of guilt on the part of the respondent. Nevertheless, even arrests that have not been pursued can provide significant information, both in terms of the circumstances of the arrest, and of the youngster's response to it. Finally, one may also wish to inquire of the youngster as to other delinquent actions or behavioral difficulties that have not in fact resulted in apprehension by a law officer or school official. In such a phase of inquiry, it is important to keep in mind that one is relying strictly on the youngster's own description; it has been claimed that such descriptions may be distorted either by a wish to brag or to consciously minimize prior history, and one must take care in drawing any judgment from such information. However, even if one does not wish to make a conclusion as to the actual validity of the youngster's statements, the narrative itself still gives a flavor for the delinquent's values and psychic reality.

The assessment of the delinquent's family life is often more difficult to obtain in these interviews than is a recounting of delinquent behavior. Some teenagers describe gratifying and appropriate interactions with other family members in a vivid and convincing manner. A number of others, however, depict an unstable or seemingly casual relationship with their families. Their parents, in turn, may complain of long histories of absconding, "disrespect," and a general pattern of lack of control of the respondent. It is important to steer a clear course between either underestimating or overvaluing the extent or importance of the youngster's stated attachment to the family. Some respondents consciously minimize their attachment to their family, because they may feel that this is not in accord with the image which they wish to give of being "independent" and "adult." One must also be careful of narratives that portray an unusually close parent–child relationship. Even when the tie is an intimate one, it may be relatively independent of the parent's ability to supervise the child, or the child's ability to respond to the parent's expectations. Some parents are ineffectual or passive in spite of a clear awareness of a delinquent's actions, and we have even seen selected instances where the parent consciously approved of the delinquent actions, or even accepted some of the financial rewards of those activities themselves.

In attempting to construct an accurate picture of the home environment, it may be useful to compare the respondent's account of the daily home schedule with that given to the clinician by the parent. One may in fact wish to put virtually identical questions to both parent and child in separate interviews. At times, there are gross discrepancies between the individual's statements. Many of our respondents' homes are quite crowded, and one sometimes achieves a clearer picture of actual home life by inquiring as to specifics of sleeping arrangements, cooking schedules, and so on. It will also be pertinent to ascertain the disciplinary methods of the family; types of punishment may vary from child to child within a family, and this can be a cue as to the role of different siblings within the home. When corporal punishment is frequently resorted to, one will explore whether or not there have been or continue to be episodes of actual physical abuse. Such data may be extremely important in understanding the juvenile's current pattern of behavior, and in placing it in the context of the general family mode of functioning.

As for the juvenile's interests, the clinician attempts to assess the quality, variety, and stability of those activities. School and its associated social functions are often described as boring and pointless, and in fact delinquency appears to be closely correlated with a history of recent truancy. Unfortunately, many youngsters in our population present a rather diffusely organized or defined range of nonschool activities. Many narratives here focus on "hanging out" with peers, casual sports or more recent video game competitions, or entertainment focusing on musical "jams" or movies. With such reports, the examiner may sense that there is little to be gained from a more detailed inquiry. However, even with a very bland respondent who seems to show little capacity for active enjoyment of meaningful activity, some conversation about the type of movies which the youngster enjoys will be helpful in understanding the teenager's point of view.

The evaluation of social ties is a critical step in the diagnostic process. Often, respondents seem to feel that the institution of friendship is in itself compromising to them. It is not uncommon that a youngster will deny having any friends at all, particularly when trying to make a good impression on the examiner. It appears that, in the minds of many of these teenagers, the maintenance of social relationships is viewed as being closely connected to the impetus for delinquent activities. This may be a reaction against the type of bonding which results in gang involvement, known in street argot as "crews." Crews vary from relatively structured organizations to more amorphous and transient relationships, and if gang membership is acknowledged, one will want to understand the youngster's position, his participation in such activities, and the degree of allegiance he maintains to the values of the group. One will always try to distinguish between those who are active perpetrators in such activities and those who follow along in a more passive way. Here, one may also choose to investigate the respondent's history of involvement with weapons. One will attempt to learn the extent to which such instruments may be carried for primarily defensive purposes, or for clearer aggressive intent.

The more recalcitrant delinquents may show even less of a sense of social connection, claiming that, "you can't trust anyone out there . . . you have to watch your back." Even when all friendships are denied, one may still be able to make some assessment of the nature of more perfunctory ties by inquiring into the respondent's "associates." This term seems to be reserved in the street vocabulary for relationships based primarily on matters of mutual convenience or need, which are enacted without any significant affective involvement.

There does not appear to be any distinct point at which a sustained social and sexual interest in teenage girls develops. Most of the youngsters we see acknowledge having girlfriends, and it is an extremely rare instance, one meriting further investigation, when an adolescent here denies any history or current involvement with girlfriends. The intensity and quality of these relationships varies greatly, as it does within the general adolescent population. Many of our respondents report a certain commonality in their opposite-sex relationships, noting in an apparently unself-conscious manner that they have a number of girlfriends simultaneously, although one is usually defined as primary.

Ultimately, one will investigate the respondent's own sense of his areas of weakness. We ask these youngsters to evaluate their own needs for academic remediation, psychotherapy, and whatever other social services they may view as important, both for directly helping to avert further delinquent behavior and for ameliorating background conditions of disadvantage. If placement outside the home is to be considered, one will explore the youth's feelings in this regard. Very frequently, no such change is felt as necessary; events are seen as having been imposed on the respondent from the beginning, and there may be at best a feeble sense of "going straight." In other cases, respondents will ask for placement themselves, and give definite reasons as to why they feel it would be helpful to them. We should note parenthetically that a certain proportion of youngsters do request placement, not for any help, but because they feel that such an intervention is a badge of maturity within an antisocial point of view.

ASSESSMENT DIFFICULTIES

The foregoing represents a survey of the more important areas of evaluation in our examinations. Although other topics will be broached in individual cases, these areas will have the greatest general relevance for the diagnostic and referral issues that confront us in delinquency cases. However, the actual process of eliciting the appropriate information can be complicated by the set of expectations that the examiner and examinee bring to the clinical setting, and we offer here our attempts to clarify some of the areas of potential miscommunication.

In our population, it is often a problem to gather unambiguous background and developmental information from parents or caretakers. Many of our delinquents come from large families, and it is frequently difficult for parents to recall discreet developmental milestones of an individual child. It is important that the clinician not "offer" his own guess or estimate to the parents as an attempt to "jog" their memory, because custodians who are insecure or unsure of their recall may accept the guess of an authority without any genuine recollection of their own. Even when developmental data is offered with apparent confidence, it must be evaluated critically. Frequently, speech and sophisticated language development are recounted by the parents as having occurred earlier than the first birthday, and this alerts the examiner to the possibility that other developmental milestones may also be distorted in recall.

Coherent histories of previous psychotherapeutic treatment, medication, or hospitalization are often difficult for the clinician to piece together. Many of our clients and their families make a distinction between emotional difficulties—which tend to be identified with internally disruptive and subjectively disturbing thought content—and disorders which are partially or largely manifested or experienced as occurring in somatic equivalents. It behooves the examiner who inquires into treatment history to explore not only the vicissitudes of the patient's "emotional problems" but also the history of any difficulties with the individual's "nerves." There appears to be a sense of opprobrium attached to frank emotional disorders which is not associated with the more egosyntonic "nerve problems." In many cases, our population appears to make a distinction between "talking cures" for emotional difficulties, and medication treatment for "nerves," and an inquiry into one area will not necessarily lead the client to automatically bring up the other. Many of these teenagers also have a history of special education, which may involve—at least theoretically—in-school treatment or counseling on a regular basis. However, even when such treatment has been mandated or offered by the school as part of the special education evaluation, funding or personnel allocation problems may make the delivery of such services problematic or sporadic at best; this only increases the parent's (and the child's) lack of clarity about treatment history. Certainly, the fact that the treatment is carried out through the school, rather than through the more active efforts of the family, will tend to create confusion in the parties' minds about the nature and purposes of such psychotherapy.

History-taking can also be obscured by differences in language, as well as by subcultural colloquialisms that are used in reference to the child's behavior. For example, it is often difficult to obtain a history of a youngster's aggressive behavior when the subject is discussed directly with the parent. This may be the case when a protective parent wishes to minimize the offspring's difficulties, but it appears more frequently than this in our interviews. In many of these cases, much provocative and aggressive behavior seems to be subsumed under the label of "playing" (e.g., "He just plays a lot with his sister"). The careful examiner is well-advised to explore in some detail several chains of activity that the parent considers "playing," in order to have a fuller understanding of the youngster's actual scope of behavior. In other circumstances, the parent's description of the youngster's early childhood activity may inadvertently exaggerate the extent of the disturbance in the child's development. One must be cautious when parents, particularly in large families, recall the hyperactivity of the respondent in his toddler years. Further discussion with the parent may reveal that the infant's behavior level was within normal expectations, but that the parent or family situation created an intolerance in the normal level of activity.

One will want to take special care in exploring the youngster's school and legal problems with the parent. Parents are usually adequately informed about the history of their child's educational deficiencies, such as holdovers, special class placement, and suspensions. However, many adults become unusually vague when asked about their youngster's history of truancy. Some extra diplomacy is helpful here, as it appears that the responses often reflect the caretaker's awareness that they have been acquiescent or tacitly cooperative with their child's truancy. From the standpoint of legal infractions, parents frequently give histories of police contacts that may be at variance with other sources of information. In such instances, the supervisory adult may only consider police contact that led to a court appearance as being worthy of note, and the examiner may have to ask further specific questions about "precinct arrests" or YD cards in order to gather a full picture of the delinquent's difficulties.

Finally, the naive clinician's assumptions about family structure, itself may complicate a reasonable understanding of the youngster's early development. Many of the respondents we interview come from extended family situations, where care of the child has been shared during the early years. This is especially likely when the mother was quite young at the time of the birth of the child. Again, a direct question is likely to elicit a direct—and possibly inaccurate—answer, nothing more. In many cases, parents conceive of themselves as primary caretakers even in situations where other adults have had the bulk of the responsibility for extended periods. It can be more informative to question the parent as to who has "helped" with the early raising of the child, rather than to bluntly ask who else may have "taken" or had responsibility for the infant. Once the parent has begun to discuss the help that they have received from others, they are likely to be more forthcoming and trustful in discussing the actual child-care arrangements. The careful examiner will also be aware of the fact that in many cases, children are routinely sent on extended vacations of 3 to 6 months with relatives, and such prolonged absences may be ignored or discounted by the parents unless the examiner takes a more active part in exploring such arrangements.

A mental status examination with these youngsters is in many ways similar to evaluations done with the general adolescent population. One will assess homocidal or suicidal ideation and history, the presence or absence of hallucinations and/or delusions, and other relevant psychiatric symptomatology. However, the specifically forensic nature of our practice establishes an obligation on the part of the clinician to "ask questions" even when he is virtually certain of the answer. For example, a generally well-related and oriented 15-year-old may provide absolutely no suggestion or evidence of any hallucinatory experience, and the examiner can intuitively feel that such a question is unnecessary, given the observed behavior and stream of speech in the interview. Because we function in a court setting, where clinical evaluations are effective and credible only insofar as they are based on facts and "statements" rather than inferences, such questions *must* be asked "for the record."

In evaluating the quality of the youngster's stream of speech and thought, one must be sensitive enough to distinguish between the impoverished thought content or illogicality of reasoning that will represent genuine psychiatric disturbance, and the youngster's assimilation or allegience to a street culture that has in many ways developed a distinctive but stereotyped vocabulary and speech pattern. "Street language" often seems designed to hinder real communication rather than to encourage it, and much of the colloquial language of some of our delinquents functions to obscure, rather than clarify, an accurate depiction of reality. For example, a youngster's speech may be repeatedly infiltrated with colloquilisms and a highly selective and arbitrary recounting of details, which ultimately obfuscates the auditor's capacity to establish a coherent sense of the delinquent's story. Even though such narratives may in fact be "tangential" or paralogical, it is important for the examiner to distinguish between the quality of speech that reflects the resistant youngster's enculturation in a specific milieu, and language that reflects deteriorative or regressive thinking processes.

On formal mental status, there are specific characteristics in the responses of our adolescents which can "shade into" thinking that, in other circumstances, would be more clearly pathognomonic of serious disorder. For example, false positives emerge when one inquires into the subject's credence in ideas of reference, thought control, and "mind reading." Even among our clearly nonpsychotic teenagers, there appears to be a genuine sensitivity for vulnerability to ideas of reference. In part, this seems to reflect the delinquent's awareness of his "outsider" status. It is also likely that in specific cases, these ideas of reference actually represent an unusually developed sensitivity or apprehension of the reaction of others; as such they may have an adaptive value within the standards of the juvenile delinquent's world. It is important that an examiner not mistake the presence of such beliefs, even when they are firmly held, as necessarily indicative of a nascent delusional system. Although it is obviously important to question the youngster's reality testing in this regard, in order to differentiate between a "cultural attitude" and a genuine state of pathology, this must be done in a tactful manner, not alienating the patient or conveying a lack of clinical understanding of behavior that may be normative within the values of the peer group.

Variations in superego development must also be considered as a factor in interview situations. Delinquents in our population rarely express remorse or empathy directly for their victims. Even in situations where the chronicity of the delinquent behavior is the obvious focus of court attention, these youngsters will easily acknowledge other similar delinquent activities with little apparent sense of culpability. On the other hand, our population is markedly reluctant to acknowledge even relatively inconsequential drug use. At times, youngsters come to their appointments when they are obviously under the influence of some substance such as marijuana, but there remains a rigid reluctance to acknowledge the drug abuse. This is particularly striking as the possession or use of small amounts of marijuana is no longer a crime in New York State. The refusal to acknowledge drug abuse, even when it is flagrant and obvious, appears to us as dynamically different from classical alcoholic denial. The latter typically represents an individual's negation of his drinking to himself. Drug abuse, on the contrary, appears to be an accepted factor in daily functioning for many of our adolescents, and much social interaction revolves around the purchase and sharing of such substances. In fact, many of our clients will eventually feel that their delinquencies are motivated by a need for cash to buy these substances, and it may be that the reluctance to admit drug use reflects some hesitancy in acknowledging the "motive" for the more readily admitted pattern of delinquency. Whatever the case, the diagnosis of substance abuse is thus commensurately more difficult to establish in our population, and it is likely that figures from similar programs are underestimates of the prevalence of drug abuse in similar delinquent populations.

One drug in particular merits special attention here: phencyclidine. Although many of the youngsters we interview make a general point of their "bravery" and lack of fear in dangerous situations, there is a striking unanimity of judgment in terms of the "street wisdom" that recognizes the dangers associated with the use of "angel dust." Doubtless, many of those who deny PCP abuse are accurate informants, but the fact remains that cases arise with some degree of regularity in which an adolescent will steadfastly deny any PCP ingestion in the face of repeated reliable reports from family members and other sources. In our experience, the grudging admission of PCP even "once in a blue moon" is often only the tip of the iceberg, and thus any acknowledgement of such drug use must be viewed with concern. The "street wisdom" about angel dust seems to focus on the "foolishness" and "craziness" that are part of the loss of control associated with the drug, and it is possible that the juvenile's reluctance to admit PCP abuse reflects some primitive or fundamental sense of embarassment at such "weakness."

THE CLINICAL PICTURE

As we have noted, the great majority of youngsters referred to us are ultimately diagnosed with conduct disorders. To some degree, the ubiquity of this category within our delinquint population reflects the "here and now" characteristics of the impairment. The criteria required by DSM-III for diagnosis of conduct disorder center on readily recognizable elements of behavior and social adjustment. The diagnostic requirements for the conduct disorder categories do not demand an unusually detailed grasp of history or self-observation from the informants, so many of the difficulties we have outlined above are unlikely to interfere with the clinician's ability to make an accurate diagnosis of a conduct disorder. In fact, objective or third-party reports from reliable observers will often provide input as significant and helpful as any reporting from the youngster or the parent.

The wider range of DSM-III disorders appears with variable frequency in our population. Among the DSM-III childhood and adolescent disorders, we see relatively fewer of such impairments, although various types of cognitive limitation are often associated with delinquency, and these have been identified in a separate publication.[2] In part, many of the childhood and adolescent difficulties noted in the DSM-III (e.g., various anxiety states and eating disorders) occur only rarely among the entire adolescent population, but there are also likely psychodynamic or developmental factors which account for an underrepresentation of these impairments among our clientel. For example, many authors have characterized the delinquent population as a whole as lacking the ability to internalize values and standards of the dominant society; such youngsters are also characterized as lacking the capacity to tolerate frustration, guilt, and anxiety.[5,6] The fact is that many of the disorders in DSM-III that pertain to children and adolescents reflect extremes of inhibition or subjectively experienced anxiety, and "action-oriented" delinquent youngsters are unlikely to experience such difficulties.

Several DSM-III disorders of childhood and adolescence present specific problems in diagnosis within our population. The diagnostic manual defines various states of attention deficit disorder. Oftentimes, listening to the parental history may encourage the examiner to think of a diagnosis of attention deficit disorder with hyperactivity, or of a residual form of the impairment. However, one must be quite cautious in establishing any such disorder for youngsters in our population. It is our experience that in many cases parents may not have provided basic levels of support and monitoring for their children, and DSM-III certainly indicates that in such conditions, "it may be impossible to determine whether the disorganized behavior is simply a function of the chaotic environment or whether it is due to the child's psychopathology."[7] Without clear confirmation in school reports or direct clinical impression, we would recommend that the approach to such diagnoses be conservative within this population.

DSM-III also provides the diagnosis of "identity disorder," for adolescents who experience serious difficulties in establishing a sense of role in various areas of family identity, sense of self, and social identity. As the manual represents it, the identity disorder appears to be conceptualized as a forerunner of the adult borderline personality disorder. Although the identity disorder diagnosis is doubtless apt for certain segments of the juvenile population, it is generally inapplicable among our delinquents. It is true that many of the teenagers we interview can be accurately characterized as experiencing *anomie,* as well as various disturbances in the consolidation of their personal identity. Superficially, such a pattern might be thought to qualify them for diagnosis as an identity disorder. However, such a diagnosis becomes problematic at best when one recalls that the sine qua non for such a diagnosis is that of "severe subjective distress." As we have mentioned earlier, few of the juveniles referred to us betray the necessary sustained quality of subjective discomfort; adolescents in our population who show profound identity disturbances are therefore more appropriately and accurately identified as borderline personality disorders, a category of diagnosis which is independent of subjectively felt difficulty.

In fact, either full-blown borderline personalities or various amalgams with borderline traits are perhaps the personality disorder most frequently encountered in this population. Borderline delinquents, in contrast to the general delinquent population before this court, make no secret of very heavy drug and alcohol abuse, as well as unusually precocious sexual contact. It is not uncommon to find that our borderline adolescents have begun the steady abuse of alcohol and various substances before the end of latency, and assorted consensual and coerced sexual encounters are often recalled with both peers and older individuals. It may be of some interest to note that whereas this paper focuses on male juvenile delinquency, a disproportionate number of the female delinquents we encounter have clear borderline trends. Such youngsters often are apprehended for acts that are actually associated with early prostitution, and in such cases there appears to be the generalized limitation of impulse control and instability of object relationship that characterizes the borderline's functioning.

Although the major mental disorders appear only rarely in our delinquent population, their presence seems to be relatively overrepresented in serious crimes of violence.[8] The identification of these disorders is a critical step in the dispositional process. It is thus all the more striking to record how often clearly psychotic youngsters have made their way through the social and educational system without any apparent effective notice or intervention in their condition. If the family of the child is unaware or insufficiently unconcerned about the youngster's condition, there may be few social agencies or institutions that have either the expertise or the legal mandate to deal with these deviations in development. Seriously disturbed youngsters may even be overlooked by the school system, which would otherwise appear to be the most likely avenue of support in such cases. In the first place, many of the teenagers we see have insufficient school attendance to allow meaningful contact to be made between them and the appropriate evaluative service. However, even when such an assessment is made of a youngster with a psychotic impairment, the legal parameters of the school system's involvement with such a disorder are limited to remediation and treatment only insofar as such aid is necessary to insure a basically satisfactory level of academic progress. Thus, it is not uncommon for us to encounter psychotic youngsters whose capacity for some normative cognitive progress has disqualified them from more intensive help through the school system. This is even more the case when the child's behavior at school is not a focus for disciplinary concern.

It is our clinical experience that many of the most violent crimes committed by adolescents reflect undetected and untreated psychotic processes. Given the characteristics of our population, the forensic clinician must take special care to investigate the symptomatology of such disorders. Against a background of disorganized home life, a lack of structured activity, and unspecified drug or alcohol involvement, the presenting picture of a schizophrenic or manic-depressive prodrome may initially be difficult to discern. With youngsters who are not particularly fluent, it can become even more problematic to differentiate expressive language difficulties, a lack of interest in meaningful communication, and the oftentimes paralogical style associated with the street patois from the more subtle positive signs of a disorder in mood or thinking. Here, psychological testing may be of value in order to establish true cognitive strengths and weaknesses, organic difficulties, and the significance of psychodynamic factors in the teenager's development.

When gross clinical features such as paranoid delusions or unambiguous auditory hallucinations are absent in this delinquent population, the quality of the affective contact made by the youngster remains as one of the most reliable "subtle" indicators of a major impairment in functioning. The experienced clinician will be able to make a distinction between the typically muted or guarded quality of many grossly normal adolescents, and the characteristic affective withdrawal noted with schizophrenic youngsters. Such youths may be described by their parents as unusually quiet, although of course such passivity is not incompatible with brief episodes of violent or sexual loss of control. Typically, when these juveniles are confronted with their actions, their own reactions will impress primarily as being confabulatory, rather than denying or malingering in quality. We have recently seen a 15-year-old adolescent who was before the court because of a purse-snatching attempt, apparently his first arrest and finding. On examination, he demonstrated the insidious blunting of affect and poor judgment that we associate with schizophrenics in our population. There was no suggestion, however, of any more outstanding symptom picture, and no history of medication or hospitalization. At the time we saw him, he disclosed a long history of similar delinquent activities, with the vagueness and confabulation that seemed to be associated with such functioning. He was in fact already in a day treatment program because of behavior problems in school, but it was apparent that the treating program was unaware of the extent of the pathology or of the behavioral difficulties outside of the classroom. Before Mental Health Services was able to intervene effectively, this youngster was involved in two more similar incidents (one within the court building itself), and the most recent of his infractions, occurring after his sixteenth birthday, may have now effectively placed him outside of the remedial capacities of the Family Court, and within the adult "punitive" system.

We have noted that many of the more catastrophic acts of violence or disorganization attributed to juveniles appear to be part of an early developing manic disorder. There is an increasing sensitivity in the psychiatric literature to the early onset of mood disorder, and our own clinical observations are consistent with this point of view. Because early occurring manic episodes may be brief, with a rapid onset and a relatively complete reconstitution, the input of a reliable informant is often critical to the establishment of such a diagnosis. Thus, at times, the best recourse may well be a period of hospital observation, mandated by the court for such purposes. The clinic had the opportunity to evaluate a 15-year-old male who was without significant psychiatric history and was appearing before the court in relation to two minor delinquent actions that did not involve confrontation with a victim. At the same time, the teenager was also before the Criminal Court system, as a result of his hitting and seriously injuring a pedestrian while the respondent was driving a car without a license. On initial mental status, he presented as having been insufficiently supervised at home, but without any significant symptomatology or contributory background. However, he was seen approximately 1 week later, and at that point displayed the full syndrome of the onset of an acute major depressive episode, with suicidal gestures and some palpable disorganization of behavior. Following a period of hospitalization, he appeared to have been suffering from an early occurring mood disorder, and the eventual reconstruction of his history indicated that the incident with the automobile had occurred during a manic swing.

We would conclude that although many episodes of violent confrontation occur within the context of the aggressive conduct disorders, an unusually large number of "senseless crimes" probably reflect the grandiosity, irritability, and specific impairments of judgment characteristic of the manic condition. Because intensive or inpatient psychiatric care is one of the dispositional alternatives available to the court, the clinician can make a valuable contribution in securing the needed treatment for a youngster whose condition, without delinquent involvement, would likely go untreated into adulthood.

Although this paper has focused on mental disorders as if they occurred relatively independently of various neurological problems, we are fully aware that the wide range of organicity can be a potent factor in the development of adolescent psychopathology and maladjustment. We note instances of mental defect associated with infection and trauma in our adolescent population, and call to the court's attention instances where epilepsy, organic brain syndrome secondary to encephalitis, and other forms of developmental defect exist and/or interact with the youngster's current level of functioning. An understanding of the degree to which organic factors contribute to adolescent maladjustment can be critical for disposition. Because the court is interested in the treatment and rehabilitation of the youngsters brought before it, the presence of neurological complications or traumatic history will at times enable the judge to mandate a level of appropriate care and treatment that the youngster may have been unable to obtain prior to his court involvement.

The forensic professional must be sensitive to the nuances of the major mental disorders and to their own particular manifestations within the delinquent subculture. We have observed such impairments in juveniles as young as 10 or 12 and have noted frank delusional formations and paranoid command hallucinations in latency-aged children charged with murderous fire settings and apparently wanton brutality. Still, this does not suggest to us that *all* young offenders necessarily suffer a major psychiatric impairment. We have also been in contact with examples of very young children who seem to function virtually devoid of conscience, and who have been responsible for acts of sexual assault or grand larceny attempts. The profiles of several of these latency-aged children are not dynamically dissimilar from those of adult "psychopaths," with a characteristic lack of remorse or anxiety, a precociously developed manipulative quality in relationships, and a lack of basic empathic needs. Such individuals display a pattern of personality organization distinctly deviant from older teenage "delinquents," although the DSM-III does not allow for a qualitative indication of the severity of such impairment. We have commented elsewhere on the shortcomings of the DSM-III in this regard.[9]

SUMMARY

The assessment of psychopathology among juvenile delinquents in a forensic clinic requires an awareness of the needs of the court system and the characteristics of the specific delinquent population. The clinical examination and mental status evaluation of these youngsters, set in the context of the general adolescent psychiatric examination, require a specific focus from the clinician to the court's referral question. The assessment process itself reflects the unique qualities of the juvenile population, as well as a sensitivity and resourcefulness on the part of the clinician to the difficulties created in such an environment. Although the conduct disorders emerge as the primary diagnostic entity in such a population, the prevalence of other mental disorders must not go unrecognized, and such impairments appear to be overrepresented among the more catastrophic or sensational aspects of juvenile crime.

REFERENCES

[1]Lewis, DO, Balla, DA: *Delinquency and Psychopathology.* New York, Grune & Stratton, 1976.
[2]Schuster, R, Guggenheim, P: An investigation of the intellectual capabilities of juvenile offenders. *J of Forensic Sci, 27*:393–400, 1982.
[3]Tanney, MF, Gelso, CJ: Effect of recording on clients. *J of Counseling Psychology 19*:349–350, 1972.
[4]Webb, ET, Campbell, DT, Schwartz, RD, Sechrest, L, Grove, JB: *Nonreactive Measures in the Social Sciences.* Boston, Houghton Mifflin, 1981.
[5]Sullivan, ML: Youth crime: New York's two varieties. *New York Affairs 8*:31–48, 1983.
[6]Jenkins, R: *Behavior Disorders in Childhood and Adolescence.* Springfield, Charles C Thomas, 1973.
[7]*Diagnostic and Statistical Manual of Mental Disorders,* ed 3, Washington, D.C., APA, 1980.
[8]Unger, LD, Lewis, GI, Cohen, E, Guggenheim, PD, Lewis, DO: Two violent adolescents. *Am J Psychiatry 140*:814–815, 1983.
[9]Garmise, R, Guggenheim, PD, Schuster, R: DSM-III. A perspective from Family Court. *J of Forensic Sci, 29*:1127–1139, 1984.

V

Scientific Truth Detection

11

Amytal and the Detection of Deception

MORRIS HERMAN

For a long time there has been an intense interest in the legal systems for developing technique to uncover malingering of mental illness or mental retardation in defendants charged with crime. This interest has led in the development of psychological tests, in polygraphy, and in the sodium amytal test.

Sodium amytal is a short-acting barbiturate that was used as a sedative and hypnotic. However, Bleckwenn[1], in 1930, demonstrated that an intravenous injection of this drug was capable of removing the catatonic state in schizophrenic patients. The catatonic state rendered the patient mute and usually immobile or rigid. These symptoms disappeared after injection, with the patient becoming talkative and able to reveal some of his problems, often in the delusional sphere. From a resistive, negativistic state, the patient would often become pliable and cooperative; when the effects of the drug wore off, the catatonic condition would reappear. This effect was a first demonstration of the potential for influencing mental symptoms directly by the means of a drug.

Because the technique enhanced communication in schizophrenic patients, Lindemann[2], in 1932, used the sodium amytal injection in normals and showed that communication was speeded up in this group as well. The pharmacological effect started with an initial euphoria, talkativeness; later nystagmus, a thick, slurred speech, ataxia; still later, with increased dosage, depression and sedation developed, leading to various grades of stupor.

MORRIS HERMAN • Department of Psychiatry, School of Medicine, New York University, New York, New York 10016.

The dosage of the drug varies individually, with a greater amount required in persons addicted to barbiturates or related compounds.

As a consequence of these psychopharmacological effects, sodium amytal was extensively used in psychiatric hospitals to reduce aggressiveness and negativistic behavior. This usage occurred in the 1940s and 1950s until the introduction and treatment by the neuroleptics.

In 1938, this author[3] used the sodium amytal technique to remove anmesias of the psychogenic type and to clear acute hysterical symptoms such as blindness and deafness. It was demonstrated on many occasions that memory that was inaccessible to a person was recoverable when the person was placed under a mild narcosis with intravenous sodium amytal. This, of course, led to the question whether the same techique would be useful to uncover simulated amnesias. This is discussed later.

A further question concerned the use of this drug in determining the differential diagnosis of organic amnesias and confusional states from the psychogenic. In a series of papers, Weinstein[4] and his group tested many patients and concluded that in the presence of organic brain disease the symptoms became worse, but in functional or psychogenic states the symptoms would often be removed. There were, however, false results, such as nonorganic states that did not improve if malingering was present or in certain psychotic patients. Another contrary result could occur in patients with organic brain disease when the confusional state is due to alcohol withdrawal syndrome or after an epileptic seizure. In these instances, sodium amytal has a positive therapeutic effect and improves rather than worsens the symptoms.

Another important area where intravenous sodium amytal came into use was during World War II. Acute war reactions[5] featuring anxiety and panic were prominent syndromes in battle zones. It was found that a rapid resolution of these reactions could be effected through the use of the sodium amytal procedure. This treatment was referred to as "narcohypnosis."

Because of the marked effects on behavior induced by giving sodium amytal in intravenous form, these led to attempts to apply the technique to problems encountered in the medico-legal field, such as

1. To determine the truthfulness of statements made by the defendant.
2. The existence of amnesis for the criminal act and for circumstances preceding and following this act.
3. The occurrence of an apparent psychotic state after arrest and during observation.
4. Reaction patterns that require a differential diagnosis between organic, possibly epileptic, and psychological states.

In the area of determining truthfulness, there have been those who have wrongfully designated intravenous sodium amytal as a "truth serum." This is an unfortunate designation as it is neither a serum nor does it necessarily result in obtaining the truth. In a rough paralled, sodium amytal, like alcohol, may loosen the tongue, but what comes out may not necessarily be the truth. However, there are some positive items that can be derived by this technique when combined with good clinical judgment and investigative procedures. For example, the sodium amytal technique may uncover or help to corroborate some events, time and place of occurrence, and aspects of the defendant's thinking and feeling at the time in the past. However, one must use this information carefully and place it in perspective with the clinical picture presented.

CASE 1

A defendant was charged with killing the mother of his girlfriend. He claimed amnesia for this event. Although not psychotic he showed a great deal of psychopathology based on strong but ambivalent reactions to women, particularly a mother figure. It was known that he was addicted to sexual sadism.

Under sodium amytal intravenously, he recounted the circumstances of a murder but indicated the victim, at different times during the examination, to be his own mother, his girlfriend, and her mother. Although this response does not lead to a firm factual decision, it is comprehensible psychiatrically and confirms the hypothesis that in essence the murder represented the killing of his own mother or women in general as represented by her.

CASE 2

A defendant was charged with killing his wife in a rather brutal fashion with an ax; a diagnosis of involutional psychosis had been made. A history revealed that the defendant has a long-standing passive dependent personality developed in relation to an overly dominant father. The defendant had made a marginal adjustment until the time came when he no longer was employed. Because he was unable to obtain work for some time, his wife obtained a job and the defendant was left to take care of the home. This role reversal brought to the surface his reaction to his passive-dependent traits.

There resulted frequent outbursts of irritation and hostility directed toward his wife. In a particularly serious quarrel, he picked up an ax and struck her numerous times. After his arrest, he was amnesic for the event and gradually went into a deep depression. Under sodium amytal, the defendant described the homicide giving the time, place and weapon but described the victim as his father. Again this is not the whole truth in a legal sense but can be understood in psychiatric terms. In the homicide, he was acting out his rage toward the figure that kept him dependent—his father.

Malingering is a form of deception where an individual assumes symptoms that are associated with illness but do not in fact exist. It is assumed that the malingerer volitionally utilizes these symptoms in order to gain an advantage. In the legal system the person is trying to avoid responsibility for his alleged criminal actions or he is trying to avoid involvement in the legal procedures. It is true that there are many complex unconscious factors that may play a role in the development of malingering and certainly this syndrome is seen clinically in nonlegal situations, for example, in Munchausen's syndrome.

One must also be aware that there are clinical states that resemble malingering but are significant of some other disease process. Such clinical states are some psychoses (such as schizophrenia), some types of Ganser syndrome, some types of hysteria, and some types of depressive illness resulting in pseudodementia. The differential diagnosis of these various states from malingering requires extensive psychiatric examination, in which the use of sodium amytal is only a part, perhaps even a small part.

There is another aspect of malingering that the clinician must keep in mind, and that is the malingering of health. Even some psychotic patients may under certain circumstances hide their symptoms and hold their behavior from revealing their disturbed mental state at least for a short time.

Still another type of malingering is the individual who reacts strongly in the passive state and in reaction to suggestion to give false answers that indicate involvement in the criminal act, when this is not true. This results in the cases that are known as "false confessions." Case 3 presents an example of malingering.

CASE 3

Mr. C. presented as mute when seen on the ward of a prison service. Under observation, Mr. C. showed no evidence of confusion or disorientation in the way he moved about the ward and carried out activities. There were no abnormal neurological findings on examination. There were also no symptoms associated with schizophrenic illness that can produce mutism. No signs of hallucinatory behavior and no signs of rigidity or catalepsy associated with catatonia. When further it was discovered that he had spoken and answered questions prior to his admission to the psychiatric unit, it became clear that the mutism was volitionally assumed and malingered. It was unnecessary to make use of the sodium amytal test because of the overwhelming evidence. The conclusion of malingering was further confirmed when it was established that after leaving the ward his speech returned and he communicated with persons in the prison setting. However, it is conceivable that had this prisoner in his mute state come to the attention of the examiner without any data or history, sodium amytal test could then be very useful in helping to arrive at an evaluation of that symptom. In general, a malingerer would tend to maintain the symptom at the usual dose.

The sodium amytal technique loosens the tongue, but it must compete against other forces such as strong volition, psychotic processes, or organic factors. Malingerers, therefore, can persist in maintaining their symptoms because of the strong need to evade. Tests performed on normal volunteers, who were directed to falsify information, were able to maintain the lie under the sodium amytal technique. The prisoner who malingers has certainly stronger reasons to maintain a position than normal volunteers and will do so.

In assessing truth or falsity of statements made by a patient population, one must be aware of delusional and paranoid mininterpretation as well as neurotic distortions. The examiner must have means of determining these changes clinically. In many instances, there is retrospective falsification of memory or appraisal of one's condition. Some patients who have been psychiatrically ill for months or even years will say, when they recover, that they had been faking their illness. This is usually not true but a manifestation of the well known mechanism of denial. This is a rationalization to explain away an unacceptable position of the self.

In some cases, a highly emotional state is associated with the criminal act, such as a serious assault or murder, particularly when the victim is closely related to the assailant. As a consequence, certain psychological responses may ensue. A depression of serious intensity may occur, which can have several roots—a reaction to the crime itself, a reaction to the fear of punishment and consequences, guilt, and sources in the person's psychopathological makeup.

Amnesia is another consequence that may be encountered. This may be complete but is usually partial and may be abetted by the use of alcohol or drugs. It is in this state that sodium amytal can be most useful in trying to recover memories. One must keep in mind that recovered memories can be fantasied as well as accurate. This means that the examiner must use clinical judgment in interpreting the results of the testing. Distortions in recall under amytal can be produced by suggestion, by fantasy formation, by conscious design, or by emerging psychopathology such as delusional ideas. This makes it all important for the examiner to have a full grasp of the clinical status of the subject and to be familiar with changes occuring under the sodium amytal.

It is important to measure the extent and details of amnesia before undertaking the sodium amytal technique. Questions should include meticulous detail, as in the following examples.

The day before the criminal act:

1. Where were you?
2. Did you eat meals, when, where, what?
3. How were you dressed?
4. Where did you go?
5. Whom did you see?
6. What conversations?
7. Did you work?
8. What day of the week and month?
9 When did you get to sleep?
10. Did you use alcohol or drugs, when, what, and how much?

On the day of the criminal act:

1. Where were you in the morning?
2. What time did you awaken?
3. Did you have breakfast and later other meals—when, where and what?
4. Did you use alcohol or drugs—when, what, and how much.
5. Where did you go prior to the scene of the crime and when?
6. Whom did you meet prior to the scene of the crime?
7. Did you carry a weapon—knife, gun, etc.?
8. Questions about the scene of the crime, depending on reports.

After the criminal act:

1. What happened after the criminal act?
2. Did you leave the scene?
3. Arrested—when, where, how?
4. Transported by police to which facility and by what means?
5. Where were you placed for examination (if in a hospital)?
6. Did you go before a court?
7. Did you make a statement?
8. Did the police and assistanct district attorney read you your rights?
9. Who was your lawyer?

This list is by no means complete but is basic to delimiting the areas of amnesia and acting as a model for future memory explorations of the subject. Often, this procedure will give important clues concerning the nature of the alleged amnesia.

These answers are checked with the reports of other observers—friends, family, bystander witnesses, etc. They are also checked with observations made by the police and with statements made to police and assistant district attorneys.

Once a decision has been made to use sodium amytal, one must become acquainted with a proper technique.[6] The drug is given intravenously either by drip or directly in a syringe. Usually 500 mg are dissolved in 10 cc saline, providing a concentration of 50 mg per cc. Others have used greater doses giving 75 mg per cc. I prefer the lower dose for more readily controlled reactions. Before starting to inject, engage the subject in conversation of a simple, light, nondirective type. Then inject slowly at a steady pace. Give the first cc in 2 minutes and observe the effect, whether speech is accelerated, or slurred, or whether there is presence or absence of nystagmus. Keep the patient engaged in conversation. If the effect required has not yet appeared, inject one cc per minute and pause 1 minute to observe effects. Continue in this way until the desired result is obtained. If the patient shows evidence of overdrugging by excessively slurred speech, yawning, extensive nystagmus, and especially drowsiness, stop the drug temporarily until the signs are reduced and communication can be reestablished. The optimum state is maintained consciousness with only mild slurring of speech and mild nystagmus.

Following the conclusion of the procedure it is wise to allow the patient to sleep—usually from half an hour to 3 hours. It is important to watch the patient to prevent falling during this sleep state.

When the patient is up and around the amount of recall of the communication during the procedure varies considerably. Some have no recall at all, some recall parts, and some recall a considerable amount!

CONCLUSION

Intravenous sodium amytal, although not a "truth serum," has many useful functions for psychiatrists in the complex task of identifying malingering, psychoses, organic mental states and the numerous psychogenic reaction patterns. It is important to recognize that the sodium amytal technique is part of a clinical pattern for appraisal and diagnosis and is not a recording instrument by itself. The need to be aware of the different possibilities and reactions within the procedure is discussed in this paper.

REFERENCES

[1] Bleckwenn, WJ: Narcosis as therapy in neuropsychiatric conditions. *JAMA* 95:1168, 1930.

[2]Lindeman, E: Psychological changes in normal and abnormal individuals under the influence of sodium amytal. *Am J Psychiatry 88:*1083, 1932.

[3]Herman, M: The use of intravenous sodium amytal in psychogenic amnesic states. *Psychiatr Q 12:*738, 1938.

[4]Weinstein, EA *et al.:*The diagnostic use of amobarbital sodium (amytal sodium) in brain disease. *Amer J Psychiatry 109:*889, 1953.

[5]Grinker, R, and Spiegel, J: *War Neuroses* Philadelphia, Blakiston, 1945.

[6]Perry, JC, and Jacobs, D: Overview: Clinical Applications of the amytal interview in Psychiatric emergency settings. *Amer J Psychiatry 139:*5 May 1982.

12

Clinical Polygraphy
Its Function within Psychiatry

BRIAN E. LYNCH

INTRODUCTION

Throughout history, humanity has been preoccupied, even obsessed, with truth and deception. We are a species of animal determined to uncover that which may not be as it seems. In recent times, this mission has resulted in the demise of many of our sacred institutions, even our high government offices. The need to know the truth has been the impetus behind development in areas such as science, medicine, psychiatry, and now clinical polygraphy. As we become increasingly reluctant to accept things at face value, we become more and more demanding of our assessment or investigative techniques. The demand for refinement of technique has been the driving force behind the development and progress of modern polygraphy.[1]

The term *polygraphy* is more commonly understood as lie detection.[1] Although the latter term may be a more precise description of the technique, it unfortunately carries with it a pejorative connotation. The term *polygraphy* is derived from the Greek meaning "many writings." This generic term is not the exclusive domain of lie detection, as there are many disciplines, including psychiatry, which utilize polygraphic devices. Be that as it may, society has come to recognize the term as synonymous with detecting deception.

BRIAN E. LYNCH • Canadian Security Intelligence Service, Ottawa, Ontario, Canada K1P 5H7.

The expression lie detection does not precisely define the many varied applications of polygraphy. It is being used in police investigations and candidate screening, in the employment process of many businesses, in laboratory studies at universities and in the practice of psychiatry and medicine.[2] Therefore, though the basic technique does not vary greatly across these applications, sufficient differences exist to warrant an array of more descriptive terms. The author suggests adopting the name clinical polygraphy to describe the use of deception detection within psychiatry.

As stated previously, we are a society which doubts virtually everything we see and hear. Therefore, a device and technique designed to assess veracity are going to be important assets in our day-to-day existence.

As a result of our perceptual doubts, we value very highly the input of science and the empirical method. Clinical polygraphy has been caught up in the middle of this melee with opposing sides arguing whether it is a science or an art. The issue is somewhat academic as the discipline is still in transition and therefore owes allegiance to both art and science.

To fully appreciate clinical polygraphy, it is essential that certain fundamental points be understood. First, in contradiction to the technique's colloquial name, there exists, at present, no observable or definable physiological response unique to lying.[3] Consequently, before anything can be discussed further, it must be stated that clinical polygraphy measures nonspecific arousal. That is to say, the display of arousal is homogenous regardless of the stimuli. For example, it is not possible to differentiate between arousal resulting from lying and arousal resulting from sexual excitation. Thus, clinical polygraphy uses an inferential model in arriving at a decision. Just as a psychiatric diagnosis is accomplished by assessing the various component parts of a disorder and inferring from these symptoms a disease, so too is deception inferred from its arousal components. The difference exists in the component parts. In polygraphy, the assessment is based on measured physiological arousal emanating from question stimulation. The measured differential between two stimuli-relevant and control questions results in the possibility of an inference or conclusion.[4]

The second important concept to understand in clinical polygraphy is the extent of the inference.[5] As we are not measuring lies directly, the inferences drawn from the data are limited to the extent of the belief system of the person being tested. For example, no one would describe a Rorschach Ink-Blot Test as a "schizophrenic detector." It merely indicates possible symptoms of psychotic thinking. In like fashion, polygraphy merely documents responses resulting from the mental processing of various stimuli. Consequently, we are measuring the belief a person holds about a certain situation. If a psychotic person holds a fantasy to be true, then a polygraphy test will document that state. It will not demonstrate that it is a psychotic fantasy. Simply stated, a *polygraph test* assesses the veracity of a statement resulting from a given belief system. It can detect only that which is believed to be true and not the absolute truth.

Once these fundamental concepts are appreciated, it becomes apparent that clinical polygraphy is far from a restrictive discipline but a vehicle for exploring many aspects of psychological functioning, such as arousal, attention, perception, motivation, memory and information processing.[6] An appreciation of the positive and negative limitations of polygraphy permit a better assessment of its potential role within a psychiatric framework.

THE PSYCHOPHYSIOLOGY OF CLINICAL POLYGRAPHY

Like psychiatry, clinical polygraphy has laboured in its progression from magic and mysticism into an empirically based discipline.[7] Additionally, polygraphy pays homage to many of psychiatry's forefathers. Polygraphy did not come into existence until the late nineteenth and early twentieth centuries. It was born out of a need for a more scientific means of assessing truth, particularly in a police context. There were also turn of the century attempts to utilize the technique in armed forces selection and in word association tests.

It took some time to marry the technological advances with those of question techniques. From very crude and simple devices there emerged the modern polygraph incorporating state of the art electronic transducers and circuitry. In concert with the technological advances was the progression of testing techniques from early open-ended narratives to the present structured test format.

Early lie detector machines were heavy, insensitive, pneumatic devices generally measuring only one physiological function. It was not until these devices incorporated measures of more than one function that the designation *polygraph* could be applied. Today, there are basically three measures that are taken. Although various physiological measures have been experimented with, the present configuration of respiratory, electrodermal, and cardiovascular functioning yields the highest accuracy and efficiency.

Respiration is routinely measured by using hollow convoluted tubes placed over the thorax and abdomen. Although these sensors give a fairly true picture of respiratory functioning, there is a growing faction of practitioners who are using lighter and more comfortable mercury-filled strain gauges. The mercury gauges are more sensitive and therefore yield a truer picture of chest activity. Both devices yield a measure of rate and extent of breathing.

Cardiovascular functioning is measured using two different devices and body locations. The first device is designed to measure relative blood pressure using a standard occlusion cuff over the brachial artery and inflated to a pressure slightly under average diastolic pressure (70mm/Hg.). This device yields an oscillation wave reflecting both blood pressure and heart rate. The second means of measuring heart activity is by using a photoplethysmograph. This device is attached to a peripheral body location, usually a finger, and yields a measure of small vessel blood flow and heart rate.

The remaining measure taken is electrodermal activity or the galvanic skin response. This measure is taken by recording palmar surface resistance changes to an imperceptible level of constant current. The resistance changes are a function of arousal and sweat gland activity. GSR is considered by many to be one of the most sensitive indices of arousal. Many polygraphists are changing over to measuring skin conductance, which is considered superior to resistance. Both measures yield useful displays of autonomic arousal.

All three measures are displayed through a series of pre- and power amplifiers connected to a moving ink writing system. This results in a real time permanent record of the bodily functions.[8]

The physiology underlying arousal is not unique to polygraphy. The functioning of the various physiological systems results in the display of reactions. There are many psychophysiological variables at play in lie detection and it is difficult to sort their respective roles within the test. Nevertheless, it can be stated that the autonomic nervous system is the primary system in the process. It is not the intention of the author to delve into the physiology of arousal; there are many texts available on the topic. It is, however, important to note that the subdivisions of the autonomic nervous system—the sympathetic and parasympathetic nervous systems—play paramount roles in the detection of deception. It is their relative dominance within the system that dictates the state of the organism. Other factors, such as attention, stimulus quality, memory, intelligence, and individual differences, are all intrinsically involved in the final product, the displayed arousal. For example, the organism or the examinee is placed in a state of readiness. Depending on the stimulus, the examinee can attend to it or disregard it. If the stimulus is sufficiently threatening, the organism is plunged into a state of "fight or flight," that is, the body readies itself to deal with the threat. This readying process is directly tied to the autonomic nervous system, which is a fast acting but short lived system. Therefore, if a part of the test such as a question, is sufficiently stimulating, the examinee will respond with autonomic arousal. It is this very arousal that becomes the key to assessing veracity.

In addition to the physiology underlying polygraphy are the host of psychological variables that impinge on the organism. There are factors which can have a positive effect on the test results, such as mental associations, imagery, internal conflict, and selective attention, to name a few. As well there are factors that if not properly controlled can have a devastating effect on the results and in the accuracy of the test. These factors are question intensity, situation novelty, question change, and habituation. They can be detrimental to the overall reliability of the technique.[9]

The ideal testing situation tries to control the level of error by judicious attention to the factors just discussed. As we have been stating all along, the level of inferential confidence will be dictated by the level of variability. If the test can be conducted with a minimum of confounding variables, then our inferential strength is increased. We are, therefore, more confident in our results and our decision.

THE THEORY OF CLINICAL POLYGRAPHY

Taking all of these positive and negative psychophysiological variables into account requires a formidable theory of lie detection. There are several theoretical explanations for the detection of deception. All are sound and yet none explains the spectrum of polygraphic situations. Davis[10] has highlighted three theories to explain polygraphy. The first theory is entitled the *conditioned-response theory*. It suggests that questions about the issue under investigation in the test would cause arousal responses because they would be perceived as conditioned stimuli. Therefore, whatever emotional state of mind developed during the commission of a crime would also develop when asked a question about that crime. This paradigm, however, does not account for high detection rates with trivial matters and lies. Therefore, conditioning appears to be only part of the explanation. Furthermore, it has been shown that too high stress levels can be detrimental to detection rates.

The second theory deals with the *psychodynamic concept of conflict*. This theory states that in the deception process we might expect a clash between two established personality tendencies. It is generally held that an individual will answer any given question in a straightforward, direct manner. This tendency comes into conflict with the state of lying as this precipitates the need for denial. This head on collision between straightforward answering and the self-preservation of denial results in conflict and thus arousal.

The difficulty here is that any significant response might easily be due to emotional problems and not the conflict just mentioned. Therefore, sensitive words or issues might instigate arousal patterns irrespective of the more diagnostic conflict information.

The third proposed basis for clinical polygraphy is the *fear or threat of punishment theory*. An individual produces large physiological responses out of a fear of possible consequences resulting from being detected in a lie. This theory suggests some of the dynamics underlying gambling. Gambling behavior increases in relationship to the possibility of reward. Therefore, in a polygraph test, it would be beneficial to reinforce the possibility of punishment but not the certainty of punishment. This offers the examinee an avenue of hope of escape. Without it, the test may produce a state of learned helplessness and thereby reduce its efficiency.

Davis postulates that no one theory accounts for the total phenomenon of polygraphy, but that elements of many theories may be at work. For example, an optimal polygraphic situation might be one where the crime questions cause conflicting reactions due to the possibility of consequences, the situation itself threatens possible but not certain punishment because of deception, and last, the questions have a past association with negative memories.

The lay person often feels that polygraphy is really a test of guilt and remorse over wrongdoing. Undoubtedly, these feelings play a role in the detection process, but as we discussed, they do not sufficiently explain the full scope of polygraphic applications. The concern over pathological liars and the possibility of them defeating the test is legendary. Psychopathic personalities are no doubt sophisticated in the art of "conning." Clinical polygraphy, however, is a situation with which they have had limited experience. This is a situation not dependent on one-on-one discussions as much as on the ability to control autonomic functioning. Raskin and Hare[11] studies a group of clinically diagnosed psychopathic inmates and compared them to a nonpsychopathic group in a mock crime paradim. The results showed that psychopaths are as easily detected by polygraph as nonpsychopaths. The author suggests that this is a perfect example of the fear of punishment theory in action. The psychopathic personality being what it is, it can not help itself from trying to beat the test and reap whatever rewards. This very exaggerated effort would in turn enhance the autonomic functioning sufficiently for detection. Therefore, by trying so hard, the psychopath causes his own defeat through detection.

Up to this point, the discussion has dealt with the psychophysiology and instrumentation involved in a polygraph test. We have only hinted at the primary element: the questioning technique. There are a plethora of questioning techniques in use today. However, they are not all equivalent in terms of reliability and validity. One of the most widely used tests is the control question technique (CQT).[9] This technique had its beginning in the 1940s and has undergone countless modifications throughout its history. Although not all CQTs are identical, they all share the fundamental ingredient of the control question, which will be discussed farther on.

VALIDITY AND RELIABILITY

The CQT and polygraphy, in general, have come under attack for supposedly inflating their claims of reliability and validity. It is not the author's intention to further confound the issue by capriciously stating unfounded estimates of accuracy. Furthermore, a chapter of this sort is not the proper arena for a prolonged discussion of detection rates. The author suggests, for a more complete discussion of reliability and validity, that the reader refer to the following references.[3,4,9,12,13]

Establishing a realistic estimate of reliability and validity for polygraphy is a formidable task. First, in real life testing, ground truth or an external criterion on which to base a decision is extremely difficult to attain. In the case of truthful individuals, there is no way of knowing if a correct decision has been made unless they are part of a group of test takers and within that group a guilty party confesses his or her deceit. Some authorities even question confessions as reliable external indications of accuracy.

Thus, estimations of accuracy in the field are simply that—estimates. It is possible to cull a significant number of studies from both laboratory and field research and examine these accuracies. Although accuracy claims have gone from chance to 100%, it is possible to pinpoint the reliability somewhere in the middle. The author suggests that clinical polygraphy has an accuracy between 85% to 95%. This estimate is dependent on the issue to be examined, namely, the information available and the experience of the polygraphist. For discussion purposes, this places polygraphic accuracy at 90%. The 10% error portion can be roughly divided into 6% false positive, finding an innocent person guilty, and 4% false negative, finding a guilty person innocent.

An accuracy rate of 90% is an impressive statistic. It does not, however, deal with all types of test takers. It is often queried, "Is it possible for an individual to beat the polygraph?" The answer is an unequivocable yes. In any empirical endeavour there is always an element of error. What should impress the scientific reader is not the 10% possibility of error but the 90% probability of accuracy. Society functions on probabilities and not possibilities. Should polygraphy be any different?

The author will concede that if society demands 100% accuracy from polygraphy, then the test should not be used. However, clinicians are routinely using many psychometric tests which are not infallible but are in fact far less reliable than polygraphy. Suffice it to say that usage of polygraphy should be applied with a realistic appreciation of its limitations and not an irrational fear of its many negative possibilities.

THE POLYGRAPH TEST

Pretest Interview

All polygraph tests are made up of three distinct phases: the pretest interview, the question, sequence administration and analysis, and the posttest interview.[1] The pretest interview, by some estimates, is the most important part of the test. It is the clinical assessment portion, wherein the polygraphist has an opportunity to assess the potential quality of the test in terms of the examinee and the issue to be examined. The pretest also permits the examinee an opportunity to become familiar with the testing process before the actual questions are asked. The pretest involves an explanation of the test, a discussion of the test issue, establishment and review of the questions to be asked, and a brief life history data collection. This phase of the test also entails an explanation of its voluntary nature and a reassurance that the examinee may terminate whenever desired. The rapport that is established during the pretest is very important in relaxing the apprehensive innocent test taker. Extraneous arousal can be a confounding variable in the test if it is not kept within tolerable limits. The pretest can also serve to exacerbate the apprehension of the guilty and enhance their test responsivity.

This portion of the test also facilitates assessment of verbal and nonverbal behavior for indicators of deception. Caution must be taken in over reading these indicators to avoid contaminating the results, but valuable information can be gained nevertheless.

The primary function of the pretest phase if to formulate and review the test questions. These questions are generally of three types: neutral, control, and relevant.

Neutral questions, as their name suggests, are designed to be non-arousing.[9] They are as devoid of emotionality as possible and are about something which is blatantly true. For example, "Is your first name Beth?" or "Are you now living in Ottawa?" Generally these questions will not elicit any type of arousal. Neutral questions are used to begin the question sequence and as possible inserts if a period of nonarousing questioning is required. They usually call for an affirmative answer.

Relevant or crime questions are the essence of the test.[9] These are the stimuli that will cause responses in guilty persons indicating deception. Relevant questions are formulated to be direct and simply stated. They cover only one concept or issue. In clinical polygraphy, reliability is a function of the distinctness and magnitude of the issue under examination. Therefore, the simpler the issue and the graver the consequences, the better the test. Nevertheless, a good test tries to deal with a single, discrete topic. The more confused an issue becomes the less reliable are the results.

An example of a relevant question would be, "On June 26, did you rob Michael Putignano." These questions are designed to be answered with a no. Good question formulation involves clarity and simplicity. The question and its meaning must be understood identically by both the polygraphist and the examinee. Therefore, the level of language and comprehension must be taken into account during the formulation of all questions.

With relevant questions, their impact will be dependent on their construction. The ideal question is one that forces the guilty person to relive the issue being examined. Its impact will be amplified by clarity and conciseness.

If relevant questions have such impact, will they not also effect innocent persons? The answer would probably be yes if there were only relevant and neutral questions in the test sequence. However, this very situation brought about the genesis and development of the control question. In the early stages of polygraphy development, there were only neutral and relevant questions being asked. This situation gave rise to the possibility of innocent people being categorized as guilty. Without some type of conflicting stimulus, the innocent person might be overly stimulated by the relevant questions. What was needed was a type of question that would be selectively stimulating to innocent examinees. In fact, a question that would be an adversary to the relevant question.

The control question was designed to tap sensitive life issues and thereby serve as a counter stimulus to the relevant question.[9] In contrast to the relevant question, the control question is deliberately broad in scope and intent, permitting a vast array of interpretations depending on an individual's personality and past. It is designed to be answered in the negative. A control question example would be, "During the first twenty years of your life, do you remember ever hurting anyone?" The general nature of this question allows it to take on any meaning an individual wishes to give it.

As with the relevant question, the control question should affect even the guilty examinees, though it is intended only for the innocent. Relevant and control questions are combative stimuli. Hypothetically, both question types may arouse both guilty and innocent persons. What seems to happen, however, is a function of selective attention. The guilty persons process the relevant questions for longer periods because they perceive them as more threatening. Likewise, the innocent attend to the controls far more. This selective attention results in a differential in arousal between the two question types and the two test groups. Simply stated, the two test groups react to the greater of two evils. This conflict of stimuli results in an abundance of reactions to control questions for the innocent and to relevant questions for the guilty.

Once all of the various questions have been formulated, they are reviewed with the examinee to eliminate any surprise element. The following question sequence is an example of a CQT presently being taught at the Canadian Police College.[14]

Mock Test Question Sequence

1. Is your first name Beth? (Neutral question)
2. Are you afraid I'll ask you a question we didn't review? (Outside issue question)
3. Do you intend to answer each question truthfully? (Stimulation question)
4. During the first 20 years of your life, do you remember ever taking something that didn't belong to you? (Control questions)
5. On Tuesday, July 15, did you rob the Acme Shoe Store on Maple Street? (Relevant question)
6. Before 1975, do you remember ever stealing something from someone who trusted you? (Control question)
7. On Tuesday, July 15, did you alone, holdup the Maple Street Acme Shoe Store? (Relevant question)
8. Were you born in Ottawa? (Neutral question)
9. Before the age of 30, do you remember ever taking something of value from someone who loved you? (Control question)
10. Last Tuesday, July 15, did you rob the Acme Shoe Store on Maple Street? (Relevant question)

There are two additional questions in the sequence that have not been discussed. The outside issue question (2) is designed to identify mistrust on the part of the examinee. If there is another issue preoccupying his thoughts or the examinee believes there will be surprise questions asked, this question will tap that concern. The stimulation queston (3) is intended to familiarize the examinee with answering relevant questions without the need to waste a scoreable question. Both of these questions and their purported usage are still under investigation and therefore are excluded in the final numerical evaluation.

Question Sequence Administration and Analysis

Question review marks the end of Phase 1 and the beginning of Phase 2, the question sequence administration and analysis. The various body sensors are attached at this point. Before the reviewed sequence is asked, a short demonstration test, known as a stimulation test, is given.[15] There are several variations of this test but the majority involve the choosing of a numbered card from an array of numbered cards. The examinee is asked not to reveal the number as the polygraphist will attempt to identify it from the polygraphic readings. The array of numbers is then asked one at a time and the examinee is instructed to answer no to each number, thereby lying to one number only. The polygraphist then examines the physiological readings and attempts to identify the correct number. It should be noted that some schools of thought advocate a "rigged" test, wherein the number is known by the polygraphist before the graph is taken. The author prefers a straight, nonrigged test, wherein the real efficacy of the exam can be shown, and the polygraphists credibility is not called into question. Nevertheless, both approaches serve the purpose of demonstrating the effectiveness of the polygraph and thereby enhancing the reactivity of the examinee.

Following the stimulation test, the reviewed test sequence is administered a minimum of three times with each administration requiring a rotation of the questions. This question rotation insures that by the end of the test, each relevant question has been paired against every control question. The obtained polygraph charts are then subjected to a numerical analysis. This analysis involves scoring Relevant Questions 5, 7, and 10 (see sequence sample) for physiological criteria indicative of deception. A score of zero through $+3$ or -3 is assigned to each parameter of respiration, GSR, and cardiovascular functioning for each question. This results in 27 separate scores that are then summed for a grand total. For example, relevant questions are always scored against their preceding control question, thus, Relevant Question 5 would be examined for arousal criteria against Control Question 4, 6, or 9 depending on the rotation sequence. Should there be greater reaction in Question 5 in the respiration channel than in Question 4, then a score of -1, -2 or

−3 would be assigned to that measure. If the reaction differential had been reversed in favour of the control question, then a score of +1, +2 or +3 would be assigned, depending on the magnitude of the difference. The greater the differential, the higher the score. Each of these scores are then tallied and the total is considered in the decision. If the total is +6 or greater the decision is technically truthful, if the total is −6 or less, the decision is technically deceptive, and if the total falls somewhere in between then no decision is rendered and a retest is scheduled.

The numerical scores contribute very highly to the final decision. However, if the test does not deal with a single issue but multiple issues, then the scores are less definitive. Many factors, including multiple issues, must be considered before a decision is rendered. The polygraphist must be confident that there was not purposeful distortion during the charts, that the arousal is consistent and not contradictory, and that the assessment of the examinee's behavior is in accordance with the numerical score. In short, the polygraphist must make a clinical assessment of all test data and then decide if the examinee is truthful or deceptive. Although the test score is not the single deciding factor in a determination of deception, it is one of the most important.

At this point, certain types of issues would call for further tests, such as a peak of tension test (POT). This test is designed to deal with the identification of critical material from an array of noncritical material. For instance, using our mock question sequence, one could formulate a POT to test if the examinee knew the type of weapon used in the holdup. The question would be structured in such a fashion that each type of weapon would be perceived equivalent for everyone but the guilty party, who would react to the critical weapon. This type of test adds further substantiation to the decision process.

Posttest Interview

Once the decision has been made, the test enters the final phase, the posttest interview. If the decision was truthful, then this finding is reported to the examinee and he/she is dismissed. If the decision is negative or deceptive, then an interview ensues in an effort to explain any possible errors or to verify the decision by a confession of guilt. The posttest interview with the deceptive requires great interviewing skills and expertise and is an excellent opportunity to externally validate the decision.

CLINICAL POLYGRAPHY AND PSYCHIATRY

Of what use, then, is clinical polygraphy to the field of psychiatry? Psychiatry is interested in understanding the human psyche through the study of behavior and personality traits. Clinical polygraphy can assist this empirical study. There are alternative means of assessing veracity, including truth serum and hypnosis, but the evidence supports the superiority of polygraphy.

Today, general and forensic psychiatrists are increasingly being asked for personality assessments for purposes of court.[5] The issues of fitness to stand trial, intent during the commission of a crime, appreciation of actions and even custody issues are becoming the domain of modern psychiatry. Unfortunately, many psychiatrists are not availing themselves of modern assessment techniques. As with most things, there are limitations to pure clinical assessment. Verbal and nonverbal behavior indicators are not the most objective means of assessing an individual. In all subjective assessments, the element of malingering plays a potential role. The elimination of this potentially confounding variable is possible through the proper use of polygraphy. The objectivity inherent in clinical polygraphy provides an excellent vehicle for assessing the worth of any given statement. Rather than a replacement of the clinical art of assessment, clinical polygraphy is an excellent adjunct to the practitioner's arsenal. With an ever increasing dependency on subspecialties, the inclusion of clinical polygraphy into the psychiatric assessment has merit.

Clinical polygraphy can be used in a host of ways as long as the limitations of the test are kept in mind. The use of polygraphy in validating delusions or hallucinations holds promise. As stated earlier, if the hallucinations or delusions are incorporated into a person's belief system, the polygraph should be able to verify that fact. If they are not, then an identification of the malingering should also be possible. In short, any mental state that depends on belief can probably be assessed by clinical polygraphy for its worth. Therefore, an individual who believes himself to be Napoleon might well be assessed as truthful by a polygraph test. If, however, it is not a genuine belief, then they might be assessed as deceptive.

Assessing a person's state of mind at the time of an offense is a particularly difficult task. Clinical polygraphy can assist the assessment by shedding light on the person's intent during the offense. Again, the polygraph will only verify that which is believed to be true. If an individual believes that they did not intend to kill a certain person but only to harm them, then the polygraph can help in validating that statement.

Memory dysfunction is another area in which clinical polygraphy can be useful. It is an impossible task with our present psychometric techniques to verify the presence or absence of a specific memory. However, polygraphy is quite capable of such a task as well as of assessing many aspects of memory functioning. The author refers to a rather unique case that he was involved with at a psychiatric institute.[1]

A male patient, charged with attempted murder, was sent by the court to the hospital on a 60-day Warrant of Remand to undergo a psychiatric examination. The patient was suspected of stabbing his brother-in-law in the throat with an ice-pick. The patient claims to have been drinking heavily and denies any memory of the offense. This patient had convinced the psychiatrist who first examined him of the genuineness of his amnesia and the necessity of further observation at the author's hospital.

During his stay at the hospital, he underwent a battery of physiological, psychological, and sociological tests. All tests results substantiated the possibility of genuine amnesia for the offense. On the day before his discharge and return to court, a polygraph test was requested. At this point in the assessment, the official report read as a probable case of automatism or reduced responsibility due to the effect of alcohol. The patient arrived for his polygraph test and promptly stated that his memory loss had been a sham. He further stated that he had been able to "snow" everyone in the clinical process but thought it would be fruitless with the polygraph.

This case highlights very dramatically the positive contribution of clinical polygraphy to the psychiatric assessment process. In this particular case, more judicious use of the technique might have guided the assessment in a more productive fashion. Polygraphy's value is in its ability to sort individuals into whatever categories are under investigation.

In addition to assessing the presence of memory, clinical polygraphy has proven valuable in delineating the extent of the memory loss.[16] The polygraph technique is useful in defining the type and extent of the amnesia. As with its other applications, it serves well in substantiating the psychiatric assessment of the amnesia. Lynch and Bradford[16] suggested that the percentage of genuine amnesia cases is quite small. Therefore, polygraphy is beneficial in assessing the existence of malingering.

Child custody cases resulting from sexual and/or physical abuse are another area that could benefit from polygraphy.[17,18] All too often, custody cases break down to a subjective assessment of which parent or party is telling the truth about the abuse. Polygraphy could be most beneficial in identifying the truthful party and thereby guiding the custody decision process. Therefore, the function of the polygraph in child custody cases is twofold. First, it may establish veracity and second, it may lead to substantial changes in the attitudes of some of the parties involved such that the best interests of the child are served. Any procedure that leads to the clarification of the contested issues and the abbreviation of the legal process deserves serious consideration.

Clinical polygraphy is not a panacea for all that ails the field of psychiatry. It is, however, a very useful technique for assessing the veracity of mental states and statements. There are as many applications of polygraphy to psychiatry as the practitioner's imagination will allow. If the limitations of this technique are fully appreciated, then the proper application of polygraphic results to the field of psychiatry can be made. Psychiatrists who might be interested in using clinical polygraphy should exert the same care in selecting polygraphists as their patients do in selecting them. There are many reputable associations at both the state and federal levels that would be most willing to help in the selection process or to answer any further questions about polygraphy.[19,20]

REFERENCES

[1]Lynch, BE: Detection of deception: Its application to forensic psychiatry. *Bulletin of the A.A.P.L., 7*(3):239–244, 1979.

[2]Lynch, BE: The Psychophysiological Detection of Deception (PDD) and Psychiatry, in *Forensic Psychiatry*, S. Smith and J. Bradford (eds), in press.

[3]Lykken, DT: *A Tremor in the Blood: Uses and Abuses of the Lie Detector.* New York, McGraw-Hill, 1981.

[4]Orne, MT, Thackray, RI, Paskewitz, DA: On the detection of deception: A method for the study of the physiological effects of psychological stimuli, in N Greenfield & R Sternbach (eds.), *Handbook of Psychophysiology.* New York, Holt, Rinehart & Winston, 1972.

[5]Lynch, BE: The polygraph; a psychiatric resource, *Polygraph, 10*(1):13–19, 1981.

[6]Barland, GH, Raskin, DC: Detection of deception, in WF Prokasy & DC Raskin (eds.), *Electrodermal Activity in Psychological Research.* New York, Academic Press, 1973.

[7]Trovillo, PV: A history of lie detection. *Journal of Criminal Law and Criminology, 29*(6):848–881, 1939, *30*(1):104–119, 1939.

[8]Podlesny, JA, Raskin, DC: Physiological measures and the detection of deception. *Psychological Bulletin, 84*(4):782–799, 1977.

[9]Abrams, S: *Polygraph Handbook for Attorneys.* Lexington, Lexington Books, 1977.

[10]Davis, RC: Physiological responses as a means of evaluating information, in the *Manipulation of Human Behavior*, A Bidderman & H Zimmer (eds.), New York, John Wiley and Sons, 1961.

[11]Raskin, DC, Hare, RD: Psychopathy and detection of deception in a prison population. *Psychophysiology, 15*(2):126–136, 1978.

[12]Ansley, N : A compendium on polygraph validity. *Polygraph, 12*(2):53–61, 1983.

[13]Markwart, A, Lynch, BE: The effect of polygraph evidence on mock jury decision-making, *Journal of Police Science and Administration, 7*(3):324–332, 1979.

[14]*Course Training Standard, Canadian Police College*, Polygraph Training Section, Ottawa, Canada, 1983.

[15]Barland, GH: An introduction to the number test. *Polygraph, 7*(3):173–175, 1978.

[16]Lynch, BE, Bradford, JM: Amnesia: Its detection by psychophysiological measures. *Bulletin of the A.A.P.L., 8*(3):288–297, 1980.

[17]Lynch, BE, Waters, BG: A polygraphy examination of a sexually molested child. *Polygraph, 9*(3):143–147, 1980.

[18]Waters, BG, Lynch, BE: *The polygraph as a facilitator in custody and access disputes and child welfare cases;* unpublished manuscript, available from authors. Canadian Security Intelligence Service, Ottawa, Ontario, Canada K1P 5H7.

[19]American Polygraph Association, PO Box 74, Linthicum Heights, Maryland, 21090.

[20]Canadian Association of Police Polygraphists, c/o Brian E. Lynch, MA, Canadian Police College, PO Box 8900, Ottawa, Ontario, K1G 3J2.

13

The Use and Misuse of Hypnosis in Court

MARTIN T. ORNE

Over the years, much of the forensic interest in hypnosis has dealt with the question of whether an individual can be compelled to carry out antisocial behavior* and the implications that such a possibility would have for the concept of legal responsibility. More recently, however, there has been a sudden upsurge of legal cases throughout the country which have involved the use of hypnosis in an entirely different context. These cases employ hypnosis (*a*) to enhance defendants' memories in order to bring out new information which might clear them of accusations against them, or (*b*) to increase the recall of witnesses or victims who have observed a crime, either to facilitate the pretrial investigation or to enhance memory sufficiently so that following hypnosis the individuals can serve as eyewitnesses in court. Finally, hypnosis has been

Reprinted from *Crime and Justice: An Annual Review of Research,* vol. 3, edited by Michael Tonry and Norval Morris, © 1981 by The University of Chicago. All rights reserved. Published by the University of Chicago Press. An earlier version of this essay appeared in the Monograph Issue of the *International Journal of Clinical and Experimental Hypnosis* on the forensic uses of hypnosis, 27(4) (1979):311–41.

*For a detailed discussion of these issues, see Barber (1961), Orne (1960, 1962), Orne and Evans (1965), and the *International Journal of Clinical and Experimental Hypnosis* 20(2) (1972), a special issue of the journal which includes relevant papers by Coe, Kobayashi, and Howard (1972), Conn (1972), Kline (1972), Orne (1972a), and Watkins (1972).

MARTIN T. ORNE • The Institute of Pennsylvania Hospital, University of Pennsylvania, Philadelphia, Pennsylvania 19139.   The substantive work carried out in our laboratory relevant to this paper and its preparation was supported in part by grant MH 19156 from the National Institute of Mental Health and by a grant from the Institute for Experimental Psychiatry.

used to help in the psychological and psychiatric evaluation of defendants, especially to determine their state of mind (Kline,1979). Although this application will not be discussed substantively in this essay, all the limitations of hypnosis for the proof of fact generally apply even more strongly to its use to document the fact of a state of mind.

Because of our laboratory's work on the nature of hypnosis, I have become involved in a number of cases where our work was directly relevant to the proposed forensic use of hypnosis. Of particular relevance were our empirical studies dealing with the nature of hypnotic age regression (O'Connell, Shor, and Orne, 1970; Orne, 1951), the potential use of hypnosis in interrogation (Orne, 1961), the question of whether antisocial behavior can be elicited by the use of hypnosis (Orne, 1962, 1972a; Orne and Evans, 1965), the nature of posthypnotic behavior (Orne, 1969; Orne, Sheehan, and Evans, 1968; Sheehan and Orne 1968), the simulation of hypnosis (Orne, 1971, 1972b, 1977), and posthypnotically disrupted recall (Evans and Kihlstrom, 1973; Kihlstrom and Evans, 1976, 1977; Nace, Orne, and Hammer 1974; Orne, 1966).

This essay reviews the major issues of some of the forensic uses of hypnosis, illustrates the difficulties which may be encountered by examining the relevant scientific evidence as well as some of the relevant legal cases, and finally proposes some general guidelines for the use of hypnosis that should minimize the likelihood of serious miscarriages of justice.

THE USE OF HYPNOSIS TO LEGITIMIZE NEW INFORMATION AND INCREASE CREDIBILITY

In the past few years there has been a sharp increase in the use of hypnosis—by prosecutors and defendants, plaintiffs and respondents alike—to enhance memory for events associated with a crime or civil suit. In most cases, the courts ultimately refused to admit hypnotically elicited material as evidence. An examination of some of these cases illustrates many problems that can occur in the forensic use of hypnosis if appropriate safeguards are not employed.

To Exonerate a Defendant

At one time, both hypnosis and "truth serum" (sodium amytal and pentothal administered intravenously) were thought of as techniques which could elicit truthful information. Since it is widely believed by laymen that there is a virtual certainty of obtaining truthful information when a subject's critical judgment is diminished by either hypnosis or a drug, it is hardly surprising that efforts have been made to introduce hypnotic testimony in court as a way for the defendant to demonstrate his innocence to a jury. The courts, however, have recognized that hypnotic testimony is not reliable as a means of ascertaining truth and appropriately have rejected both these techniques as means of determining factual information.

Although these early decisions were usually accompanied by gratuitous deprecatory remarks about hypnosis, the wisdom of the decisions themselves is supported by scientific data. Thus, experience with a research design where deeply hypnotized subjects and unhypnotizable subjects instructed to feign hypnosis are seen by hypnotists who are unaware of the subjects' actual status (Orne, 1959, 1971, 1972b) has shown that it is possible to deceive even highly experienced hypnotists (Hilgard, 1977; Orne, 1977; Sheehan, 1972). Not only can individuals fake hypnosis, but even subjects who are genuinely in deep hypnosis are nonetheless able wilfully to lie (Orne, 1961).

Although the courts have usually rejected the use of hypnosis as a truth-telling device, recognition of hypnosis as a valid therapeutic method by the American Medical Association and the American Psychological Association has contributed to a new trend in the use of hypnosis in legal cases. Hypnosis has been widely used in a therapeutic context to help individuals remember material they had forgotten. Many defendants claim to be unable to remember the events for which they are being tried, and so it seemed reasonable to consider that hypnosis might help refresh their memories so that they might better assist in their own defense. In other cases it has been proposed that hypnosis could be useful in ascertaining the defendant's state of mind at the time of the crime. By this back door, then, the role of hypnosis in facilitating the recall of otherwise "forgotten" facts or memories of the state of mind was reintroduced into the courtroom, and efforts were made to introduce hypnotically elicited testimony to juries.

An excellent example of this strategy occurred during the retrial of a convicted murderer in Ohio (State v. Papp, No. 78-02-00229, Com. Pleas Ct., Summit Co., Ohio, 3/23/78). The defendant claimed to be unable to remember some of the events at the time of the crime, and the court ordered that he be hypnotized to assist in his defense. Using the procedure of hypnotic age regression, the defendant apparently relived the period of the crime and exonerated himself, leading the press throughout the state to proclaim his innocence. After viewing the videotape record of the hypnotic session, which, according to the prosecution experts, revealed some anomalies in Papp's response to hypnosis, the hypnotist hired by the defense was persuaded to administer specific tests to assess possible simulation. The defendant behaved in a manner typical of those who are pretending to be hypnotized, and the result recorded on videotape was sufficiently clear that it was not effectively disputed by the defense. Consequently, no attempt was made to introduce the videotape recording purportedly demonstrating the defendant's innocence in court.

Criminal defendants have a clear self-interest in the outcome of hypnosis; accordingly great care must be taken in the interpretation of hypnotic material. It must also be kept in mind that the hypnotic session, which may involve displays of considerable feeling, is extremely arousing and compelling to the untrained observer. For example, in the case of People v. Ritchie, No. C-36932, Super. Ct., Orange Co., Calif., 4/7/77, the defendant was accused of killing a 2½-year-old child. When confronted with an overwhelming amount of circumstantial evidence, the defendant requested that he be hypnotized to enable him to remember details which he could not recall. Under hypnosis he relived the experience in an exceedingly dramatic fashion, remembering material indicating that his wife committed the murder and clearing himself. Through an analysis of the videotape recording of the hypnosis session, it was possible to document how the defendant had inadvertently been led by the hypnotist and also to demonstrate a number of intrinsic inconsistencies which clearly indicated that the version the defendant relived under hypnosis was either confabulated or a conscious lie designed to serve the needs of his case. After extensive testimony, the court excluded the hypnotic evidence because of its unreliability.

To Cause a Defendant to Confess

Confessions are regularly obtained by interrogators without the use of force, the threat of force, or even any obvious form of mental coercion, and even individuals who know that they would be better off not confessing often do so. There is general consensus that hypnotized individuals will not carry out activities which are morally unacceptable or inherently self-destructive. One would expect, therefore, that hypnosis should not cause a guilty individual to confess to a crime, since it is rarely if ever advantageous for a defendant to confess. The situation here is considerably more complex, however, since good interrogators frequently obtain confessions from defendants who know that they jeopardize their position by confessing. Somehow it is possible for the interrogator to make the relationship in the here and now seem more important than the eventual, detrimental consequences of having confessed. It seems clear that there are psychological needs which will be served by confessing, and that even in the usual waking state the relationship with a skilled interrogator may tap that psychological balance. It would hardly be surprising, therefore, that in some instances confessions have been obtained in a context of hypnosis. In the New York case of the People v. Leyra, 302 N.Y. 353, 98 N.E. 2d 553 (1951) the defendant was accused of the hammer murder of his mother and father. A psychiatrist retained by the district attorney's office saw him in jail and elicited a full confession. A tape recording of the session was available which showed that the psychiatrist identified himself as a physician there to help the defendant, massaged his forehead and temple repeatedly, demanded the defendant look into his eyes, told him that he was not morally responsible for what he had done, suggested that he had picked up the hammer and struck his parents, and even threatened to give him an injection if he failed to cooperate. The confession was introduced at the trial and the defendant convicted. On appeal, the judgment was reversed on the grounds that the confession was involuntary and coerced. The defendant was retried and again convicted. On appeal to the U.S. Supreme Court, the defendant prevailed (Leyra v. Denno, 347 U.S. 556 [1954]). While hypnosis is not explicitly mentioned, Justice Black's opinion in writing for the majority points out that "suspect's ability to resist interrogation was broken to almost *trance-like submission* by the use of the arts of a highly skilled psychiatrist. Then the confession petitioner began making to the psychiatrist was filled in and perfected by additional statements given in rapid succession to a police officer, a trusted friend, and two state prosecutors" (emphasis added; *id.* at 561).

It is worth noting that false confessions may also be elicited under hypnosis for the same kind of complex reasons that cause innocent individuals to assert their guilt whenever there is a well-publicized crime. It is important to recognize that merely because certain individuals, originally seen as witnesses, begin to relive the events of a crime during hypnosis and clearly implicate themselves one should not accept their actions as necessarily indicating guilt. An example of this kind involved a distinguished physician, an authority on the use of hypnosis, who at the request of the police department sought to facilitate the recall of a purported murder witness. Surprisingly, under hypnosis incriminating statements were made which would have implicated the witness as the perpetrator of the crime. The witness then became a suspect. Fortunately, subsequent investigation did not corroborate any of the statements made under hypnosis, including the location of the possible murder weapon, and the case turned out to be an inadvertent false confession obtained under hypnosis (see Kroger, 1977).

In every instance where the courts have become aware that hypnosis has been used in an effort to obtain confessions, such confessions have been excluded. Consequently, everyone agrees that hypnosis should not be used in such a manner. While the likelihood of obtaining false confessions is not widely understood, it is a moot issue because care is taken to avoid the use of hypnosis with any possible suspect. Indeed, most prosecutors recognize that if they hypnotize a witness who later turns out to be implicated as a defendant, they will significantly complicate his or her ultimate prosecution.

To Recall Relevant Details in Civil Suits

Hypnosis has been used to help plaintiffs in accident cases remember details of the incidents. For example, in a Canadian case (Crockett et al. v. Haithwaite et al., No. 297/73, Sup. Ct., British Columbia, 2/10/78), a woman and a male passenger were found in a car which had run off the road and hit a tree. The passenger was dead and the driver seriously injured. British Columbia law is such that if the driver had been careless or distracted, her insurance would be liable to the estate of her dead passenger and she herself would have no substantial claim; however, if another car caused her to run off the road, her insurance company would not be liable and she herself would be able to recover very substantial damages from a special fund set up to compensate those injured by unidentified drivers. At the time of the accident, however, the woman reported no recollection of such a car. Some time later her attorney referred her to a psychiatrist for help with emotional difficulties stemming from the accident, and also requested that he might seek to facilitate her memory of the accident. There is little doubt that the driver and her lawyer were clearly aware of the substantial difference it would make whether or not another vehicle had been involved in the accident; thus it is hardly surprising that under hypnosis she remembered a van coming toward her and forcing her off the road. If the driver had simply stated that one day she suddenly remembered that a van had forced her off the road, a jury would be likely to reject such "spontaneous" memories as self-serving and not trustworthy. Memories which are recalled via the use of hypnosis, however, are more apt to be taken at face value. This case was ultimately settled on the courthouse steps. Even so, it represents a use of hypnosis closely analogous to hypnotizing a defendant and open to all the caveats involved in such a use.

THE NATURE OF HYPNOTIC RECALL

When hypnosis is used with a defendant or plaintiff who has much to gain by recalling one set of memories rather than another, motivational factors are superimposed upon the basic mechanisms involved in hypnotically aided recall. While these motivational factors complicate the picture, the basic facts about the phenomenon of hypnosis and its effects on recall apply to all circumstances where hypnosis is employed. The unreliability of hypnotic recall is due both to factors inherent in the nature of hypnosis and properties of the human memory system. This section reviews relevant research findings concerning the nature of hypnotic age regression, the effect of direct suggestions to remember material that was apparently forgotten, some aspects of memory as they are relevant to hypnotically aided recall, and the mental mechanisms which may account for the apparent increase in recall, including the tendency to confabulate, that is, to make up plausible pseudo memories for those portions of an event that the person is unable to recall. Finally, some aspects of the hypnotist's behavior characteristic of the hypnotic context which tend to alter the quality of recall are discussed.

Age Regression

Although direct suggestion is sometimes used to facilitate recall in hypnosis, the procedures most widely employed involve some form of hypnotic age regression. This dramatic phenomenon appears to enable individuals to relive an event which might have occurred many years past. It is also a method that can be equally effective in helping an individual relive recent events, particularly if they involve some trauma leading to motivated forgetting manifested by the inability to recall significant events. Not only are extensive clinical observations available concerning hypnotic age regression, but it has also been studied systematically in the laboratory, providing data which shed much light on the nature of the process, and on the critical issue of the historical accuracy of hypnotically elicited recall.

When a hypnotized individual is told that he is 6 years old and at his birthday party, for example, he will begin to act, talk, and to some degree think like a child. He may play as a child would; address the friends who apparently were at his birthday party; and describe in detail the room where the party is occurring, the people who are in attendance, and the presents he is receiving. The naturalness with which these descriptions are given and the conviction that is communicated by the individual are compelling even to trained observers. The feelings which are expressed appear appropriate to a child more than to an adult, and the entire phenomenon is such that it is generally described as beyond the skills of even a professional actor. In a therapeutic setting, the material that is recovered during hypnotic age regression is often of great importance to a patient's treatment. As Breuer and Freud (1895) discovered at the end of the nineteenth century, the reliving of traumatic events may result in the cure of troublesome pathological symptoms, lending credence to the historical accuracy of these events. For these reasons, there is a widely held belief among both laymen and practicing clinicians that the events relived during hypnotic age regression are historically accurate.

Typically, age regressed individuals will spontaneously elaborate a myriad of details which apparently could be produced only by someone actually observing the events as they occurred. It is these details which sophisticated clinicians find most compelling and occasionally cause them to testify that they know with certainty that the individual was truly regressed. It is rare indeed, however, for the clinician to have the time, energy, or need to be certain that would cause him to attempt to verify the accuracy of an individual's description of events that actually happened many years ago in childhood. Unfortunately, without objective detailed verification, the clinician's belief in the historical accuracy of the memories elicited under hypnosis is likely to be erroneous. Freud's early "infantile seduction" theory of hysteria gives dramatic evidence of this.

Freud originally believed that seduction in childhood by an adult, usually the father, was the etiological factor in hysteria (see Ellenberger, 1970) because in hypnosis his patients dramatically relived such an event and typically showed considerable subsequent improvement. It was some years later that Freud realized the seduction scene that the patients relived in treatment accurately reflected the fantasies of the patient but did not accurately portray historical events. Often the relived episodes combined several actual events and many fantasies. This is no way detracted from the usefulness of reliving these events in treatment where the purpose is to help the patient gain relief from his symptoms. Consider, however, the catastrophe which would have resulted if Freud had acted upon his patients' recollections and had urged the authorities to imprison the fathers for incest!

Experimental work with hypnotic age regression is possible because hypnosis is a phenomenon that can readily be induced in normal individuals. It is sometimes possible to obtain materials that an individual has not seen since the age of 6, then to age regress him back to that time, and while the subject is talking, acting, and writing like a child, to elicit these same materials—for example, childhood drawings. Characteristically, the productions superficially resemble those of a child. One tends to accept them as "typical" of what a 6-year-old would have done, *unless* they are compared to what the individual had actually drawn as a child. In an early study (Orne, 1951), however, an expert in children's drawings examining a series of age regressed productions indicated that these were not done by children but showed "sophisticated oversimplification."

Since that time, other experimental studies have sought to document the historical accuracy of material produced during hypnotic age regression. The best known is an interesting monograph by Reiff and Scheerer (1959) who compared five highly responsive subjects age regressed to ages 10, 7, and 4 with three groups of role-playing subjects instructed to act as if they were 10, 7, and 4 respectively. The results seemed to document cognitive processes characteristic of children of the appropriate age in the age regressed subjects, but not in the controls. In our laboratory, this study was extended and replicated (O'Connell, Shor, and Orne, 1970). With larger samples and controlling for subtle experimenter bias, it became clear that both modest increase in recall as well as increased confabulation occurred within the same subject in the same age regression session. There were many times that subjects provided us with what appeared to be factual material relating to events that occurred many years ago such as their school's name, their teachers' names, and the names of schoolmates who sat next to them in the fifth and second grades. The subjects would describe their classmates so vividly and with such conviction that we were surprised indeed to find, when we went to the trouble of checking the actual school records, that some of these individuals had not been members of the subject's class; nor was the factual recall better than that of the unhypnotized controls.

The hypnotic suggestion to relive a past event, particularly when accompanied by questions about specific details, puts pressure on the subject to provide information for which few, if any, actual memories are available. This situation may jog the subject's memory and produce some increased recall, but it will also cause the subject to fill in details that are plausible but consist of memories or fantasies from other times. It is extremely difficult to know which aspects of hypnotically aided recall are historically accurate and which aspects have been confabulated. The details of material that is confabulated depend upon the subject's total past experience and all available cues relevant to the hypnotic task. Subjects will use prior information and cues in an inconsistent and unpredictable fashion; in some instances such information is incorporated in what is confabulated, while in others the hypnotic recall may be virtually unaffected.

As a consequence of these limitations, hypnosis may be useful in some instances to help bring back forgotten memories following an accident or a crime while in others a witness might, with the same conviction, produce information that is totally inaccurate. This means that material produced during hypnosis or immediately after hypnosis, inspired by hypnotic revivification, may or may not be historically accurate. As long as this material is subject to independent verification, its utility is considerable and the risk attached to the procedure minimal. There is no way, however, by which anyone—even a psychologist or psychiatrist with extensive training in the field of hypnosis—can for any particular piece of information determine whether it is an actual memory or a confabulation *unless* there is independent verification. Thus, there are instances when subsequently verified accurate license plate numbers were recalled in hypnosis by individuals who previously could not remember them. In the Chowchilla kidnapping case (Kroger and Doucé, 1979), the license plate number was helpful in the initial investigation of the case (although ultimately not required in the courtroom because of the abundance of other evidence available). On the other hand, a good many license plate numbers that have been recalled under hypnosis by witnesses in other cases in fact belonged to cars and drivers none of which, as it turned out after investigation, could have been involved.

Hypermnesia by Direct Suggestion

Another approach which has been used to increase memory is to give direct suggestions to the hypnotized individual that he will be able to remember crucial events which occurred some time ago. While generally used to enhance recall for recent events, it can also be employed to induce hypermnesia for the distant past.

Stalnaker and Riddle (1932) used direct suggestion to facilitate recall of long forgotten memories, shedding light on the mechanism of hypermnesia. It was suggested to deeply hypnotized subjects that they would recall prose and verse that they had committed to memory in grade school. In hypnosis, these subjects appeared to remember the material far more easily, with far better recall, than they otherwise could. Careful analysis, however, showed that, while some additional material was recalled in hypnosis, the amount was far less than it first seemed; in fact, subjects showed a pronounced tendency to confabulate so that many of the new phrases "recalled" had simply been improvised in a style that superficially resembled the author's. Often these confabulations were sufficiently good so as not to be easily recognized as such on casual examination. This study clearly established two tendencies in hypnotic hypermnesia: (*a*) a modest increase in the amount of material available to memory, and (*b*) a tendency to confabulate—to fill in those aspects which the subject cannot remember, in an effort to comply with the suggestions of the hypnotist. More recent studies, such as those of White, Fox, and Harris (1940), Sears (1954), and Dhanens and Lundy (1975), appear to show increased recall of meaningful, though nontraumatic, material in hypnosis. (No such effect has been demonstrated with nonsense syllables.) However, when the effects of hypnosis on increased memory are compared with those of increased motivation (Cooper & London, 1973), and procedures analogous to hypnosis with unhypnotizable subjects (Dhanens & Lundy, 1975), there is no significantly greater increase in recall with hypnosis. Thus, the widely held belief that hypnotic suggestion can not only increase the amount but also the reliability of the material recalled ignores motivational factors on the one hand, and the concurrent dramatic increase in the "recall" of inaccurate information on the other. This is illustrated in the Stalnaker and Riddle study (1932). Depending upon how they scored their material, these investigators could observe a 65 percent increase in memory for material learned many years earlier when recalled during hypnosis. Such a figure is obtained if one simply looks at the number of more accurate memories that are produced. At the same time, however, subjects in the hypnotic condition vastly increased the amount of inaccurate details that were "remembered."

The apparently increased recall in hypnosis can in large part be understood if one takes into account the deeply hypnotized individual's tendency to manifest a decrease in critical judgment. The same process that increases suggestibility by permitting subjects to accept counterfactual suggestions as real also makes it possible for subjects to accept approximations of memory as accurate. When not hypnotized they are unwilling to consider approximate or fragmentary memories as acceptable recall; in hypnosis, however, they alter their criterion of what is acceptable and express accurately recalled fragments mixed with confabulated material. When hypnosis is used in the context of gathering investigative leads, such a change in criterion is desirable since it will cause witnesses to produce bits of information which they would not otherwise have felt confident enough to report—*provided*, of course, one recognizes that these fragments are made available at the cost of adding other details which are likely to be inaccurate. Further, neither the subject nor the expert observer can distinguish between confabulation and accurate recall in any particular instance. This can be done only by corroboration extrinsic to the hypnotic situation.

Confusion of Memories during Hypnosis with Waking Recall

When subjects are hypnotized and told to remember the events of a particular day (and awakened without amnesia suggestions), they may be able subsequently, and not under hypnosis, to describe their recollections in hypnosis and clearly differentiate them from their earlier recollections before being hypnotized. It is another matter, however, if subjects are convinced before being hypnotized that they will have the "true facts" that they are now unable to remember, or if prior to awakening, they are given the suggestion that they will wake up and remember everything, including the details of what actually occurred on a particular day, and that they will be able to recall all details as vividly and clearly as in hypnosis. Under these circumstances, they will typically awaken and confound the hypnotic memories with their waking memories. Such suggestions, which are now widely used for forensic purposes, result in individuals' tending to accept the events relived in hypnosis as if they were what actually happened. The previous gaps or uncertainties in memory are now filled in, and the events as they were relived in hypnosis become recollections of what actually occurred on the day in question.

Witnesses who testify following such a procedure may even fail to be able to distinguish which memories occurred in hypnosis and which came about as part of the normal waking recollection. Instead of differentiating between earlier fragmentary recall and the gaps later filled in—perhaps by pseudo memories created during hypnosis—they experience the totality as their recollection of what had originally occurred. It is this new recollection that is convincingly reported when the individual is asked what happened. Even though prior to hypnosis they had been very uncertain about their memory, had changed their stories many times, and had not reported many of the details that emerged only during hypnosis, they will now report their "memories" consistently and with conviction. As a consequence, memories which occurred only during hypnosis may be incorrectly presented in court as though they represented recollections based on original memory traces of the events that actually occurred on the day in question, and of course they will be presented with the credibility attributed to sincere beliefs.

Hypnotic Recall as Part of Basic Memory Processes

The idea that one can in hypnosis somehow reactivate original memory traces stems from a popular view (shared among lay hypnotists) that memory involves a process analogous to a multi-channel videotape recorder inside the head which records all sensory impressions and stores them in their pristine form. Further, there is a belief that while this material cannot ordinarily be brought to consciousness, access to it can be obtained through hypnosis; this mechanism is presumed to make possible the phenomenon of age regression or revivification. Suffice it to say that such a view is counter to any currently accepted theory of memory and is not supported by scientific data (Hilgard and Loftus, 1979; Jenkins, 1974; Putnam, 1979; Roediger, 1979). As Bartlett (1932) pointed out many years ago, memory is continuously changing and is *reconstructive* as well as reproductive. It is possible that highly traumatic, emotional material that is repressed could be less subject to the kind of continuing changes seen with relatively neutral material, but even this is doubtful since, as has been pointed out earlier, many of the memories recovered in psychotherapy include material which is not historically accurate.

Particularly relevant to our consideration here, however, are the observations discussed by Hilgard and Loftus (1979) indicating that free narrative recall will produce the highest percentage of accurate information but also the lowest amount of detail. Conversely, the more an eyewitness is questioned about details, the more details will be obtained—but with a marked decrease in accuracy. This observation, based on research with unhypnotized individuals, is virtually certain to apply to hypnotized subjects as well.

From Hypnotic Enhancement of Recall to the Creation of Memory

Although the laws that govern memory inevitably apply to hypnotic recall, it is difficult to disentangle which aspects of hypnotically enhanced memories represent accurate recall and which represent fantasies that are confabulated to approximate what might have occurred. The extent to which the process of confabulation may be stimulated by hypnosis becomes obvious when, instead of being asked to relive a prior event, the subject is given suggestions to experience a future event—about which no memories could possibly exist. For instance, in age progression (Kline & Guze, 1951), a subject is given the suggestion that it is the year 2000 and asked to describe the world around him. Such a suggestion, given to the deeply hypnotized individual, will lead to a vivid and compelling description of all kinds of new, as yet unseen, scientific marvels. Obviously, the plausibility and the precise nature of a subject's description will depend upon the scientific knowledge, the reading, and the intelligence of that subject.

The same process that allows hypnotized individuals to hallucinate the environment of the year 2000 can also be involved when they are urged to recall what happened six months ago, especially if they lack clear, waking memories to permit them to recall details accurately. Unfortunately, such pseudomemories can and often do become incorporated into individuals' memory stores as though they had actually happened. It is worth noting that this can occur even with bizarre memories such as when people "recall" their past lives and become convinced that these events really took place or, in other instances, when individuals under hypnosis remember encounters with flying saucers and become convinced they have actually communicated with beings from another galaxy. In such instances, the sophisticated listener smiles about the subject's assertions as it is obvious that they represent pseudomemories. Unfortunately, if such pseudomemories relate to events which occurred six months ago and are plausible, there is no way for either the hypnotist or the subject or a jury to distinguish between them and actual recall of what occurred.

The content of pseudomemories when they are wittingly or unwittingly induced during hypnosis is, of course, not random. If the subject has just seen a science fiction film, one can usually recognize elements of that film in the subject's description of what is going on about him or her in the year 2000; similarly, if a witness is hypnotized and has factual information casually gleaned from newspapers or inadvertent comments made during prior interrogation or in discussion with others who might have knowledge about the facts, many of these bits of knowledge will become incorporated and form the basis of any pseudomemories that develop. Furthermore, if the hypnotist has beliefs about what actually occurred, it is exceedingly difficult to keep from inadvertently guiding the subject's recall so that the subject will eventually "remember" what the hypnotist believes actually happened.

A simple experimental demonstration which I have often carried out is directly relevant to the circumstances of attempts hypnotically to enhance recall. First, I carefully establish and verify that a particular subject had in fact gone to bed at midnight on, say 17 February, and had arisen at 8 a.m. the following morning. After inducing deep hypnosis, it is suggested that the subject relive the night of 17 February—getting ready for bed, turning out the light, and going to sleep at midnight. As the subject relives being asleep, he is told that it is now 4 a.m. and then is asked whether he has heard the two loud noises. Following this question (which is in fact a suggestion), a good subject typically responds that the noises had awakened him. Now instructed to look around and check the time, he may say it is exactly 4:05 a.m. If then asked what he is doing, he may describe some activity such as going to the window to see what happened or wondering about the noises, forgetting about them, and going back to sleep.

Still hypnotized, he may relive waking up at 8 a.m. and describe his subsequent day. If, prior to being awakened, he is told he will be able to remember the events of 17 February as well as all the other things that happened to him in hypnosis, he readily confounds his hypnotic experience with his actual memory on awakening. If asked about the night of 17 February, he will describe going to sleep and then being awakened by two loud noises. If one inquires at what time these occurred, he will say, "Oh, yes, I looked at my watch beside my bed. It has a radium dial. It was exactly 4:05 a.m." The subject will be convinced that his description about 17 February is accurately reflecting his original memories.

The subject's altered memory concerning the night of 17 February will tend to persist (unless suggestions are given to the contrary), particularly because the subject was asleep at the time and there are no competing memories. The more frequently the subject reports the event, the more firmly established the pseudomemory will tend to become. In the experimental demonstration, we are dealing with an essentially trivial memory about which the subject has no strong inherent motivations. Nonetheless, the memory is created by a leading question, which, however, on casual observation seems innocuous.

In a life situation where hypnosis is used to enhance recall, the same mechanisms which we have purposively employed in the laboratory to create plausible pseudomemories which subjects accept as their own may easily occur inadvertently. It must be emphasized that one is not usually dealing with a conscious effort on the part of the hypnotist to distort witnesses' memories; on the contrary, the process by which hypnotized subjects are affected typically occurs outside of the hypnotist's awareness. Thus, if the hypnotist knows that two shots have been fired at approximately 4 a.m. on the night of 17 February, what seems more natural than to inquire of a witness whether he or she had heard any loud noises? Further, since usually the witness also knows something about the case and the kinds of memories which would be relevant and important, it may be sufficient simply to inquire at critical times, "Did you hear anything?" in order to lead the responsive hypnotized subject to create the desired "memories."

Lifting of Amnesia versus "Refreshing Memory"

Traditionally, hypnosis has been a widely used procedure to treat spontaneous amnesia. Similarly, when hypnosis has been used to treat traumatic neuroses, previously amnesic material would suddenly become accessible to consciousness, usually accompanied by profound affect as the patient relives the experience. As these internal emotions are relived, the patient's sudden awareness of a myriad of details becomes clear from the manner in which the events are reexperienced. The therapist, seeking to help the patient become aware of feelings, encourages the process of reexperiencing and allows the expression of affect to run its course. The therapist is careful to avoid interrupting the largely spontaneous experience of the patient; although he or she may well want to know more about some important details, questions are postponed in order not to interfere with the process.

It is characteristic of repressed memories that they suddenly come to consciousness as an entire experience rather than emerging detail by detail. In short, the procedure leads to a narrative exposition as the patient relives the experience. While there is no certainty about the historical accuracy of these memories, when they emerge largely spontaneously and without undue pressure, they are more likely to have been kept out of consciousness because of emotional reasons. To the extent that one is not dealing with the usual processes of forgetting but with material that is being kept out of awareness without having been forgotten, the likelihood of obtaining some accurate and important information seems greater. When the emotional blocks to recall are circumvented, one is more likely to obtain the important, and possibly accurate, information which had been remembered but kept out of consciousness than would be the case with neutral or irrelevant material that is forgotten over time.

Because these instances involved pathological conditions, the approach—even when legal issues were at stake—was essentially therapeutic, and hypnosis was carried out by psychologists or psychiatrists in the context of a traditional doctor–patient relationship. In contrast, hypnosis has more recently been used in circumstances where there is no evidence of pathological memory loss. Here, on the assumption that every memory is somehow recorded, hypnosis is purported to be simply a means of "refreshing memory." As such, it is claimed that there is no issue of therapy involved.

As a consequence, hypnotic technique is typically altered to prevent subjects from expressing intense feelings that would raise therapeutic issues and would tend to be frightening to lay observers. Thus, it is suggested to the subjects that they can visualize the events that they seek to recall on a special television screen; this screen can, as in televised sports events, move forward or backward through time, allowing events to be seen in instant replay, slow motion, or frame by frame. Further, it is explained to subjects that they need not experience any discomfort, that they are merely to observe the screen and see the events unfold—as if they were spectators rather than participants (e.g., Reiser, 1974). Suggestions are given, such as "It is just like watching a television show except that you not only can see it but you can control and even stop the motion; you can be there, but you need not experience pain or fear." Since hypnotic subjects who have been emotionally affected are wont to take the opportunity to relive the experience, there is often some struggle between the hypnotist attempting to keep the affect bottled up and the subject seeking to express it.

This type of "objective" reliving, rather than the "subjective" reliving generally encouraged by trained therapists, seems to bring forth fragmentary recall based not so much on the subject's reliving the experience as upon the hypnotist's detailed questions about what is occurring. Typically, the subject is repeatedly asked to "stop the film and look at the face carefully," and is then asked further questions about the details of the face. The same is generally done in relation to all potentially important details. Since this type of procedure involves a great many questions about details, it will, of course, elicit many more details than a narrative. By the same token, as the work summarized by Hilgard and Loftus (1979) has indicated, it will result in vastly lowered accuracy of the material obtained. Further, such a procedure maximizes the potential input of the hypnotist about what is wanted, making it even more likely that the subject's memories will more closely resemble the hypnotist's prior conceptions than would ordinarily be the case.

It is, of course, quite useful at times to use metaphors such as "stopping a videotape" and "instant replay" when working with hypnosis. However, no competent hypnotherapist would, in using such a metaphor, confuse it with the manner in which memory is organized. The therapist would also recognize that great pressure is thus being put on the subject to produce something, and the greater the pressure, the more likely the development of guided confabulations.

Unfortunately, no meaningful research is available to document the relative merit of facilitating the reliving of a traumatic event versus attempting to prevent the affect from being relived by using specific suggestions and questions to increase the amount of memory-like material being brought forth. Considerable experience in the clinical and forensic use of age regression and related techniques suggests that patients have a higher likelihood of producing uncontaminated memories if allowed initially to relive the events without much questioning by the hypnotist. Further details can then be elicited by questioning the second or third time the material is brought forth. It is interesting that the interrogation technique advocated by Loftus (1979), based on an entirely different body of data with waking eyewitnesses, is remarkably similar to that which evolved with hypnotic subjects.

The Effect of the Hypnotic Context on Refreshing of Memory

Although the effect of hypnosis is most clear-cut in the realm of memory when one is dealing with circumscribed areas of pathological amnesia, a dramatic lifting of amnesia (with which most laymen are familiar from its portrayal in films, novels, and the media) is the exception rather than the rule. With the increasing use of hypnosis, particularly with individuals *without* any obvious memory disturbance and *without* the ability to enter profound hypnosis, the clear demarcation between effects specific to hypnosis and what may occur in everyday interrogation with unhypnotized individuals becomes blurred. While there is no doubt that the kind of processes involved in hypnosis can also be shown to occur under many other circumstances and that the basic laws governing human memory are not negated because the individual is hypnotized, it would be quite wrong to assume that the hypnotic *procedure* brings about no important changes.

Some advocates of the wide use of "forensic hypnosis" have argued that we need not be concerned about the kinds of issues that have been described earlier, because these problems occur even in the waking state and are certainly negligible if the subject is only relaxed and not deeply hypnotized. It is ironic that this kind of disclaimer is made by the very persons who tout the unique effectiveness of hypnosis as an aid to criminal investigation. They cannot have it both ways! The reason hypnosis is used as a forensic tool is that it is effective in eliciting more details. This is so even with persons who are not particularly hypnotizable but who cooperate in the hypnotic situation. It is being in the hypnotic situation itself that may profoundly alter some aspects of the subjects' behavior and experience (London and Fuhrer, 1961). Thus, there is a strong expectancy that hypnosis will facilitate recall. Subjects in the hypnotic situation feel relaxed and less responsible for what they say since they believe that the hypnotist is both an expert and somehow in control. The hypnotist in turn makes certain that subjects cannot "fail." Hypnotic technique involves the extensive use of reinforcers through frequent verbalizations, such as, "Good," "Fine," "You are doing well," and so on, which are novel, satisfying, and reassuring, particularly in a police interrogation situation. Not surprisingly, subjects want to maintain the level of approbation; consequently, when the hypnotist stops the expressions of approval (simply by not saying "Good"), he or she clearly communicates that something else or something more is wanted. It requires only a modest decrease in the level of support to alter subjects' behavior, after which there is a return to the previous frequent level of reassurance. Similarly, in the relaxed and apparently benign context of hypnosis, subjects may be generally less anxious and less critical—allowing themselves to produce bits of information about which they are uncertain but which may in fact be accurate and important—information that would not be forthcoming in contexts where the subjects are made to feel responsible for their memories and challenged about their consistency. Thus, one might say that the hypnotic situation itself serves to change the subject's "guessing strategy."

To date, little systematic research has sought to distinguish between different kinds of effects that the hypnotic situation may exert on recall. Some mechanisms may require a profound level of hypnosis and relate primarily to the recall of material which is actively kept out of awareness; other mechanisms may be involved in the recall of meaningful details in emotionally neutral contexts.

Finally, there are aspects of the hypnotic situation that are not related to hypnotic depth, but nonetheless facilitate the increased reporting and acceptance of detailed information. For example, once a series of details is reported and accepted as valid by the hypnotist, that very fact serves to help convince the subject about the accuracy of these memories—memories that might previously have been extremely tentative and about which the subject had little or no subjective conviction. While there has not been much systematic exploration of the means by which the hypnotic context itself may alter the experience of persons who are only lightly hypnotized, from a pragmatic point of view it is necessary to recognize that these effects exist and may be profound. While careful research will be needed to clarify precisely which kinds of subjects— under what circumstances, relating to what kinds of memories, and in response to which specific techniques—will be more or less likely to yield reliable information, in the absence of such data it seems best to illustrate these issues in a life context by a selective review of relevant legal cases.

The Use of Hypnosis with Witnesses or Victims to Enhance Memory

Given the limitations of the hypnotic technique to facilitate recall, it becomes crucial to distinguish between apparently similar applications which in fact are very different and which consequently range from entirely appropriate to completely misleading. The key issue is not only the possible benefits that material obtained under hypnosis might accrue but also the need to assess the potential harm that would be caused by erroneous information. The use of hypnosis in an investigative context, with the sole purpose being to obtain leads, is clearly the area where hypnotic techniques are most appropriately employed. We will contrast the investigative use of hypnosis with other uses where the purpose is oriented not to the task of providing leads subject to verification but more to providing witnesses who can testify in court. We will show that as emphasis shifts away from the search for clues that will lead to reliable independent evidence and focuses more on helping to prepare witnesses to give eyewitness testimony, the difficulties that hypnosis creates for the administration of justice become increasingly greater. Thus, we will distinguish between (1) the situation where hypnosis is used exclusively to provide leads in a context where facts are not known, (2) a superficially similar situation insofar as the witness was originally hypnotized ostensibly for investigative purposes but where, in fact, he or she became an eyewitness and the only real evidence against the defendant, (3) the circumstances where there is no concern with the uncovering of details unknown to the investigating officer but only to help the witness remember what happened so that he or she is able to give eyewitness testimony, and (4) yet a different situation where a witness may have given a number of conflicting statements where hypnosis is utilized to "help the witness remember what really happened," but the search is not for the facts nor is the emphasis on independent verification. Rather there is an effort to use the hypnotic session itself as a means of verifying a witness's statement. The overall effect is to help the witness become reliable in his statements while reassuring both the authorities and the witness himself about the validity of these statements.

When Facts Are Not Known or Presumed

There are many cases involving victims or witnesses to crimes who cannot recall potentially important details and where the enforcement authorities are equally in the dark. In cases of assault, for example, hypnosis has made it possible for the victim to recall the assailant's appearance, enabling police artists to draw a reasonable likeness. To the extent that the victim or witness, police, artist, and hypnotist alike share no preconceived bias about what might have occurred, the situation approaches the ideal case for hypnosis to be most appropriately employed: to develop investigative leads.

Hypnotic suggestions may directly or indirectly enhance memory by providing contextual cues, and the relaxed environment of a sensitively conducted session may help diminish the anxiety which otherwise interferes with attempts to recall. Several cases of this type are described by Kroger and Doucé (1979). Many of the limitations of the technique—even in such circumstances—have been emphasized earlier, and other pitfalls are described by Kroger and Doucé. Given appropriate care, however, hypnosis has provided important new information to the authorities in many instances. If the sole purpose of the hypnotic session is to provide clues which ultimately lead to incriminating evidence, the fact that hypnosis was originally employed becomes irrelevant. However, if there is even the vaguest possibility that hypnotically enhanced recall is to be used in court, it is essential that the entire contact of the hypnotist with the subject be recorded on videotape to allow an independent assessment of the events preceding, during, and following the hypnotic session to determine whether the memories might have inadvertently been guided by cues in the situation.

When Witness Hypnotized to Obtain Facts Becomes Eyewitness

The investigative use of hypnosis involves helping a witness or victim remember additional details in an investigation, perhaps even to make eyewitness identifications. Sometimes additional information produced during hypnosis does not result in verifiable leads, though it may result in an eyewitness identification. In these circumstances, the temptation to utilize the witness as the basis for an indictment and prosecution often proves irresistible. The problems here transcend even the very difficult issues involved with all eyewitness testimony since the hypnotic procedure makes the hypnotized individual unduly responsive to suggestions, a process which can result in the creation of memories. A recent case in Illinois (People v. Kempinski, No. W80CF352, Cir. Ct., 12th Jud. Cir., Will Co., Ill. 12/21/80) illustrates this problem nicely. A young man was stabbed to death by two assailants in a residential suburb. By systematic canvassing, the police were able to determine that a young man had been sitting in a pickup truck facing in the right direction when the murder occurred at approximately 9:30 in the evening. When questioned, the young man indicated that he saw a man running toward him from a distance to a point which was approximately 250 feet away. He was being pursued by two others. The witness heard the sounds of a struggle when the three men were not in sight and then saw two figures running away. He was, however, unable to identify them because of the distance and the poor light. When hypnotized, he was told that he would be able to remember accurately everything that his visual system had seen, that he would be able to see things occurring on a screen which was like the videotape of a sporting event. It would allow him to speed up, slow down, or bring to a total stop what had happened. He could reverse and zoom in on all events. The subject described the scene and was asked to stop the motion while one of the presumed assailants was turned toward him. While he said he could not identify him initially, he then zoomed in on the assailant and brought him right up to where he was sitting; at that point he indicated that he could identify him. In fact, he first described him as ugly, then as short, later as normal, and then as tall, and eventually said he had known the individual in high school, that the assailant was a senior when he was a sophomore. He also indicated approximately where he lived. He then picked the presumed individual out of some mug books. Although there was no other apparent independent evidence to indicate that the suspect had been at the scene of the crime or was the actual murderer, he was nonetheless indicted and brought to trial.

This case is unusual because it was possible to demonstrate with the aid of a research ophthalmologist, appropriate weather charts, and studies of the available light at that time of the evening that the only kind of vision possible would be the relatively inefficient achromatic rod vision. The ability of the eye to resolve an image is sufficiently limited that it would be virtually impossible to identify a face beyond 30 feet, whereas the assailants had never been closer than well over 200 feet!

Thus, while in all instances hypnotically aided recall is an amalgam of actual recollection and confabulation, the extent to which one or the other factor predominates is all but impossible to determine outside of a laboratory experiment. In this situation, however, since true visual perception could not have taken place, the identification must have been based on confabulation, a point that was acknowledged by both the prosecution and defense experts. It was also possible for me to point to other clear inconsistencies of the apparent recall. The defendant had dropped out of high school in his sophomore year and could not have been the individual whom the witness remembered as having been a senior when he was a sophomore. His home also was in a very different area from where the witness had said he lived.

This case is particularly striking because of the fortuitous circumstances which made it obvious that the witness could not be testifying from his memory of the original event. It is worth noting, however, that he claimed to be testifying from his waking recall of the original events, obviously demonstrating the fallacy of accepting a witness's assurances in this regard after a hypnotic session. Further, the defendant was brought to trial solely on the unverified eyewitness identification which had occurred only during hypnosis. While in this instance it was possible to prove that the hypnotically created pseudomemory could not possibly be true recall, if by chance the assailant had run past the pickup truck where the witness was sitting, precisely the same psychological processes could have taken place but it would have been considerably more difficult to show the inherent problems created by the hypnotic session. In fact, no unverified hypnotic testimony should ever be permitted in court, and assertions by the waking individual that he actually had remembered the events prior to hypnosis are worthless because the witness is not in a position to determine whether that is or is not the case.

When Significant Facts Are Known or Presumed

An increasing number of instances are finding their way into law courts where hypnosis is used to help "refresh" the memory of a witness or victim about aspects of a crime which are known to the authorities, the media, or the hypnotist and may involve presumed facts that in one way or another have been made available to the subject. Of course, witnesses or victims cannot testify on such matters unless they are able to remember them personally. Particularly when the interrogation focuses on some relevant detail and involves leading questions is there the greatest likelihood of mischief. A "memory" can be created in hypnosis where none existed before. While cases of this type were once rare, there has been a dramatic increase in recent years. Although the sources of the factual information may vary widely, all these cases have the quality that information is somehow introduced into subjects' memories which causes them to testify to the facts as if they were based on prior memories.

A Pennsylvania case, United States v. Andrews, Gen. Ct. Martial No. 75-14, N.E. Jud. Cir., Navy/Marine Corps Judiciary, Phila., Pa., 10/6/75, illustrates the kind of problem that may occur. Two seamen recuperating from illness were working in an office when a sailor appeared in the doorway, aimed a pistol at one of the sailors, shot at his head, and fled the scene. Fortunately, the intended victim moved quickly and suffered only a grazing wound to the ear. When the seamen were shown pictures of persons who might fit the description and could have been in the area, the victim was unable to identify anyone. The witness, however, identified one of the pictures as that of the assailant. Subsequently, at a preliminary hearing, the victim was present when the witness identified the defendant as the assailant. The victim, however, indicated that the accused looked like but was not the assailant. The victim was then hypnotized on two occasions by an experienced Navy psychiatrist to facilitate his recall. During the first session, he was still unable to make an identification; however, during the second session he claimed to recognize the defendant who had previously been identified by the witness as the assailant.

At the general court-martial, the issue of the role of hypnosis was raised by the defense and I was asked to testify as an expert. My testimony pointed out that the victim's reaction to hypnosis would probably have been the same whether or not he could actually remember the assailant. Thus, if he continued to be unable to remember him—which was highly likely considering the difficulties encountered in eliciting the recollection—he would have been prone to confabulate an individual who appeared to be the most likely candidate. He had seen the defendant accused during the preliminary hearing, was aware that the witness had identified him with certainty, and knew also that it was the general belief of the prosecution that the defendant was guilty. The hypnotic session altered the victim's memory and, while he would now testify to what he erroneously believed his original memory to have been, he was in fact testifying on the basis of what he had been led to recall during hypnosis, which was quite different from his actual earlier memories.

In this instance, the military judge ruled as a matter of law that the victim could testify to those things that he had previously testified to but that since his memory was altered by hypnosis he was not permitted to identify the defendant. In the weeks following this event, two persons who had left for overseas the evening of the incident returned from Germany and independently corroborated the defendant's alibi, making it extremely unlikely that he was the actual assailant. In this case, it is interesting that the effect of hypnosis on the victim's memory persisted, and well over a year after the event he still asserted his conviction that the defendant had in fact fired the shot which nearly killed him.

Another example is a recent capital case in Milwaukee, Wisconsin, State v. White. No. J-3665, Cir. Ct., Branch 10, Milwaukee Co., Wis.,

3/27/79. A 20-year-old Indian girl nicknamed "Sweetie Pie" had been found strangled several years before. The case had not been solved but had raised considerable attention and concern and had not been closed. Sometime later, another girl reported to the police that her boyfriend had beaten her several times and she wanted him to seek psychiatric help. When questioned, she admitted that on occasion he had choked her, presumably in an attempt to frighten her. The authorities became more interested at that point, particularly when it turned out that the boyfriend, also an Indian, had known "Sweetie Pie." At that point, the girlfriend became uncooperative because she had wanted only to induce the boyfriend to seek treatment and had no wish to have him become involved with the police. On further investigation, however, it was found that the boyfriend did not have an alibi for the time in question, and the authorities talked at length with his former wife, from whom he had been separated about a year, and her sister. Both women had lived with the defendant and had children by him.

The wife, who maintained some relationship with the defendant, was not particularly helpful to the authorities, but the sister, who was felt to be more willing to discuss matters, was interviewed on several occasions by police officers. She was asked whether she had been beaten up and indicated that there were times when this had occurred but claimed that she could not remember much else. When it was suggested that she and the former wife participate in a hypnotic session, they agreed to do so. The hypnotic session was carried out by a well-trained psychologist. Prior to hypnosis, he showed a gruesome picture of the dead body to the sister, who had also been a close friend of the murdered girl. He then induced hypnosis, and shortly thereafter said,

> For the moment I want you to think about just you and me and Sweetie Pie, who got strangled, thrown out on the road, taken to the morgue, put in a box, and buried in the ground. Now somebody did that. I don't know who, but you know that Joe White is a suspect in this case, don't you? Do you think that there is any reason why Joe White should or should not be a suspect in this case?

At the end of the session, which included an age regression-like procedure that did not work very well despite the subject's otherwise good response to hypnosis, there was a posthypnotic suggestion given that she would be thinking about telling the truth, how good it would feel to tell the truth, and that she was going to tell the truth. Within a week after the session, the sister called the police and told them how the defendant had often choked her, that he seemed to enjoy it, and that one time shortly after the murder he was choking her and said something to the effect, "If you don't behave, the same thing can happen to you that happened to Sweetie Pie." When she asked whether he had killed "Sweetie Pie," he allegedly broke down crying and said that he had not intended to but admitted that he had.

The case against the defendant was primarily based upon the sister's hearsay testimony which became available shortly after the hypnotic session. After a lengthy hearing, the court ruled that as a matter of law she could not testify before a jury because, thanks to the hypnotic session, the presumed memory was likely to have been created rather than remembered. It is unlikely that anyone will ever know for certain whether the defendant was or was not responsible for the murder. There was no doubt in the sister's mind, however, as to the kind of memory which was wanted, and the sister was amply motivated to testify against the defendant. She had continued to live with the defendant, supposedly knowing that he was a murderer, for many months until he rejected her. Consequently, her testimony would have been totally discounted if it had not come after the hypnotic session. The court recognized the danger of permitting hypnosis to be used in a context where it is more likely to create a memory than to refresh it.

Whereas in the first case the identity of the defendant became known to the victim during a pretrial hearing, and in the second case the nature of the memory was shaped by conversations with the police officers, with the sister, and particularly by the way the hypnotic session was conducted, it is equally possible for the suggestion about what to recall to come from entirely different sources unrelated to and long before hypnosis. For example, in the Minnesota case of State v. Mack, Dist. Ct., 4th Jud. Dist., Hennepin Co., Minn. (1979), a physician insisting that a laceration must have been made by a knife led to a total reorganization of an apparent victim's memory about how she had acquired an internal wound. In other cases, the media have provided the critical information, while in still others, the manner in which a lineup was conducted facilitated the creation of "memories" at hypnotic sessions conducted at a later date (e.g., State v. Peterson, No. CCR 79-003, Cir. Ct., Hamilton Co., Ind., 7/12/79).

In addition to criminal cases, it is not uncommon to find something of this kind in civil cases where persons are helped by hypnosis to remember details of accidents they had been unable to recall previously. By the time hypnosis is carried out, it is generally clear to subjects which of possible events that might have occurred would be most helpful to their particular cases. Although accurate information may be recovered, the important effects that motivation can exert on memory—hypnotically enhanced or otherwise—must be taken into account in assessing the "memories" obtained.

When Reliability of Witness's Statement Is to Be Affirmed

Many witnesses are unreliable in the sense that they tell somewhat different stories each time they are asked to tell what occurred. These differences may relate to important details of the crime. The adversary system upon which Anglo-Saxon justice is based relies upon cross-examination as the means of unmasking the unreliability of witnesses before the finder of fact.

The effect of hypnotizing witnesses of this kind, presumably to help refresh their memories, is generally dramatic. Even if the subject is not particularly responsive to hypnosis, reviewing the events in the hypnotic context and having the memories legitimized by the hypnotist generally fixes one particular version of the testimony in the witness's mind which is then faithfully and reliably reproduced every time. In these cases, hypnosis does not serve to produce any new information, but the procedure can bolster a witness whose credibility would easily have been destroyed by cross-examination but who now becomes quite impervious to such efforts, repeating one particular version of the story with great conviction.

To appreciate the effect of hypnosis in these kinds of cases, it is important to view the use of the technique in its broader perspectives. Often it will involve a witness about whom the prosecution has considerable doubts. In one California case (*In re Milligan*, No. J-17617, Super. Ct., Monterey, Calif., 6/29/78), for example, the prosecution's star witness was a 14-year-old girl who had told many different stories to the police at different times and readily changed her story during early depositions. Indeed, she repeatedly stated that it was impossible for her to say whether her recollections were a dream or represented actual events. The case involved the murder of the witness's aunt, sister, grandmother, and cousin, and there was some serious question as to the degree of possible criminal involvement of the witness herself.

The witness was hypnotized and again told her story to the district attorney and the police. However, now it was during hypnosis, which everyone agreed would reliably help her recall and she would know whether her memories related to real events or to her dreams. Simply carrying out the hypnotic session committed the prosecution to the view that the witness was not criminally involved since it would not be permissible for the state to hypnotize a defendant—especially a minor. Somehow the witness became reassured that she would be safe and her story became remarkably stable, virtually unshakable on cross-examination.

In a real sense, the hypnotic procedure also helped change the prosecution's attitude toward the witness. She was accepted as having no part in the crime, and instead of being considered an unreliable juvenile, became an exceedingly effective witness whose testimony led to the conviction of the other individuals involved. This was so despite the fact that the story she produced under hypnosis and on subsequent occasions contained a number of incorrect statements recognized as such by the hypnotist but ignored. Hypnosis had not resulted in accurate memories, but rather had served to produce consistent memories. Further, the technique served to reassure the law enforcement officials that the witness was in fact telling the truth, an aspect which was perhaps as important as the effect the hypnotic session had in stabilizing the witness's recollections.

The confounding effects of hypnosis in altering the views of the law enforcement agencies as well as the perceived credibility of the witness testifying before the finder of fact makes it essential that the use of hypnosis be disclosed to the other side whenever a witness has been hypnotized. Below I will spell out some relatively simple safeguards that must be adhered to in order to be able to assess the effect of hypnosis in a given case. Thus, unless proper videotape recordings are available of the hypnotic session as well as the interviews preceding and immediately following it, no witness who has been hypnotized should be allowed to testify.

The Consequences That Follow from the Inappropriate Use of Hypnosis

The attitude of law enforcement agencies toward the use of hypnosis is an important factor in the problems that may arise. In the case of State v. White (1979), referred to earlier, a senior law enforcement official was asked under oath about his views of hypnotically aided testimony and he succinctly expressed widely held beliefs when he testified that hypnosis lends "credibility and strength to your investigation." Perhaps the most interesting, as well as the most frightening, consequence of this belief is illustrated by a New Jersey case (State v. Douglas 1978). A woman was stopped at a light and two black men entered the car and forced her at gunpoint to drive to a deserted place on the outskirts of town. When they arrived there, the man in the front seat attempted to rape the woman. When she protested that she was pregnant, the man on the back seat with the gun told the attacker to stop. They took the woman's purse, made her leave the car, and threatened her that if she contacted the police, terrible things would happen to her family. On getting back to her home, the woman immediately reported the attempted rape, as well as the theft of her car and valuables. At the police station, she was shown mug shots and she identified one man and picked out another as a look-alike. Subsequently, she received several threatening notes which were turned over to the police. She continued to be unable to identify the second man involved in the crime, and finally the police persuaded her to undergo hypnosis. Although the police had videotape as well as audiotape recording equipment available, it was claimed that the equipment would not work, and hypnosis was carried out without any objective record of what occurred. During the hypnotic session, however, the victim identified the look-alike as the man who was involved in the crime.

It turned out that the district attorney had been quite skeptical about the case but was finally convinced to prosecute by the hypnotic session. It was only after the hypnotic session that indictments were brought against the two suspects. However, it was impossible for the defense to find out the details of what had occurred during the hypnotic session. As one might anticipate, the descriptions by the investigating officer and the district attorney of the events were quite different, and there was simply no way of ascertaining what had actually occurred. Nonetheless, when the district attorney learned that the use of hypnosis would be vigorously challenged and that the public defender's office was prepared to use this case as a vehicle to prevent the use of hypnosis by the police, she decided to have another look at the facts of the case. She was struck by the peculiarity of the handwriting in the threatening notes, and for the first time submitted these to a handwriting expert who identified the writing as that of the woman who had filed the charges. When the alleged victim was confronted with this fact, she confessed that there had never been an attempted assault, that she had never met the two men whom she had accused, and that she had generated the complaint and the threatening notes in an effort to reawaken the interest of her husband, who was in the process of filing divorce proceedings against her.

The appalling aspect of this case is that it was the hypnotic sessions that initially prompted the district attorney to cast doubt aside and proceed with the prosecution. The hypnotically enhanced memories would have been the basis for the victim's testimony and might well have led to the conviction of two innocent, individuals who happened to have been in the collection of photographs available to the police and did not have excellent alibis. It was only when the district attorney became aware that the defense would have apppropriate expert help to challenge the totally inappropriate way in which hypnosis was employed in this case that a more careful review of the evidence, uncovered the true state of affairs. Far from being helpful to the prosecution, the manner in which hypnosis was employed actually served to confuse the authorities.

THE ROLE OF THE EXPERT IN FORENSIC HYPNOSIS

It is not possible in a single essay to more than touch upon the complex issues involved in the forensic use of hypnosis. However, it behooves those of us experienced in the clinical use of hypnosis to exercise extreme care when we use our skills in a forensic context. We should keep in mind that psychologists and psychiatrists are not particularly adept at recognizing deception. We generally arrange the social context of treatment so that it is not in the patient's interest to lie to us, and we appropriately do not concern ourselves with this issue since in most therapeutic contexts it is helpful for the therapist to see the world through the patient's eyes in order ultimately to help him view it more realistically. (See Lindner, 1955, for a superb description of the kind of countertransference which leads to the uncritical acceptance of the patient's views that, on the one hand, makes treatment possible but, on the other, can be a source of serious difficulties.)

As a rule, the average hotel credit manager is considerable more adept at recognizing deception than we are. Not only does his livelihood depend upon limiting errors of judgment, but he is in a position to obtain feedback concerning those errors of judgment, whereas in most treatment contexts the therapist is neither affected by being deceived nor even likely later to learn that he or she has been deceived. While military psychiatrists and other health professionals who are required to make dispositional judgments on a daily basis do become adept at recognizing manipulation and deception, only a few health professionals who are experienced in the use of hypnosis have had this type of background. Consequently, they have little experience or concern about being deceived or used. On the other hand, a defendant in a murder trial or, for that matter, a witness or a victim in a crime of violence may well have an axe to grind, and it is essential for us to recognize that in a forensic context the unwary expert witness may become a pawn either for the prosecution or for the defense. With the increasing popularity of hypnosis in the courts, it is essential that those of us who have an interest in these matters develop the necessary sophistication and judgment in the forensic context, much as we have had to acquire it in the therapeutic context. It would be foolhardy indeed to assume that familiarity with one context is sufficient to allow us to function effectively in the other. On the contrary, the ground rules governing the two situations are vastly different, and we must guard against being co-opted—wittingly or unwittingly—by prosecution or defense.

The use of hypnosis and related techniques to facilitate memory raises profound, complex questions, and it is likely that the individual will be protected only if these issues are dealt with at the highest level of our court system. There are instances when hypnosis can be used appropriately provided that the nature of the phenomenon is understood by all parties concerned. It must be recognized, however, that the use of hypnosis by either the prosecution or the defense can profoundly affect the individual's subsequent testimony. Since these changes are not reversible, if individuals are to be allowed to testify after having undergone hypnosis to aid their memory, a minimum number of safeguards are absolutely essential. Based upon extensive review of the field and my own experiences in a considerable number of circumstances, I have proposed the following minimal safeguards in an affidavit (Orne, 1978) in the case of *Quaglino v. California* which was filed with the Supreme Court of the United States (*cert. den.*, 99 S. Ct. 212 [1978]).

1. Hypnosis should be carried out by a psychiatrist or psychologist with special training in its use. He should not be informed about the facts of the case verbally; rather, he should receive a written memorandum outlining whatever facts he is to know, carefully avoiding any other communication which might affect his opinion. Thus, his beliefs and possible bias can be evaluated. It is extremely undesirable for the individual conducting the hypnotic sessions to have any involvement in the investigation of the case. Further he should be an independent professional and not responsible to the prosecution or the investigators.

2. All contact of the psychiatrist or psychologist with the individual to be hypnotized should be videotaped from the moment they meet until the entire interaction is completed. The casual comments which are passed before or after hypnosis are every bit as important to get on tape as the hypnotic session itself. (It is possible to give suggestions prior to the induction of hypnosis which will act as posthypnotic suggestions.)

Prior to the induction of hypnosis, a brief evaluation of the patient should be carried out and the psychiatrist or psychologist should then elicit a detailed description of the facts as the witness or victim remembers them. This is important because individuals often are able to recall a good deal more while talking to a psychiatrist or psychologist than when they are with an investigator, and it is important to have a record of what the witness's beliefs are before hypnosis. Only after this has been completed should the hypnotic session be initiated. The psychiatrist or psychologist should strive to avoid adding any new elements to the witnesses's description of his experience, including those which he had discussed in his wake state, lest he inadvertently alter the nature of the witness's memories—or constrain them by reminding him of his waking memories.

3. No one other than the psychiatrist or psychologist and the individual to be hypnotized should be present in the room before and dur-

ing the hypnotic session. This is important because it is all too easy for observers to inadvertently communicate to the subject what they expect, what they are startled by, or what they are disappointed by. If either the prosecution or the defense wish to observe the hypnotic session, they may do so without jeopardizing the integrity of the session through a one-way screen or on a television monitor.

4. Because the interactions which have preceded the hypnotic session may well have a profound effect on the sessions themselves, tape recordings of prior interrogations are important to document that a witness had not been implicitly or explicitly cued pertaining to certain information which might then be reported for apparently the first time by the witness during hypnosis. (Orne, 1978, pp. 853–55)

Guidelines based upon these safeguards have been adopted by the courts in the State v. White (cited earlier), and in the *State of New Jersey v. Hurd,* 173 N.J. Super. 353, 362–63 (1980), and judicial notice has been taken of these guidelines by the Supreme Court of Minnesota in *State v. Mack* (cited earlier), and by the Supreme court of Massachusetts (Commonwealth v. A Juvenile, S.2160, Supreme Judicial Court [1980]).

SUMMARY AND CONCLUSIONS

An effort has been made to outline some of the major issues that must be considered for the forensic use of hypnosis, and particularly if hypnotically enhanced recall is to be used in court. It is possible to document, as has been done here, some of the circumstances where hypnosis has worked against the judicial process. Much of what has been said about memory and hypnosis in this essay has already been documented empirically; however, further rigorous research is needed. Future work will need to direct itself to the task of spelling out the circumstances under which the likelihood of confabulation is maximized, the specific effects which result from the hypnotist's preconceptions, the consequences of allowing the reexperiencing of relevant affect as opposed to suppressing it during the process of recall, the different effects which hypnosis may have on the recall of different kinds of material on the one hand and on the other to assess whether hypnosis has different effects in facilitating recall of material that was purposively learned as opposed to that incidentally noted. At the present state of knowledge, it is relatively easy to point to some clear-cut abuses and try to identify some relatively safe and appropriate applications of hypnosis. As serious research addresses the question of the effect of hypnosis and the hypnotic context on memory, it will become possible to be increasingly specific about other circumstances where hypnosis may play a legitimate role as opposed to those where its use will serve only to further confuse an already blind justice.

ABSTRACT

Hypnosis may be helpful in the context of criminal investigation and under circumstances involving functional memory loss. Hypnosis is not useful in assuring truthfulness since, particularly in a forensic context, subjects may simulate hypnosis and are able to lie wilfully even in deep hypnosis; most troublesome, actual memories cannot be distinguished from confabulations—pseudomemories where plausible fantasy has replaced gaps in recall—either by the subject or by the hypnotist without full and independent corroboration. While potentially useful to refresh witnesses' and victims' memories to facilitate eyewitness identification, the procedure is relatively safe and appropriate only when neither the subject nor the authorities nor the hypnotist has any preconceptions about the events under investigation. If such preconceptions do exist, hypnosis may readily cause the subject to confabulate the person who is suspected into his "hypnotically enhanced memories." These pseudomemories, originally developed in hypnosis, may come to be accepted by the subject as his actual recall of the original events; they are then remembered with great subjective certainty and reported with conviction. Such circumstances can *create* convincing, apparently objective "eyewitnesses" rather than facilitating actual recall. Minimal safeguards are proposed to reduce the likelihood of such an eventuality and other serious potential abuses of hypnosis.

ACKNOWLEDGMENTS

For their help in clarifying the issues involved, I wish to thank especially my colleagues at the Unit for Experimental Psychiatry: Emily Carota Orne, David F. Dinges, William M. Waid, William H. Putnam. Special appreciation is due to John F. Kihlstrom and Robert A. Karlin for their substantive suggestions. I am particularly grateful to Nancy K. Bauer, Lani Pyles MacAniff, Joanne Rosellini, and Mae C. Weglarski for their assistance in the editing, formatting, and referencing during the preparation of this manuscript.

BIBLIOGRAPHY

Barber, Theodore X. 1961. "Antisocial and Criminal Acts Induced by 'Hypnosis': A Review of Experimental and Clinical Findings," *Archives of General Psychiatry* 5:301–12.

Bartlett, Frederick C. 1932. *Remembering.* Cambridge: Cambridge University Press.

Breuer, J., and S. Freud. [1895] 1955. *Studies on Hysteria.* Vol. 2. *The Standard Edition of the Complete Psychological Works of Sigmund Freud,* ed. and trans. J. Strachey. London: Hogarth Press.

Coe, William C., K. Kobayashi, and M. L. Howard. 1972. "An Approach toward Isolating Factors that Influence Antisocial Conduct in Hypnosis," *International Journal of Clinical and Experimental Hypnosis* 20:118–31.

Conn, Jacob H. 1972. "Is Hypnosis Really Dangerous?" *International Journal of Clinical and Experimental Hypnosis* 20:61–79.

Cooper, Leslie M., and P. London. 1973. "Reactivation of Memory by Hypnosis and Suggestion," *International Journal of Clinical and Experimental Hypnosis* 21:312–23.

Dhanens, Thomas P., and R. M. Lundy. 1975. "Hypnotic and Waking Suggestions and Recall," *International Journal of Clinical and Experimental Hypnosis* 23:68–79.

Ellenberger, Henri F. 1970. *The Discovery of the Unconscious.* New York: Basic Books.

Evans, Frederick, and J. F. Kihlstrom. 1973. "Posthypnotic Amnesia as Disrupted Retrieval," *Journal of Abnormal Psychology* 82:317–23.

Hilgard, Ernest R. 1977. *Divided Consciousness: Multiple Controls in Human Thought and Action.* New York: Wiley.

Hilgard, Ernest R., and E. F. Loftus. 1979. "Effective Interrogation of the Eyewitness," *International Journal of Clinical and Experimental Hypnosis* 27:342–57.

Jenkins, James J. 1974. "Remember that Old Theory of Memory? Well, Forget It!" *American Psychologist* 29:785–95.

Kihlstrom, John F., and F. J. Evans. 1976. "Recovery of Memory After Posthypnotic Amnesia," *Journal of Abnormal Psychology* 85:564–69.

Kihlstrom, John F., and F. J. Evans. 1977. "Residual Effects of Suggestion for Posthypnotic Amnesia: A Reexamination," *Journal of Abnormal Psychology* 86:327–33.

Kline, Milton V. 1972. "The Production of Antisocial Behavior Through Hypnosis: New Clinical Data," *International Journal of Clinical and Experimental Hypnosis* 20:80–94.

Kline, Milton V. 1979. "Defending the Mentally Ill: The Insanity Defense and the Role of Forensic Hypnosis," *International Journal of Clinical and Experimental Hypnosis* 27:375–401.

Kline, Milton V., and H. Guze. 1951. "The Use of a Drawing Technique in the Investigation of Hypnotic Age Regression and Progression," *British Journal of Medical Hypnotism* Winter:1–12.

Kroger, William S. 1977. *Clinical and Experimental Hypnosis.* 2d ed. Philadelphia: Lippincott.

Kroger, W. S., and R. G. Doucé. 1979. "Hypnosis in Criminal Investigation," *International Journal of Clinical and Experimental Hypnosis* 27:358–74.

Lindner, Robert. 1955. *The Fifty-Minute Hour.* New York: Rinehart and Farrar.

Loftus, Elizabeth F. 1979. *Eyewitness Testimony.* Cambridge, Mass.: Harvard University Press.

London, Perry, and M. Fuhrer. 1961. "Hypnosis, Motivation and Performance," *Journal of Personality* 29:321–33.

Nace, E. P., M. T. Orne, and A. G. Hammer. 1974. "Posthypnotic Amnesia as an Active Psychic Process," *Archives of General Psychiatry* 31:357–60.

O'Connell, Donald N., R. E. Shor, and M. T. Orne. 1970. "Hypnotic Age Regression: An Empirical and Methodological Analysis," *Journal of Abnormal Psychology* 76:1–32 (Monograph Supplement no. 3, pt. 2).

Orne, Martin T. 1951. "The Mechanisms of Hypnotic Age Regression: An Experimental Study," *Journal of Abnormal Psychology* 46:213–25.

Orne, Martin T. 1959. "The Nature of Hypnosis: Artifact and Essence," *Journal of Abnormal and Social Psychology* 58:277–99.

Orne, Martin T. 1962. "Antisocial Behavior and Hypnosis: Problems of Control and Validation in Empirical Studies." Paper presented at Colgate University Hypnosis Symposium, Hamilton, N.Y., April 1960.

Orne, Martin T. 1961. "The Potential Uses of Hypnosis in Interrogation." In *The Manipulation of Human Behavior*, ed. Albert D. Biderman and H. Zimmer, pp. 169–215. New York: Wiley.

Orne, Martin T. 1962. "Antisocial Behavior and Hypnosis: Problems of Control and Validation in Empirical Studies." In *Hypnosis: Current Problems*, ed. George H. Estabrooks, pp. 137–92. New York: Harper and Row.

Orne, Martin T. 1966. "On the Mechanisms of Posthypnotic Amnesia," *International Journal of Clinical and Experimental Hypnosis* 14:121–34.

Orne, Martin T. 1969. "On the Nature of the Posthypnotic Suggestion." In *Psychophysiological Mechanisms of Hypnosis*, ed. Leon Chertok, pp. 173–92. Berlin: Springer-Verlag.

Orne, Martin T. 1971. "The Disappearing Hypnotist: The Use of Simulating Subjects," *International Journal of Clinical and Experimental Hypnosis* 19:277–96.

Orne, Martin T. 1972a. "Can a Hypnotized Subject be Compelled to Carry Out Otherwise Unacceptable Behavior? A Discussion," *International Journal of Clinical and Experimental Hypnosis* 20:101–17.

Orne, Martin T. 1972b. "On the Simulating Subject as a Quasi-Control Group in Hypnosis Research: What, Why and How." In *Hypnosis: Research Developments and Perspectives*, ed. Erika Fromm and R. E. Shor, pp. 399–443. Chicago: Aldine-Atherton.

Orne, Martin T. 1977. "The Construct of Hypnosis: Implications of the Definition for Research and Practice," *Annals of the New York Academy of Science* 296:14–33.

Orne, Martin T. 1978. Affidavit of Amicus Curiae, *Quaglino v. California*, U.S. Sup. Ct. No. 77–1288, *cert. den.* 11/27/78. In *16th Annual Defending Criminal Cases: The Rapidly Changing Practice of Criminal Law*, chm. E. Margolin, 2:831–57. New York: Practising Law Institute.

Orne, Martin T., and F. J. Evans. 1965. "Social Control in the Psychological Experiment: Antisocial Behavior and Hypnosis," *Journal of Personality and Social Psychology* 1:189–200.

Orne, Martin T., P. W. Sheehan, and F. J. Evans. 1968. "Occurrence of Posthypnotic Behavior Outside the Experimental Setting," *Journal of Personality and Social Psychology* 9:189–96.

Putnam, W. H. 1979. "Hypnosis and Distortions in Eyewitness Memory," *International Journal of Clinical and Experimental Hypnosis* 27:437–48.

Reiff, Robert, and M. Scheerer. 1959. *Memory and Hypnotic Age Regression: Developmental Aspects of Cognitive Function Explored Through Hypnosis*. New York: International Universities Press.

Reiser, Martin. 1974. "Hypnosis as an Aid in a Homicide Investigation," *American Journal of Clinical Hypnosis* 17:84–87.

Roediger, H. L. 1979. "Implicit and Explicit Memory Models," *Bulletin of the Psychonomic Society* 13:339–42.

Sears, Alden B. 1954. "A Comparison of Hypnotic and Waking Recall," *International Journal of Clinical and Experimental Hypnosis* 2:296–304.

Sheehan, Peter W. 1972. *The Function and Nature of Imagery*. New York: Academic Press.

Sheehan, Peter W., and M. T. Orne. 1968. "Some Comments on the Nature of Posthypnotic Behavior," *Journal of Nervous and Mental Disease* 146:209–20.

Stalnaker, John M. and E. E. Riddle. 1932. "The Effect of Hypnosis on Long-Delayed Recall," *Journal of General Psychology* 6:429–40.

Watkins, John G. 1972. "Antisocial Behavior Under Hypnosis: Possible or Impossible?" *International Journal of Clinical and Experimental Hypnosis* 20:95–100.

White, Robert W., G. F. Fox, and W. W. Harris. 1940. "Hypnotic Hypermnesia for Recently Learned Material," *Journal of Abnormal and Social Psychology* 35:88–103.

VI

Special Topics in Forensic Psychiatry

14

The Problem of the Malingering Defendant

DANIEL W. SCHWARTZ

The title of this chapter may be somewhat misleading, for the malingering defendant really poses numerous problems. Such problems include, but are not limited to, the following: the identification of the malingerer; the proper handling of him in a correctional or detentional institution; the appropriate psychiatric treatment; an understanding of why certain people malinger and why those who do choose certain specific symptoms; and, last but not least, the problem of proving in a court of law that a defendant is, in fact, malingering. A discussion of all these problems would fill a good-sized book. Moreover, we would still not have an adequate understanding of the psychodynamics and ego psychology of the malingerer. In this chapter, then, I shall try briefly to present a picture of the malingerer, raise some legal problems, and suggest some practical solutions.

DEFINITION

The word *malinger* has been defined in various ways. According to *Webster's Third New International Dictionary,*[1] it comes from the French "malingre," meaning sickly or ailing. This in turn is assumed to derive from the Old French "mal" and "haingre," meaning badly and thin, lean. For many years it applied primarily to men who sought to evade

DANIEL W. SCHWARTZ • Department of Psychiatry, Downstate Medical Center, State University of New York, Brooklyn, New York 11203.

military duty. In recent times it has acquired a more general meaning. Thus, *Webster's* gives the following definition: "To pretend to be ill or otherwise physically or mentally incapacitated so as to avoid duty or work," with a malingering soldier as only one of several examples.

Webster's offers a second meaning, which involves more than mere fakery: "to deliberately induce, protract, or exaggerate actual illness or other incapacity so as to avoid duty or work." One well-recognized special dictionary, however, restricts its definition solely to pretense. *Black's Law Dictionary*[2] defines *malinger* as, "to feign sickness or any physical disablement or mental lapse or derangement, expecially for the purpose of escaping the performance of a task, duty or work." Campbell, in his *Psychiatric Dictionary*,[3] includes both concepts but in a more concise form than *Webster's:* "To feign or protract one's illness; to simulate, with intent to deceive."

DSM-III[4] classifies *"Malingering"* as a diagnostic entity under the heading, "Conditions Not Attributable to a Mental Disorder That Are a Focus of Attention or Treatment." Like *Webster's* and Campbell it includes in the meaning both pretense and exaggeration: "The essential feature is the voluntary production and presentation of false or grossly exaggerated physical or psychological symptoms." Having already classified the term "Factitious Disorder" as a genuine mental disorder and having defined it as the voluntary production of symptoms for the sole purpose of assuming the role of a patient, DSM-III now goes to great lengths to distinguish Malingering from Factitious Disorder. In *Malingering,*

> the symptoms are produced in pursuit of a goal that is obviously recognizable with an understanding of the individual's circumstances rather than of his or her individual psychology. Examples of such obviously understandable goals include: to avoid military conscription or duty, to avoid work, to obtain financial compensation, to evade criminal prosecution, or to obtain drugs. . . . The differentiation of Malingering from Factitious Disorder depends on the clinician's judgment as to whether the symptom production is in pursuit of a goal that is obviously recognizable and understandable in the circumstances. Individuals with Factitious Disorders have goals that are not recognizable in light of their specific circumstances but are understandable only in light of their psychology as determined by careful examination. . . the diagnosis of Factitious Disorder excludes the diagnosis of the act of Malingering.

IDENTIFICATION

The malingerer, then, is voluntarily pretending to be ill or exaggerating an already present illness with the intent to deceive others for obviously recognizable and practical reasons.

Although in the military and in work situations malingerers may often simulate physical incapacitation, the overwhelming majority of criminal defendants who malinger pretend to be mentally ill. The problem of identifying the malingering defendant as such is, therefore, primarily a psychiatric problem. It may be that he has actually fooled the court or the prison psychiatrists, or simply that they want an expert opinion to resolve any doubts or to confirm their own beliefs. In either case, the malingerer's simulation usually creates reasonable grounds for the ordering of a psychiatric examination.

The psychiatrist's task of identifying the malingerer is generally not an easy one. It requires, first of all, a reasonable degree of suspicion. For those of us in forensic psychiatry, it is almost incredible how easily the psychiatrists in civil hospitals can be fooled by a bare minimum of alleged symptomatology, as related, for example, in "On Being Sane in Insane Places."[5] The psychiatrist must also have a good knowledge of the signs and symptoms of genuine mental illness, for this is the yardstick against which he must measure the clinical picture presented by the defendant. In addition, he should have proper training and experience with criminal defendants and must know the criteria for the legal issue at hand. Whether a defendant is malingering or genuinely mentally ill is immaterial if he can meet these legal criteria. On the other hand, certain criminal defendants may undergo Adjustment Disorders due to the special combination of their personality disorders and the particular stresses involved in being a criminal defendant, and the form their illnesses take may not fully coincide with the classic pictures of mental illness. Nevertheless, they may be genuine and must be distinguished from malingering.

Exactly how one goes about examining a suspected malingerer is a very difficult question to answer. Like all psychiatric examinations it undoubtedly must vary from one psychiatrist to another, depending on the psychiatrist's personality and his ability to tolerate what he believes is malingering. Some psychiatrists, whether they realize it or not, will be offended by the attempted fakery and will be harsh and punitive toward such a defendant. Others will enjoy the challenge and will react in a soft and seductive manner. If a psychiatrist is retained by the court or the prosecution, he must be able to examine a defendant in the presence of defense counsel, for in most jurisdictions counsel has every right to be present. (Actually, if the defendant consults with and obeys counsel during a fitness to proceed examination, this is one of the best arguments that he can assist in his defense. Similarly, if on advice of counsel he conceals certain aspects of his life in a criminal responsibility examination, this will cast great doubt on the genuineness of a psychiatric issue.)

Most psychiatrists are probably unaware how often they ask leading questions in the early stages of the examination, but this is a definite error. To ask a defendant at this point if he hears voices, if people are trying to kill him, if his thoughts are being broadcast, if he feels like taking his own life, etc., is to give him too early in the examination a clear example of psychiatric pathology. The best way to conduct such an examination is to ask open-ended questions about his present legal situation (e.g., "What's this all about?" "What's a nice guy like you doing in a situation like this?") and his past history (e.g., "Tell me whatever you can about your past life," "What do you think is important about your past?"), and leave it to him to make the first statements of possible pathology. Then one can ask further questions along this line to see if there are signs and symptoms that substantiate the alleged pathology. Only after all this has been done should one ask, for the sake of completeness, what amounts to a Review of Systems of possible mental illness. If pathology shows up for the first time at this point, one can legitimately question how genuine or incapacitating it really is. Whenever possible, one should inquire of other, reliable sources, for example, nurses, correction officers, as to the defendant's daily functioning and whether it conforms with his alleged pathology.

Occasionally, the evidence that a defendant is malingering will be discovered fortuitously.

> A young man who had been arrested for a series of robberies of Park Avenue dentists' offices presented himself as though he were facing charges of rape. (It is probably not mere chance that he was pretending to have been arrested on such charges; quite likely it reflected his unconscious, or perhaps even conscious, fear of the homosexual environment that prison represented.) He also claimed that he had been acting under the command of a certain angel, the angel of either patience or patients, for as he spoke the word it was impossible for me to tell which. In my desire for accuracy, I asked him how it was spelt, with a *ce* or a *ts*. Believing that I had seen through his act, he angrily responded with a "f--k you," terminated the examination, and pled guilty the next day.

There will always be some malingerers who will succeed in fooling psychiatrists, and any psychiatrist who thinks otherwise is himself a fool. It is this very fact that makes it impossible to estimate how often malingering occurs. Conversely, in order to avoid the shame of being labeled mentally ill, a certain number of those whom we have so diagnosed will later claim that they were only malingering, but whether or not they were really voluntarily simulating symptoms at the time of the examination, we shall never know. The problem becomes even more complex because, DSM-III notwithstanding, some defendants undoubtedly are both mentally ill and malingering.

To diagnose a defendant as malingering is, in substance, to accuse him of lying. Doing this may seem distasteful and unprofessional to many psychiatrists, and in most cases there are alternatives. When the legal issue is criminal responsibility, that is, a state of mind in the past, one can just as easily conclude that the apparently psychotic picture he now portrays of himself at that time is the result of a faulty, wish-fulfilling memory, what I call retrospective falsification. In other words, without intentionally fabricating, the defendant, like any of us, is prone to recall things in a more favorable, self-serving light. If the legal issue is fitness to proceed, very often the professed mental illness does not really impair the defendant's competency. One can then make a diagnosis of Adjustment Disorder, usually the type known as "with Mixed Disturbance of Emotions and Conduct" or "with Atypical Features," and can then explain in the body of the report or the discussion why this defendant's symptoms do not impair his fitness to proceed, without directly calling him a liar.

PROOF

If the psychiatrist identifies a defendant as a malingerer, he is faced with a second, even more difficult problem, that of convincing the court. Although competency hearings are not true trials, there are reasonable rules of evidence and logic. The psychiatrist cannot expect the court to accept his conclusion that a defendant is malingering simply because he says so. He must also be prepared to present some kind of evidence, that is, the observations on which he bases his opinions. Moreover, this evidence must be sufficient to convince a layman, namely, the court. Sometimes this can be quite difficult. The experienced psychiatrist may "feel" that a defendant's illness is feigned, if for no other reason than that the picture the defendant presents is unlike that of the hundreds of thousands of truly mentally ill patients he has seen before. But how is he to demonstrate this satisfactorily to the court? The psychiatrist's problem here is quite similar to that of the district attorney who "knows" that a defendant has committed a certain crime but has no evidence that will stand up in court. What both of them have to find is "hard evidence." Otherwise, they have no case. There are times when the psychiatrist may be forced to report to the court that a defendant is incompetent, even though he knows in his heart that the man is malingering.

These two problems—identifying the malingerer and proving it in court—are two coordinates that we may use in presenting a picture of the malingerer and in classifying malingerers into different categories. Neither of these coordinates, of course, has discrete elements within it; rather, the degree of difficulty ranges in a continuum for both problems. Nevertheless, we can assign malingerers to approximate categories on both coordinates and come up with some rough system of classification. What to call these different categories is still another problem. Because malingerers are playing a kind of game, sports terminology would seem as appropriate as any other, and I would classify the malingerer on the basis of how well he plays the game: amateur, semipro, minor leaguer, and major leaguer.

The *amateur* malingerer is someone who plays the game so poorly, so obviously, that the problem of proving it in court will seldom arise. Typically, he is a young offender who has heard from other prisoners that it would be to his advantage to be found incompetent. He has had very little experience with true mental illness. As a result, his pretense is usually an outlandish one and often quite amusing.

> Such a case was a 17-year-old boy who decided to pretend blindness, partial paralysis and an inability to speak. The fact that none of these things had anything to do with the legal definition of competency to stand trial had not dawned on him. So he groped and limped his way in and out of my office, somehow managing, despite his "blindness," to avoid bumping into anything, including the doorway and the prison gates. It so happened that, as soon as he got back into the dayroom, he saw a cigarette lying on the floor. As he bent down to pick it up, the ward clerk said to him, "I thought you were blind." Unable to sustain the act any longer, he burst out laughing and the next day was talking normally to the examining psychiatrists.

Another type of amateur is the one who is more sophisticated about mental illness but still quite naive about the criteria for legal competency. He is well aware of the difficulties involved in faking present symptomatology. Accordingly, he does not even try. What he does instead is claim amnesia for the time of the alleged crime, something he mistakenly believes will preclude his standing trial. The fact that it is very easy to feign retrograde amnesia—after all, unless a person reveals his memory to someone else, how can you possibly prove that he does recall something?—makes it quite appealing as a symptom. Unfortunately for this type of malingerer, amnesis *per se* does not make him incompetent to stand trial.[6] Occasionally, however, defense counsel also does not appreciate this aspect of the law. Accordingly, he will insist on a hearing, and it will remain for the court to instruct him on the law.

> Such a patient was a 39-year-old man who was examined by us 5 months after he had been arrested for stabbing his paramour to death. At the age of 23, while serving a 5-year term in prison for robbery, he had apparently become psychotic and had been transferred to a Department of Correction

psychiatric hospital. He remained there for 14 years until, in accordance with Baxtrom,[7] he was transferred to a civil state hospital. Even though there was no evidence of mental illness at the time of his transfer, he was kept in the hospital for about a year until he walked away. Nine months later came the stabbing.

When we first saw him, he gave a detailed account of the crime, explaining that the victim had been a drug addict for whom he had made many sacrifices. When he found her in bed with another man, his anger got the better of him. Even though there was no indication of psychosis at the time of our examination, he naively asked to be returned to the state hospital. When we informed him that because of both his indictment for murder and his history of having escaped from that hospital he would probably have to go to another state hospital, one with maximum security, he said he preferred to return to court.

Six months later he changed his mind. Now he claimed amnesia for the time of the alleged crime and even for his previous admission to my service. These were isolated, sharply demarcated periods of "amnesia," and he was both willing and able to discuss the remainder of his entire life history in a perfectly rational, coherent, relevant and non-psychotic manner. He fully understood and appreciated the fact that a woman was dead and that he was charged with her murder. Although we could not, of course, prove positively that his amnesia was feigned, his own spontaneous statements about it were quite suggestive: "I don't remember when the crime took place. If you don't remember, that's in your favor. I don't believe they will put a man on the stand who doesn't remember the crime he commits." Suffice it to say that at the hearing, the court, in the absence of any other symptoms of mental illness, even according to the testimony of the defense psychiatrist, ruled him competent.

A somewhat more difficult defendant is the *semipro* malingerer. His choice of symptoms is much better designed to fool the layman. Moreover, it is wisely directed specifically at the question of his ability to stand trial. He usually adopts a pose somewhere between that of the mental defective and the catatonic. During the examination his bodily movements are minimal, and he usually looks around the office with a bewildered expression on his face. His statements are sparse, and whatever he does say is usually delivered in a dull, emotionless, monosyllabic manner. Very often he pretends ignorance of having been arrested and insists that his wife (or mother) brought him to the hospital. When shown the arraignment affidavit or the indictment papers and confronted with the arm patch of a uniformed correction officer, he usually develops a sudden loss of his previous ability to read.

What distinguishes the semipro from the amateur is his ability to impress the nonpsychiatrist. Although his malingering is fairly obvious to the forensic psychiatrist, the doctor knows that he will have to develop a certain amount of objective proof. It will probably be too difficult simply to convince the court that this set of sumptoms does not correspond to any known psychiatric illness. Fortunately, this proof is usually not too hard to obtain. The semipro seldom thinks beyond his appearance in court or the actual interviews with the psychiatrists. There he is prepared to put on his act. What he is not prepared to do is to sustain this act throughout his entire period of hospitalization. Once he is back on the ward, he thinks he can safely drop his pretense. What he does not realize is that we always ask the nurse and correction officers about the behavior of any such patients on the ward. And here is where we get our "hard evidence." We find, in the case of the semipro malingerer, that this man who in our office allegedly could barely move or talk and could not understand the simplest questions, that this same man on the ward can converse rationally with nurses, correction officers and fellow prisoners, can understand directions, can move about normally, can feed himself, can clean up, can watch television, can play cards, ping pong, checkers or even chess, can read newspapers and books, etc.

One such patient was a 33-year-old man who had malingered his way into a state hospital on two of his numerous previous arrests. This time, we insisted that he was able to stand trial, particularly in view of the fact that his two previous state hospitalizations had resulted in two of the most fantastic "recoveries" known to man: The first time he had escaped after 33 days, the second time after only 5. His behavior during the interviews, and its contrast on the ward, was typical of the semipro. Even the defense psychiatrist was forced to acknowledge at the hearing that this patient's symptomatology was unlike that of any functional psychosis he had ever seen. Still, there was his strange, withdrawn behavior in court. And the defense psychiatrist did suggest that possibly there was some brain damage. So a further examination was ordered to rule out this last possiblity.

Both the skull x-rays and the electroencephalogram were, of course, normal. It was his performance on the psychological tests that demonstrates most graphically the type of behavior so often seen in a semipro malingerer. He was, naturally, very resistant to taking any tests. He did them in any old way and definitely did not apply himself. The inconsistencies in his test performance defied belief. On the one hand, he was able to copy a square on paper, an act which indicates a mental age of at least 4. On the other hand, he did not know what a bed was, something the average two-and-one-half-year-old knows. Nor did he know, he said, what a penny was. On the other hand, he kept asking the psychologist for a light for his cigarette, a much more advanced, abstract concept than either a penny or a bed. When asked to draw a human figure, he at first refused. However, when told to draw a circle and then told to put in the eyes, nose and mouth, he was able to insert these anatomical parts in a fairly sophisticated way. As a matter of fact, when told to draw a second figure, he did so, and the form on that figure, without specific instructions, definitely ruled out the possibility of mental deficiency or brain damage.

The *minor leaguer* presents a much more difficult problem. His choice of symptomatology is usually either severe agitation or depression. Furthermore, in order to make his act convincing, he is willing to go to great lengths, even to the point of endangering his own life. Often, he will slash himself repeatedly in jail or attempt to hang himself but in a way that is carefully timed for rescue. Or he will behave so violently on the ward that he has to be placed in restraints. On examination, he either behaves in a belligerently uncooperative manner or simply maintains that he does not care what happens to him, that all he wants to do is die. The minor leaguer is sophisticated enough to know that, in order to be competent to stand trial, he has to be able to participate in his defense. Unlike the semipro, he does not pretend ignorance of the charges against him or the fact that he is under arrest. He simply acknowledges these facts and shrugs them off, as if he were indifferent to them. Moreover, he maintains his act fairly consistently on the ward.

About the only way we can get "hard evidence" on a minor leaguer is to check his past record. Such a person has often put on an act following previous arrests and has been committed to state hospitals. When we check with the state hospitals (a rather lengthy procedure), we often find that this allegedly psychotic defendant, like the semipro just described, has "recovered" quite rapidly and escaped. Although this type of behavior does not prove beyond a reasonable doubt that he is malingering, it at least raises sufficient doubt so that the burden is now on the defense (or, at least, should be) to substantiate the claim of incompetency.

Sometimes we can convince the court, from the fact that he eats and sleeps well on the ward, that the minor leaguer's symptoms are not genuine. Most of the time, however, his malingering is very hard to prove to a layman. And even if we could, there would always be the danger that he might accidentally injure himself quite seriously in one of his suicidal acts. We also know that it would be a major struggle to convince the jail authorities to keep him. Very often, then, we declare him incompetent to stand trial because there is no other practical alternative.

Such a patient was a 19-year-old who, when apprehended in a stolen car, ran into an alleyway and held the arresting officer at bay by threatening to cut himself with a hunting knife. He finally did, slashing his left arm, the left side of his neck and both legs.

On examination, soon after his initial arraignment, he was mildly depressed and quite bitter about the way life had treated him. His mother had been in a state hospital for 14 years, his alcoholic father was impossible to get along with, and he had no one to turn to. He discussed the details of the present offense quite adequately, stating that he had done it so that he might get away from his father. There was no evidence of psychosis or incompetency, although we were aware of the possibility that he might act up in court.

Eleven days after discharge he was sent back for reexamination with a gaping wound across his right forearm. While in detention, he had also swallowed a razor blade, which somehow passed through his body without doing any harm. Now the picture was much more confusing. On several examinations, he appeared depressed and was breathing rather heavily. He complained of people making fun of him and laughing at him and at times would dramatically cry out, "Why did they take my mother away?" At times, he knew the charges but insisted on his innocence, even claiming that he must have been in the hospital at the time of the alleged offense. At other times, he professed ignorance of the charges, even after they were told to him. In either event, he would never really address himself to the charges but always seemed preoccupied with the idea that his mother had been taken away from him.

Throughout this entire period of apparent depression and severe mental anguish, he slept well every night. In fact, the ward personnel reported him "as normal as anybody else," stating that he would begin to put on an act as soon as he approached the gates for an interview in the doctor's office. When confronted with these reports, this rather rigid, staring, barely responsive young man became quite excited and began shouting, "They've been doing this to me since I'm small. First they take my mother, then my brother. Now they want to get rid of me." Still later, he discussed his unhappy life in a much more reasonable and subdued way, obviously trying to elicit sympathy. However, he continued to threaten suicide, shouting that he would do what he wanted and that nobody could make him stand trial if he didn't want to. It was felt that, although he had a long-standing depression, he was deliberately exaggerating his feelings whenever it suited his purposes.

About the *major leaguer*, there is very little one can say. By definition, he is do adept at feigning mental illness that he succeeds in fooling the examining psychiatrists. The problem of proving his malingering in court, therefore, never arises. The major leaguer puts on an act which is quite compatible with a well-recognized psychosis. He does not try for outlandish extremes or for illnesses that it would be impossible for him to feign. Moreover, he maintains this act consistently on the ward. Finally, he has not undergone miraculous "recoveries" every time he has been committed to a state hospital. Rather, he has been willing to wait until it has been reasonable for him to recover and then be properly discharged.

If such defendants put on such convincing acts, how do I know they are actually malingering? How do I know that such major leaguers really exist? In the first place, humility and logic tell me so. Forensic psychiatrists, even the best, are not infallible. There must exist defendants who can fool us. Secondly, other defendants often tell us that so-and-so fooled us and got himself committed to a state hospital. Granted that these informants are not the most reliable sources, it happens often enough that they must be correct and truthful some of the time. Thirdly, there is the rare case of a major leaguer who changes his mind in the midst of his hospitalization.

Such a patient was a 19-year-old who had been indicted for Robbery II and Assault I. He had snatched a purse from an elderly lady on the street and had made his escape; but then, for some unknown reason, he had returned and gratuitously beaten her within an inch of her life. The patient had a past history of psychiatric hospitalization in St. Albans Naval Hospital and, for a while, after his discharge from the Marines, had been receiving a disability pension.

When I first saw him, he was the classic picture of a psychotic schizophrenic. His statements were bizarre, and his feeling tone was quite shallow and inappropriate. He insisted in a very pleasant manner that he had been arrested for Disorderly Conduct. When told that it was actually Robbery II, he replied, "That's what I'm saying now." When asked why he called Robbery II Disorderly Conduct, he responded, "That's the way I pronounce it." His understanding of what court procedure and this hospitalization involved was, to say the least, different: "My lawyer told me to tell you I would be released in your custody on $50.00 bail. I don't know how you would arrange that. I swear I know nothing about how much you are making off the deal." Actually, this was said in a much more garbled manner than I could possibly record. Some of his spontaneous statements give an even clearer picture of his disordered thinking: "I mortgaged the house of the Virgin of the King. See, I can sing like Nat King Cole. Elizabeth Taylor is making me do all the dirty work. I went down there and pressed the charges with Elizabeth Taylor. She's trying to get one million dollars for her eyes." This was followed by a series of incomprehensible numbers and then some kind of unintelligible reference to Sugar Ray Robinson.

Three days later, when seen by another psychiatrist on my service, he was a different person. He talked quite normally, understood and appreciated the charges against him, told a detailed story about his arrest, insisted on his innocence and wanted to return to court. When I aksed him about our previous interview, he insisted, with a twinkle in his eye, that he had never seen me before and that I must have him confused with another patient. During all interviews, including the initial one where he was patently psychotic, he always presented himself as a sweet, lovable person. On the other hand, there was the unnecessarily brutal nature of his crime.

Furthermore, he was the ringleader on our ward in an attempt to beat up and rob another patient. It seemed in retrospect that he had been putting on an act and playing with me for his own amusement. But what an act! Had he not decided that he had had enough of our hospital, we would never have been able to detect his malingering.

PSYCHODYNAMICS AND MOTIVATION

This, then, is a rough picture of the various types of malingerers. It is, however, only a surface picture. For a variety of reasons we really have very little in-depth understanding of what kind of person chooses to malinger and what kind of person does so with any degree of success. Perhaps the successful malingerer has been exposed to mental illness in his immediate family or during a previous period of psychiatric hospitalization. Perhaps, as some have boasted, he has intentionally studied about delusions and hallucinations in a publicly available psychiatry textbook. Perhaps at another time he himself has undergone some degree of mental illness, and it is his recollection of this experience that makes him so familiar with the signs and symptoms. If this is so, then the difference between this type of defendant and the truly incompetent is the former's conscious intentional choice to use his illness in a self-serving manner.

Defendants decide to malinger for a variety of reasons. Explanations given by confessed malingerers include the hope that feigning mental illness will somehow help them in later pleading out or being found not criminally responsible on the grounds of mental disease or defect. Probably the most common incentive is simply the wish to be temporarily transferred to a mental hospital from their present jail situation. The professed motive for such a transfer can be as mundane as the fact that they have heard that the hospital has better food or that, bored with their prolonged confinement, they just want a change of scene. At times they may decide to exaggerate their symptomatology in order to receive the psychiatric attention or "tender loving care" for their depression and/or anxiety that is not available in jail. Sometimes they have a fear of being homosexually assaulted in the general jail population, a fear which may be conscious or unconscious and, even if conscious, they may not acknowledge. Regardless of what the defendant tells us, the psychodynamics are undoubtedly overdetermined, and even if the defendant were revealing all the motives of which he was consciously aware, there would undoubtedly be other, unconscious factors. Nevertheless, when a defendant "drops the act," it still behooves us, as supportive psychotherapists, to try our best to discuss all the relevant motives with this defendant, for we may be able to help prevent any further incidents. For instance, if he despairs because his family and defense attorney seem to have abandoned him, contact with them by a member of the therapeutic team can go a long way towards helping the defendant. Or if he has good reason to fear a homosexual assault in a particular jail location, arrangements can often be made to transfer him elsewhere.

One motive is worth discussing in particular, namely, escape. There was a time in New York State (and perhaps still in other states) when there was no civil psychiatric hospital devoted to the care and treatment of criminal defendants. The only defendants transferred to a hospital that had sufficient security, because it was operated by the Department of Correction, were those who had been indicted by a Grand Jury. All nonindicted defendants, regardless of the severity of their charges, were committed to general civil psychiatric hospitals, the choice depending solely on their place of residence. By that time civil hospitals were becoming ever increasingly places of treatment, with more and more emphasis on voluntary admissions, and very few, if any, security measures. The result was the creation of excellent opportunities for criminal defendants to escape if they could malinger their way into such hospitals prior to indictment.

The solution was the creation of a special, maximum-security civil state mental hospital (Mid-Hudson) operated by the Department of Mental Hygiene for the care and treatment of those dangerous, incompetent felony defendants who had not yet been indicted. (Theoretically, another solution would have been the indictment of all felony defendants within a few days of their arrests but especially in heavily populated counties, except for a few notorious cases, this is a practical impossibility and in all counties in many cases is simply not in the best interests of justice.) With time the criterion of dangerousness was dropped, the Department of Correction facility was closed, and virtually all incompetent felony defendants, regardless of whether or not they had been indicted, were sent to this special facility. Eventually, if the defendant's incompetency persists but he is deemed reasonably safe, he may be transferred to the high-security unit of a regular civil state mental hospital or even discharged,[8] but the likelihood that this will be accomplished through malingering is remote. The result of the creation of such a special hospital has been a significant reduction of malingering of incompetency for the purpose of escape.

PRACTICAL ASPECTS

In almost all cases, when a psychiatrist openly presents the diagnosis of malingering, he is a psychiatrist who has been appointed by the court or retained by the prosecution. Very rarely will a psychiatrist called on by the defense report to counsel that his client is malingering. Counsel may or may not be able to convince his client to drop the act. If he cannot, he will have to decide whether to continue to represent the defendant, whether to call on another psychiatrist, etc. All these are decisions to be made by the defense attorney and do not directly concern the psychiatrist, for whom this chapter is written. His obligation is to report his findings to the attorney who has retained him for the examination.

If the prosecution expert concludes that the defendant is malingering, the next step to be decided is whether there is any practical value in making such a diagnosis. If the prosecution's contention, either fitness to proceed or criminal responsibility, can be well argued without getting into this area of malingering, it is probably to the prosecution's best advantage to avoid it. A skilled defense attorney can at times evoke even greater sympathy for his client when the prosecution's psychiatrist can be portrayed as a person who will stop at nothing, even calling a defendant a liar, to achieve a conviction. This question of strategy should be discussed with the prosecutor before the formal report is written. The vast majority of cases in which the prosecution psychiatrist concludes that the defendant is fit to proceed or criminally responsible does not require the diagnosis of malingering. Only a few do. Once that diagnosis is placed on the record, the prosecution psychiatrist has exposed himself to one more area of cross-examination.

A psychiatrist who has testified for the defense that a defendant is mentally ill and therefore incompetent (or was mentally ill and therefore not responsible) must always be prepared to acknowledge on cross-examination that (a) psychiatry is not an exact science, and (b) the defendant may be malingering. However, if allowed, he will add at that point, or, if not allowed, later on re-direct (having discussed this beforehand with defense counsel) that it is always theoretically possible that the defendant is (or was) malingering, but that a psychiatrist must deal in probabilities, not mere possibilities, and the probability is that the defendant is (or was) genuinely mentally ill, etc.

CONCLUSION

Malingering is usually a diagnosis of exclusion, that is, one that is reached when the psychiatrist is reasonably satisfied that the clinical picture is not attributable to a mental disorder. As such, it should be used sparingly. Once having made such a diagnosis, the examiner must be reasonably flexible, that is, confronted with new, satisfactory evidence, he must be willing to acknowledge true mental illness. Conversely, he must also be prepared to recognize when a formerly malingering defendant, usually after conference with his attorney, has decided to cease the pretense or exaggeration. Finally, he should not be surprised if, despite his best arguments, the court or jury disagrees when a malingerer and skilled counsel have raised reasonable doubts.

REFERENCES

[1]*Webster's Third New International Dictionary, Unabridged.* Springfield, MA, G & C Merriam, 1965.

[2]*Black's Law Dictionary,* Revised 4th Ed. St. Paul, Minn., West Publishing, 1968.

[3]Campbell, RJ: *Psychiatric Dictionary,* Fifth Edition. New York, Oxford University Press, 1981.

[4]*Diagnostic and Statistical Manual of Mental Disorders,* 3rd Ed. Washington, DC, Amer Psychiatric Assn, 1980.

[5]Rosenhan, DL: On being sane in insane places. *Science 179:*250–258, 1973.

[6]Wilson v U.S., 391 F.2d 460 (1968) and People v Francabandara, 354 N.Y.S.2d 609; 33 N.Y.2d 429 (1974).

[7]Baxstrom v Herold, 383 U.S. 107 (1966).

[8]Jackson v Indiana, 406 U.S. 715 (1972).

15

Premenstrual Syndrome (PMS) and the Law

"It happens without warning and I have no control over it. I will suddenly feel tired with such heaviness that it's as if I'm bearing the weight of the whole world. It starts with feeling irritable but then this dark feeling comes over me where almost anything that wouldn't otherwise bother me makes me fly into a rage. When that happens, I don't care what I destroy or who I hurt. I really get angry and I'm mortified with guilt and shame afterwards but nobody seems to understand."

These are the words of a PMS sufferer. With only minor variations the same feelings have been expressed by women who, on a regular and predictable basis, will experience extreme mood changes as well as physical and behavioral changes that for some will take the form of violence towards themselves or others.

SYMPTOMATOLOGY AND DIAGNOSIS

Psychological symptoms are the commonest manifestations of PMS. They are generally described as tension, depression, irritability and lethargy. *Lethargy,* for example, has been described as a "crushing and overwhelming heaviness that makes simple and ordinary tasks virtually impossible." This feeling has been known to lead to abandonment of maternal responsibility and industrial absenteeism.[1] Though these sub-

NORMAN WEISS • Department of Psychiatry, New York Medical College, Valhalla, New York 10595.

265

jective complaints cannot be precisely defined or measured, it is in the context of these complaints that behavior disorders occur that can, in extreme cases, take the form of child and spouse abuse, antisocial behavior including crimes of violence and for the borderline or prepsychotic woman, overt psychosis and suicide.

Almost invariably physical symptoms accompany the psychological ones and can contribute to the deterioration of mood and behavior. Many of these symptoms appear to be on the basis of fluid retention. Weight gains during this period of 4 or 5 pounds are not uncommon and for some women a gain of more than 10 pounds may not be uncommon. Abdominal bloating, breast pains, joint and muscle pain, headache and acniform rashes are the commonest complaints. Less frequently reported are seizures, asthmatic attacks, and migraine headaches. Subtler symptoms can include clumsiness, herpes, styes, and disequilibrium. This is by no means a comprehensive listing of symptoms as more than 150 have been identified and cover the widest range of symptomatic possibilities.

But what do all of these varied symptoms have in common and why are they called a syndrome? The common denominator is their regularity in relation to the menstrual cycle. Symptoms are experienced every cycle virtually unchanged, for the same number of days, or will change gradually with age. The periodicity rather than the symptoms *per se* is necessary for the diagnosis of PMS to be made.

The usual age of onset for women is early 30s but can begin in puberty or with approaching menopause. It can start following a difficult pregnancy, surgical procedure, life stress, or for no reason that is obvious. It is usually relieved by pregnancy and generally disappears 2 or 3 years after menopause.

Classically, symptoms recur 5 to 7 days before the onset of menses and relief is experienced by the first or second day of the menstrual flow. Variations of this pattern include symptoms at mid-cycle, the time of ovulation, persisting for 2 days and then either remitting or continuing and increasing in severity until the onset of menses brings relief. Because for many women symptoms extend a number of days into menses, a more accurate designation for the disorder would be Paramenstrual Syndrome[2] as the paramenstruum includes those days prior to and following the onset of the menstrual flow.

HISTORY AND BACKGROUND

Premenstrual Syndrome, or PMS, has been described as the world's commonest disorder. Dr. Dalton,[3] who gave it its name and has been studying and treating the syndrome in London since 1948, estimates that 40% of women suffer some PMS symptoms and perhaps 5% experience it to a severe and disabling degree.[4]

Ancient writers such as Hippocrates made reference to the periodic and changeable moods in women in terms similar to those expressed today.

The association between phases of the menstrual cycle and disturbed or antisocial behavior has also long been observed, and Dr. William Healy[5] referred to it in 1915 when he wrote, "Premenstrual restlessness may be correlated with sex offenses and also other delinquencies."

In 1931, Frank[6] described "premenstrual tension" and related it to high estrogen levels in the blood secondary to defective renal excretion. Since that time, much has been written to establish a cohesive pathophysiological formulation, but to date, much of the data has been anecdotal and often contradictory.[7] Hypotheses have included hypoglycemia, vitamin deficiency and specific allergies. Dr. Dalton[4] has been the chief proponent of progesterone treatment, believing that an absolute or relative deficiency of progesterone during the luteal phase of the menstrual cycle, in relation to estrogen, results in the varied symptomatic picture described. This hypothesis, to date, appears to possess the greatest number of adherents, and Dr. Dalton claims to have successfully treated thousands of women in England with good results. Others dispute the efficacy of such treatment and believe that a placebo effect is present. A most comprehensive recent paper by Reid and Yen[7] defines the syndrome as "a major clinical entity affecting a large segment of the female population" and suggest that the pathophysiological disorder is of neuroendocrine origin within the hypothalamic-pituitary axis, which influences neurotransmitter function.

Yet, to date, despite growing interest in the syndrome, virtually no controlled research has been reported and most of what we know has been based on anecdotal references. It is hoped that with greater attention by both the general public and the medical community, the next few years will produce scientifically valid research that will more precisely define the syndrome by elaborating causes.

To be sure, PMS is more than a medical issue but a social and political one as well. With the feminist movement and its emphasis on equality, there was the fear that any condition that underscored female disability could be used to suppress women. This fear was realized by the 1970 statement made by Dr. Edgar Berman,[8] an appointee to the Democratic Party's Committee on National Priorities, that women were unfit for responsible positions because of "raging hormonal imbalances." The attitude expressed by this statement has caused considerable ambivalence on the part of the Women's Rights movement towards PMS. But most recently, with the greater attention paid by the media to PMS, the focus has been on the suffering of so many women and the need to awaken the medical community to the need for help.

PMS AND ANTISOCIAL BEHAVIOR

The relationship between PMS and antisocial behavior had been studied and commented on prior to Dr. Healy's 1915 reference. It was in the 1890s that criminologists in Europe began to write about this phenomenon.[9]

It was in 1945 that Cooke[10] examined police records and found that 84% of violent crimes committed by the women he investigated were during the days just prior to and just following the onset of menstruation (paramenstruum). In a later study by Dalton,[4] she investigated the relationship between crime and the menstrual cycle in 156 new female prisoners and found that about half had committed their crimes during the paramenstruum. Oleck,[11] in 1953, was the first to raise the issue of "premenstrual tension as a form of temporary insanity." In pressing this recommendation, he referred to the French courts that had for some time accorded PMS such a defense. Perhaps the most interesting findings in relating criminal behavior to the menstrual cycle was the work of D'Orban and Dalton[12] in 1980, who found in their sample of 50 women charged with violent crimes that 44% committed their offenses during the paramenstruum with a significant diminution during the ovulatory and post ovulatory phase. They further concluded that the association to the paramenstruum was not related to psychosocial factors and that no relationship existed between the crimes and any subjective symptoms usually associated with PMS. The only symptoms experienced by some of the women in their study, then, were those associated with antisocial behavior unrelated to conscious mood change or "tension." They further concluded that women who were violent during the paramenstruum had similar tendencies during other phases of their menstrual cycle.

PMS AND PSYCHIATRIC ILLNESS

Numerous investigators have reported on the relationship between psychiatric symptoms and crisis during those times of the month associated with PMS. Coppen and Kessel[13] found significant evidence of mood changes that included irritability, depression and tension states.

Mandell and Mandell[14] reported an increase in the frequency of calls to a suicide prevention center by paramenstrual women, and Jacobs and Charles[15], in a study of 200 women, found that the menstrual phase, premenstrual phase and midcycle (ovulatory) phase of the menstrual cycle were times of peak psychiatric contact. Both Dalton[16] in 1959 and Abramowitz et al.[17] in 1982 described an increase in the hospital admission rate. Dalton found the highest incidence during the first 4 days of menstruation followed by the 4 days prior to menstruation and finally the midcycle. Abramowitz, in reviewing the hospital admissions of depressed women over an 18 month period, reported that 41% were admitted on the day prior to and the first day of the menstrual flow. Other sources[18] have also suggested that periodic crises may be associated with the paramenstruum, with an increase in the relapse rate among women with manic and schizophrenic disorders during the premenstrual and menstrual phases of the cycle.[19]

Ribero[20] confirmed the cross-cultural nature of premenstrual behavior disorder by reporting on 22 Hindu women who commited suicide by immolation and found that 19 had been menstruating at the time of the act.

The relationship between physical illness, marital and sexual maladjustment, and suicide attempts during the paramenstruum was explored by Glass et al.[21] They found that women seen in a psychiatric emergency room had a positive correlation for the above.

The plethora of studies relating PMS to both antisocial behavior and psychiatric illness raises the most important forensic question of the capacity of these women to control the behavioral manifestations of PMS. Ribero's work[23] suggests that the disordered behavior is not exclusively a Western cultural phenomenon. An inability to control behavior may indeed exist for severe sufferers, not withstanding the fact that many of these women may, at other times of the menstrual cycle, be prone to antisocial behavior or psychiatric illness.

PMS AND THE CIVIL LAW

On May 17, 1983, at a Social Security Disability Hearing in Brooklyn, N.Y., a 31-year-old woman was awarded disability for PMS. Her symptoms, which began in puberty, included mood changes with depression, tension, irritability and violent behavioral outbursts. Physical symptoms included fluid retention which resulted in abdominal bloating and breast tenderness. These symptoms were severe and interferred with her functioning approximately 1 week out of every month. Her legal aid attorney brought the matter to my attention for the purpose of evaluation. By charting her sumptoms with the help of a menstrual calendar and noting their regularity in relation to her menstrual cycle, and excluding other medical conditions, the diagnosis was made. Corroborative medical documentation going back a number of years supported her story and demonstrated the degree of severity. It described her incapacity as a student to take exams when premenstrual, marital strife resulting in divorce, and a loss of work days every month. This had resulted in the loss of numerous jobs despite an otherwise satisfactory work record.

Because Premenstrual Syndrome (PMS) does not exist as an official diagnostic entity in the official Social Security Regulations Manual, the basis for the finding was a psychiatric diagnosis (12.04 Functional Nonpsychotic Disorders). Though this diagnosis served a practical bureaucratic purpose, it misrepresented her true condition. According to her attorney, this was the first instance of a woman being awarded social security disability based on PMS. If this is so, it represents an important legal precedent for women whose PMS may be of a disabling degree and interfere with their ability to work.

Because stress can be a factor in the onset or exacerbation of PMS symptoms, it can become a very serious issue for Workers Compensation cases as well.

With greater social awareness of PMS and less tolerance of physicians who disregard it as a medical entity will come malpractice suits. Lawyers are reported to be studying the entity and collecting data to demonstrate misdiagnosis.[22] We* have collected examples of women treated for a variety of conditions where the diagnosis was clearly PMS. Women have had hysterectomies and 1 woman seen recently had ECT for her depressive symptoms.

PMS AS A CRIMINAL DEFENSE

In London in 1980, a barmaid by the name of Sandie Craddock faced sentencing for manslaughter in the killing of a co-worker.[22] This woman, in her late 20s, had been sentenced at least 30 times before for crimes ranging from theft to arson and assault. Instead of the severe sentence expected, she was released on probation after her lawyer pleaded that "she suffered a hormonal imbalance related to her menstrual cycle and that this imbalance known as premenstrual syndrome, had turned Ms. Craddock into a raging animal each month forcing her to act out of character."

*Martorano, JT, Weiss, N, work in progress.

The expert medical witness for the defense was Dr. Kathrina Dalton, who testified that Ms. Craddock was suffering from "an extremely aggrevated form of premenstrual physical condition." Dr. Dalton[2] had been involved in three other cases of PMS with charges of manslaughter, arson, and assault respectively. In each case, Dr. Dalton claimed to have successfully treated the condition with daily injections of natural progesterone. The condition of Ms. Craddock's probation was that she be treated with progesterone. But the story of Sandie Craddock, or Sandie Smith as she then became known, did not end here. She was re-arrested less than a year later for threatening to kill a police officer. At this second trial, Dr. Dalton testified that regular injections of progesterone had allowed the patient to become less symptomatic, but at the time of her arrest for threatening the police officer, her progesterone dose had been reduced, renewing her earlier antisocial behavior pattern. At trial, the judge refused to allow the jury to consider PMS as a substantive defense but did, once again, allow Dr. Dalton's testimony to be considered at the time of sentencing. The "Jekyll and Hyde" effect on Sandie Smith's life was again accepted by the Court, progesterone treatment was more carefully monitored with the hope that it would keep her "safe and benign."

In another British court on the very next day, another woman who had killed her lover by running him down in a car was acquitted of murder based on the plea of "premenstrual tension."

Following these cases, attempts were made to relate them to other cases where "physical states" resulted in antisocial or criminal behavior and where substantive defenses were established.

In 1973, a precedent was established for the defense of "automatism" in the case of *Queen v Quick*.[23] In that instance, the court quashed a guilty verdict against a diabetic male nurse working at a mental hospital. The nurse was given an improper dose of insulin, became hypoglycemic, assaulted a patient and was convicted. The Court of Appeals, in reversing the conviction, said that the lower court had not considered "the defendant's criminal responsibility and intent under the circumstances and that the defendant should have been allowed to show that he acted as an automaton because of the effect of the improper dose of insulin."

Similarities to the Sandie Smith case are obvious where her "prior pattern of antisocial behavior was related to an improper dose of progesterone."

Following the cases in England, it was not long before PMS was raised in a criminal proceding in the United States.[24] The defense was raised in a motion to dismiss assault charges against Shirley Santos, a woman accused of abusing her 4-year-old daughter.[25] Stephanie Benson, the Legal Aid attorney for Ms. Santos, said that the case "was crying out for the PMS defense." Judge Becker adjourned the case six months pending completion of the Family Court proceedings and in the interval the defense was dropped. In his opinion from the bench, Judge Becker said that "since eruptions of the mind are admissible on the criminal intent issue, should not proof of physiological eruptions of the body likewise be admitted." PMS research has yet to establish such proof.

In recent years, British and Canadian Courts have introduced criminal defenses for medical conditions.[26] These have included automatism,[27] epilepsy,[23] and diabetic hypoglycemia.[28]

Feldman[29] discusses the legal status of illness or conditions that are episodic in nature, resulting in antisocial or criminal behavior, but are not among the primary psychiatric disorders. He locates these "in an uncertain, indefinite and inconsistent legal area somewhere between insanity and an involuntary act." PMS, with its periodicity, secondary manifestations of mood and behavior disorder and evidence of underlying endocrine disorder, would fall into this category. Its greater prevalence would distinguish it from the others.

How PMS would fit into the traditional legal defenses, that is, the Insanity Defense, would depend on several factors. These would include the definition of the defense in that jurisdiction, the nature of the symptoms that resulted in the criminal behavior and the prevailing societal attitudes about PMS.

Though it is an accepted principle of the criminal law that a person should not be punished for acts over which they have no control, the M'Naghten Rule[30] takes the position that insanity is a cognitive rather than a behavioral disorder and emphasizes appreciating the significance of behavior rather than the defendant's ability to control conduct. Because PMS is primarily a mood and behavior disorder rather than a cognitive one, an insanity defense would not in all likelihood be successful.

The Model Penal Code[31] excludes certain behaviors that are considered involuntary from criminal responsibility. Though no universally acceptable definition of involuntary behavior has been put forth, it is viewed as lacking intent or purpose. An actor would be exonerated when evidence can be demonstrated that a criminal act was committed in an altered state of consciousness when that state was not self-imposed. The presumption would be that the act was involuntary and behavior control was not possible. Although, for the PMS sufferer, an altered state of consciousness would not be certain, the second arm of the American Law Institute (ALI) rule referring to the "lack of capacity to conform conduct to the requirements of the law"[32] could be the basis for a successful insanity defense.

Because the law recognizes gradations of impairment, "partial responsibility" or "diminished capacity" could be more likely invoked than the insanity defense for PMS related crimes. This may be a more acceptable approach for society considering the fact that PMS is not a primary psychiatric disorder and the semantic association of insanity and psychosis would be abhorrent to the large number of PMS sufferers.

Indeed, efforts have been ongoing to provide a conceptual basis for a mitigating defense. Goldstein[33] proposed the idea of "subjective liability," whereby the subjective state of the defendant may be a mitigating factor in both the offense charged as well as the sentence. According to Stone,[34] the Model Penal Code permits a reduction in a homicide charge from murder to nonreckless manslaughter if "committed under the influence of extreme mental or emotional disturbance for which there is reasonable explanation or excuse."[35] What is weighed in such cases is not what the defendant felt but what a normal person in a similar position and with similar beliefs may have felt.[34] Considering the number of women with PMS symptoms, it would be interesting to consider the effect of such a defense on a jury that could itself include PMS sufferers.

Another standard exemplified by the so called Wells–Gorshen doctrine[36] takes into account the peculiar personal characteristics of individuals that would include the capacity for self control. In California as well as several other states, "if the capacity of the accused to form specific intent essential to constitute a crime" is found to be lacking, a finding of partial responsibility can be made.

The essential issue for the majority of PMS sufferers charged with crimes is not an altered state of consciousness that could lead to a defense of "automatism" or a pathological misperception of reality that could evoke an insanity defense, but a loss of control. The capacity to excercise control or maintain acceptable standards of behavior is impaired. To date, capacity to control behavior is no more testable than the altered state of consciousness of a temporal lobe seizure or the delusions of a schizophrenic. Nevertheless, given a longitudinal history, society will accept the "reality" of delusion or altered states of consciousness to the extent of making them the basis for a substantive criminal defense. Society, on the other hand, has been hard nosed about matters related to "lack of control" that are not based on a primary psychiatric disorder or an altered state of consciousness.

For PMS to become the basis for a substantive defense, two conditions need to be met. Firstly, the condition needs more medical recognition and acceptance that will most likely happen when more clinical experience has been shared and research has provided scientific data that addresses etiology. When this happens there will be fewer voices that attribute PMS to female neuroticism or view it as a medical myth.

Secondly, the public needs more education. It would be a mistake to leave this task primarily to the media. Grass roots organizations of women and men have been established in order to get help for sufferers by sharing information and putting them in contact with physicians or clinics who treat PMS. Sadly, it has been lay groups rather than the medical community that have brought PMS out of the closet.

DISPOSITION

Many chapters have been written about the disposition of those found "not guilty by reason of insanity" (NGI). Society has never been comfortable with either incarcerating such individuals, who no longer show evidence of a dangerous mental disorder, or releasing them with the many uncertainties inherent in such a choice. Because one function of the Law is rehabilitation, the imprisonment of women shown to suffer with PMS would be cruel and pointless. Despite some medical views to the contrary, many PMS sufferers are treatable.[4,*] Hospitalization for the purpose of establishing a treatment plan could become a condition of probation and thereby minimize recidivism. Such a plan would, of course, depend on the cooperation between the courts and the medical community.

SUMMARY

With the ever increasing attention paid to PMS by the lay public, the media, and the legal and medical professions, there is little doubt that PMS will be raised as an issue for women charged with crime, confronted with the loss of employment or misdiagnosed by the medical community. For those who claim to be unable to work, standards to establish disability will need to be developed that recognize the uniqueness of PMS. The medical profession will need to expand its awareness and understanding of PMS or face an ever more challenging response on the part of women who for years have been neglected. To what extent the issue will be raised in the criminal courts only time will tell.

Not to be overlooked are the opportunities for abuse of the PMS issue, either for personal or political purposes. Some see the possibilities of a bandwagon effect if a new criminal defense or basis for civil redress is established. Others fear that certain elements in the legal community might attempt to turn PMS into a major malpractice issue against physi-

*Martorano, JT, Weiss, N, work in progress.

cians. Added awareness on the part of the public could provide an all purpose excuse for some women who would use it in the workplace or in the courts. In England, cartoons have begun to poke fun at PMS following the court cases discussed, and concern has been voiced that to use PMS at the present time as a defense or as a mitigating factor at time of sentencing may bring the concept into disrepute. The next several years will tell the story.

REFERENCES

[1]Parker, AS: Premenstrual tension syndrome. *Med Clin North Am 44:*339, 1960.

[2]Dalton, K: Cyclical criminal acts in premenstrual syndrome. *Lancet 2:*1070, 1980.

[3]Greene, R, Dalton, K: The premenstrual syndrome. *Br Med J 1:*1007, 1953.

[4]Dalton, K: The premenstrual syndrome and progesterone therapy. London, William Heinemann Medical Books, 1977.

[5]Healy, W: The Individual Delinquent. Monclair, N.J., Patterson Smith, 232, 1915.

[6]Frank, RT: The hormonal causes of premenstrual tension. *Arch Neurol Psychiatr 26:*1053, 1931.

[7]Reid, R, Yen, S: Premenstrual syndrome. *Am J Obstet Gynecol 139:*85, 1981.

[8]Stephens, B: Premenstrual stress: Let's control the issue. *Daily News,* July 25, 1982.

[9]Icard, S: La femme pendant la période menstruelle. Paris, Felix Alcave: 1890.

[10]Cooke, WR: The differential psychology of the American woman. *Am J Obstet Gynecol 49:* 457, 1945.

[11]Oleck, HL: Legal aspects of premenstrual tension. *Intern Record of Med & Gen Pract Clinics 166:*492–501, 1953.

[12]D'Orban, P, Dalton, J: Violent crime and the menstrual cycle. *Psycho Med 10:*353, 1980.

[13]Coppen, A, Kessel, N: Menstruation and personality. *Br J Psychitry 109:*711–721, 1963.

[14]Mandell, AJ, Mandell, MP: Suicide and the menstrual cycle. *JAMA 9:*792–793, 1967.

[15]Jacobs, TJ, Charles, E: Correlation of psychiatric symptomatology and the menstrual cycle in an outpatient population. *Am J Psychitry 126:*10, 1970.

[16]Dalton, K: Menstruation and acute psychiatric illness. *Br Med Psyc* 148–149, 1959.

[17]Abramowitz, E, Baker, A, Fleischer, S: Onset of depressive crises and the menstrual cycle. *Am J Psychitry 139:*474, 1982.

[18]Endo, M, Daigujl, M, Asano, Y *et al.:* Periodic psychosis recurring in association with menstrual cycle. *J Clin Psychitry 39:*456–466, 1978.

[19]Ota, Y, Mukai, T: Studies on the relationship between psychotic symptoms and sexual cycle. *Folia Psychi Neurol Jap 8:*207–217, 1954.

[20]Ribero, AL: Menstruation and crime. *Br J Med 1:*640, 1962.

[21]Glass, GS, Henninger, GR, Lasky, M *et al.:* Psychiatric emergency related to the menstrual cycle. *Am J Psychitry 128:*705, 1971.

[22]Tybor, J: Women on trial: New defense. *Nat'l Law J,* Feb 15, 1982.

[23]Queen v Quick 2 All E.R. 347 (1973).

[24]Tell, L: PMS' U.S. court debut: hint of future success. *Nat'l Law J,* May 10, 1982.

[25]People v Santos, 1K046229.

[26]Taylor, L, Dalton, D: Premenstrual syndrome: a new criminal defense? *Cal West Law Rev 19:*276, 1983.

[27]Rubey v Queen, 114 D.L.R. 3d 193 (1980).

[28]Bratty v Attorney-General for Northern Ireland,A.C.386 (1963).

[29]Feldman, WS: Episodic cerebral dysfunction: a defense in legal limbo. *J Psych and Law 9:* 193, 1981.

[30]M'Naghten Case, 10 Clark & F. 200, 211, 8 Eng Rep 718, 722 (1843).

[31]Model Penal Code 2.01 (official draft 1962).

[32]Model Penal Code 4 (1955).

[33]Goldstein, A: The Insanity Defense. New Haven, Yale Univ Press, 1967.

[34]Stone, A: Mental health and the law: a system in transition. *N.I.M.H.* 1975.

[35]American Law Institute Model Penal Code sec. 201.3, Tent. Draft no. 9 (1959).

[36]People v Wells, 202P2d53, 62–63 (Cal 1949) cert. denied 337 U.S. 919; People v Gorshen, 336P2d 492, 503 (Cal 1959).

16

Education and Training in Forensic Psychiatry

RICHARD ROSNER

There are two principal approaches to education and training in psychiatry and the law in the United States today, each with its own attractions and liabilities. The dominant mode is self-training by reading, participation in periodic continuing medical education programs, and the acquisition of personal experience by doing work in the field. Another approach that is becoming increasingly attractive, largely appeals to those physicians who are relatively recent graduates of residency training programs in clinical psychiatry: the formal, full-time fellowship training program under the auspices of a medical school. This article will characterize each of these two approaches and will provide information for those who seek further education and training in forensic psychiatry.

THE TRADITIONAL ROUTE INTO FORENSIC PSYCHIATRY

The great majority of practitioners in psychiatry and the law are probably self-taught through on-the-job training. Typically, a psychiatrist may have started in a general practice, then have been referred several cases related to the law. With interest stimulated sufficiently to

Reprinted by permission from *Psychiatric Clinics of North America*—Vol. 6, No. 4, December 1983.

RICHARD ROSNER • Department of Psychiatry, School of Medicine, New York University, New York, New York 10016.

have done some elementary reading on mental health law and by virtue of willingness to see the forensic cases that colleagues may have avoided, the psychiatrist then begins to gradually build a local reputation as a forensic psychiatrist. This leads to more cases, more reading, and more sophisticated knowledge. Eventually, a practitioner may become aware of the opportunities for learning in a continuing medical education program. The next step would be to join one of the national organizations of forensic psychiatrists, engage in further study, more varied clinical-legal practice, and perhaps seek certification by The American Board of Forensic Psychiatry. Alternatively, the self-taught practitioner might have started with part-time work in a hospital or clinic where administrative pressures made it necessary to become aware of some issues in mental health law. This could have led to the same outcome of informal study, clinical-legal experience, awakening to the richness of the field, and a commitment to gain deeper knowledge, wider practice, and excellence. Some of the most respected educators and practitioners of psychiatry and the law are products of this type of informal education and training.

SPECIAL CONSIDERATIONS FOR A CAREER IN FORENSIC PSYCHIATRY

The best distinction between clinical and forensic psychiatry was made by Pollack,[1] who noted that forensic psychiatry was the application of psychiatric expertise for *legal ends*, whereas clinical psychiatry was the application of psychiatric expertise for *therapeutic ends*. Forensic psychiatry entails the *application* of psychiatric expertise; forensic psychiatry is a "hands-on" field. Some psychiatrists are attracted to the ideas, issues, and philosophic excitement of psychiatry and the law, but never make the transition from thinking to doing, from learning to practicing, and are content to be onlookers, rather than participants.

The ends of law are often inconsistent with the ends of psychiatric treatment. To cite an extreme example, a military psychiatrist may be obliged to put the ends of society and law above the well-being of his patient; the military psychiatrist may be required to state a soldier is suited to return to active duty (where he might be killed), rather than assist with the soldier's desire to be demobilized and return to the safety of a home-based hospital. The tradition of doctor-patient confidentiality might not apply in such military settings, because the overall good of the nation is predominant over the good of the individual soldier. There are many instances in which the forensic psychiatrist must put the good of society above the good of the individual he has been asked to evaluate and confidentiality will not apply. The court-appointed psychiatrist who reports to a judge that a given defendant does not meet the legal criteria for exculpation for a criminal offense is, like the military psychiatrist, performing a valued service to society, even though the individual defendant may then be subject to punishment. Whereas it must be emphasized that not all the work of the forensic psychiatrist necessarily conflicts with the traditional therapeutic ends of clinical psychiatry, the possibility of such conflict is the foundation for an ethical tension between competing values that may make some psychiatrists reluctant to pursue a career in forensic psychiatry.

Pollack's definition implies psychiatric expertise, as opposed to psychiatric speculation, aspiration, and good intention. In the course of clinical psychiatry, the practitioner of a therapeutic modality may not have to distinguish clearly between what he or she genuinely knows or does not know. This "knowing" is the possession of evidence sufficient to compel the assent of the majority of raional individuals. Often the therapist is guided by a metapsychologic theory that has great explanatory power, but which has never been proved by any scientific data. The type of "knowing" that is required to answer a patient who asks, "Doctor, will I really get better?" is different from the type of "knowing" that is required when a judge asks a forensic psychiatrist to tell a jury whether a man will be dangerous if he is released from a mental hospital and permitted to return to his community. Often, in the court setting, there will be a lawyer whose task it is to demonstrate that the psychiatrist does not really "know" what he or she is talking about. In clinical psychiatry it is often sufficient for effective therapeutic work, for a psychiatrist to practice what is sincerely believed, but not actually "known." In forensic psychiatry the practitioner must be able to provide proof. The pressure to be that precise, that clear, that logical, relevant, consistent, and coherent in articulation of reasoning processes may seem overwhelming to some psychiatrists.

This distinction between forensic psychiatry and clinical psychiatry may explain the reason why not many psychiatrists have chosen to become specialists in the practice of psychiatry and the law. Some introspection and honest assessment of personal resources is appropriate for any psychiatrist who is considering entering this field. If one is a doer (rather than a thinker or talker or observer), if one is able to accept the ethical burden of sometimes having to place the good of society ahead of the good of the individual person, and if one is intellectually able to commit one's self to a more rigorous standard of "knowing" than clinical practice requires, then forensic psychiatry may be an exciting, rewarding challenge, and a source of ongoing professional satisfaction.

Two refinements of the traditional route can be considered. The first, Systematic Independent Study, is closely related to the traditional route. A coordinated plan of reading and practical experience exists from the start, so that integrated learning and practice are pursued in the most time-efficient and training-effective manner. The second, Fellowship Training, is a new approach. Each route has its own unique assets and liabilities that must be considered so that the forensic psychiatrist in training can make an informed choice.

SYSTEMATIC INDEPENDENT STUDY

For the psychiatrist who wishes to become more informed and attain practical competence in the practice of forensic psychiatry, but who is either unable or unwilling to make a commitment to full-time education and training in a postgraduate fellowship program in forensic psychiatry, it has become easier than ever to proceed. A wide range of excellent books are now available and, through the efforts of organized psychiatry, it is relatively simple to locate short lecture sequences in the form of continuing medical education. Nonetheless, a guide to systematic independent study may prove useful, if only to assist the psychiatrist in choosing among the many options.

A distinction must be made between academic information that is essential to provide a foundation of essential information, and practical experience that gives empirical reality to the principles and issues that are dealt with in the books. Both are essential.

Core Readings for Systematic Independent Study

There are three classes of books that may be of use to the independent student of forensic psychiatry: discussions of issues, "how to do it" manuals, and cases and materials collections. In the first type, the psychiatrist is presented with someone else's assessment, explication, and interpretation of some or all of the core concerns in psychiatry and the law. These are the books that provide the best introduction to the field, presenting forensic psychiatry at its most exciting and thought-provoking.[2]

For every beginning student of medicine the time comes to progress from the fundamentals of anatomy, biochemistry, physiology, pharmacology, microbiology and pathology, to subjects of clinical medicine, surgery, pediatrics, psychiatry, gynecology, and obstetrics. In the same fashion, the prospective forensic psychiatrist must move from the theoretic, issue-oriented texts to the practical manuals of techniques and procedures. These are the books that will assist the student to cope with the other major component of his training, the "hands-on" work, the actual case experiences.[3]

For the more advanced student who has acquired a modicum of direct experience in the work, the collections of cases and materials provide a deeper level of understanding of psychiatry and the law. These books are compilations of important case law decisions by the courts, specialized law review journal articles, memorable extracts from psychiatric writings, and editorial commentaries.[4] Here will be found the materials that were presented in a easily digested form, filtered through someone else's mind, in the first type of books, the issues and overview books. The more advanced student can then come into direct contact with the sources and examine them directly, perhaps agreeing or disagreeing with the interpretations of the authors of the introductory books. It is similar to the difference between reading primary sources in the work of an historian, or reading secondary or tertiary sources in a college class on a survey of history. One could not readily understand the third level of books, the cases-and-materials books, if one had not previously gone through the introductory books. However, to stop at the introductory books is to stop at a second-hand level of understanding.

The advanced student can not neglect the current materials that are being developed in the progress of the field. It may take 2 years for a book to move from idea to reality, so almost all books are out-of-date as soon as they are available. To be truly up-to-date, it is necessary to read current articles in journals related to psychiatry and the law. In some instances, it is necessary to read the law and medicine notes of the major national newspapers, where the first reports of judicial decisions may appear. The librarian of the local medical school or law school can be remarkably helpful in getting access to full copies of major court determinations in both past and current cases. Much of the latest material will not appear in the psychiatric press, but will be found in publications directed to attorneys. The law library is an excellent resource. A call ahead to the librarian of the law school for an appointment to have the resources of the library explained will be an introduction to an intellectual treasure-trove. If a law library is not available, the medical school's librarian can often arrange for interlibrary loans.

As in every growing field, book learning is never completed. It is advisable to read the latest books and journals in the field. One should never presume that one knows all that is required.

Supervised Practice for Systematic Independent Study

More difficult to obtain, through systematic independent study, is the range of case experience that is necessary to become a competent practitioner. It is difficult to obtain good supervision from an experienced forensic psychiatrist outside of an organized training program. It can be done if one is willing to put in the time and to make the required arrangements.

The initial step, particularly in a larger urban community where a university medical school might be located, is to look through the "want-ads" for part-time opportunities in psychiatry and the law. The most likely jobs will be in an emergency room of a hospital; in a State hospital for the involuntarily admitted patients; as a consultant to a local jail or prison; as a staff member of a court-related psychiatric clinic or specialized municipal hospital psychiatric ward; as a liaison psychiatrist in a general hospital, or as a member of a community psychiatric professional standards review organization (PSRO). These positions will bring the neophyte into contact with the issues and practice of forensic psychiatry, often in association with more experienced practitioners who are on-the-job supervisors and professional colleagues. No one job will provide the necessary well-rounded experience, but will provide an initial toe-hold on the reality of practice in forensic psychiatry.

There are several types of practical experience to acquire: experience in civil forensic psychiatry, in criminal law forensic psychiatry, in the legal regulation of psychiatry, and in correctional psychiatry.

A job in a psychiatric emergency room admitting office or as a liaison psychiatrist in a general hospital should provide experiences related to some of the laws that regulate the practice of psychiatry. Problems related to involuntary hospitalization criteria, patients' rights to refuse treatment, patients' competence to consent to treatment, and the confidentiality of patients' communications will be endemic in such settings.

A position in a court-related clinic or municipal hospital's court-related psychiatric ward will provide experience in some areas of the criminal justice system. Problems such as competence to stand trial, competence to waive representation by counsel, competence to confess, exculpation from criminal responsibility, and the safe release of once-violent patients back to the community, will be addressed in court-related settings.

Alternatively, a Family Court clinic or the child and adolescent psychiatry wards of the municipal hospital will introduce the doctor to such issues as child abuse, child neglect, spouse abuse, juvenile delinquency, abrogation of parental rights, adoption, divorce, and child custody. Sometimes it is possible to contact the Public Defender's Office and be registered as a psychiatrist willing to do such Family Court/Domestic Relations Court psychiatric work, rather than to be employed in a specialized clinic or ward.

By registering with the Workers' Compensation board, by contacting the local Social Security disability claim office, or by contacting local offices of private insurance companies that offer disability policies, it is possible to obtain experience in personal injury litigation, assessment of vocational impairment consequent to psychiatric illnesses, as well as learning about administrative regulations and their implementation.

At a PSRO committee on psychiatry, one can get experience related to administrative and legal regulation of psychiatry and develop an understanding of the range of competent practice (thereby preparing for future work in cases involving psychiatric malpractice).

It is important to think in systematic terms from the very beginning if one is to succeed in independent efforts to become a competent practitioner of psychiatry and the law. Thus, an aspiring forensic psychiatrist could plan to work in a civil law setting for 2 or 3 years, then in a criminal law setting for the next 2 or 3 years, then in a correctional setting for the next 2 or 3 years. Simultaneously, one might want to explore volunteer work in some of the other settings that have been outlined. The goal would be to have obtained "hands-on" experience in a balanced series of psychiatric-legal settings, rather than to have a wealth of experience in any one setting, and none in any other type of forensic psychiatric work.

Competent supervision is extremely important. Immediate supervisors on psychiatric-legal jobs are not necessarily competent in forensic psychiatry. Supervisors are often experienced in their narrow area of psychiatric-legal work, but lack in-depth understanding of the issues, the legal criteria that determine the resolution of the issues. Sometimes they do not have relevant psychiatric-legal data or the capacity to reason cogently about psychiatric-legal issues. It may be possible to contact the local chapter of the American Psychiatric Association or the local university medical school's Department of Psychiatry, to learn who is genuinely knowledgeable about psychiatry and the law. Alternatively, one can inquire as to which local practitioners are Diplomates of The American Board of Forensic Psychiatry. In much the same way that students of psychoanalysis buy supervisory time from senior analysts, students of forensic psychiatry can pay for private supervision by a competent practitioner of psychiatry and the law.

Whereas a great deal may be learned from working closely with lawyers, from attending public lectures, or auditing courses at a law school, a lawyer is *not* a good supervisor for a fledgling forensic psychiatrist. A lawyer can help a physician to understand the legal issues and the legal criteria that will be used to determine legal issues. However, lawyers are not trained in the collection of relevant psychiatric-legal data and they do not have the clinical experience necessary to guide the physician. Forensic psychiatry is a *medical* subspecialty. A forensic psychiatrist is *not* merely a clinical psychiatrist who has learned something about the law. Rather, forensic psychiatry has its own specialized body of data, its own conceptual framework for the organization of psychiatric-legal information, and its own specialized methods and procedures. A piano maker can no more teach a student to become a concert artist than a lawyer can teach a physician to become a forensic psychiatrist. The important educational factor that is provided by a role model is best filled by an experienced practitioner in the field of psychiatry and the law. Surgeons are best trained by surgeons and forensic psychiatrists are best trained by forensic psychiatrists.

Integrating Reading and Practice to Attain Competence

It is through the integration of the systematic readings and the planned work experiences that the self-taught, independently trained practitioner can develop well-rounded competence in forensic psychiatry. Each case experience should be made into an opportunity for learning. The specific law related to the specific legal issue should be read, along with those pertinent case law determinations that have interpreted the specific law. Compilations of the State and Federal laws, along with commentaries and major case law decisions, can be found at a law library or obtained by interlibrary loans. Alternatively, the attorney who has requested the help of the forensic psychiatrist should be able to provide a clear, written statement of the applicable law and its case law interpretations. Although the forensic psychiatrist is not a lawyer, he or she should gradually become familiar with the State mental health law and with those Federal laws that apply to the practice of the sub-specialty. Such basic legal knowledge should permit the forensic psychiatrist to work more intelligently with attorneys and be a more effective practitioner.

A major additional resource, both in the form of didactic lectures and in "hands-on" experiences, exists in continuing medical education postgraduate courses. These may be available at the major annual conventions of the American Psychiatric Association, the American Academy of Psychiatry and the Law, and the Psychiatry Section of the American Academy of Forensic Sciences. Alternatively, they may be through local programs of State psychiatric societies or of university medical schools' Departments of Psychiatry. Some of these post graduate training programs offer one teacher to one student intensive tutorial experiences, such as would otherwise only be found in formal full-time fellowship training programs in forensic psychiatry. Because the didactic programs may be compressed within one week or less, they are ideally designed for the busy practitioner who can not set aside clinical responsibilities for an extended period. The intensive tutorial programs may require longer blocks of time, such as 5 hours per week for several months, and may not be readily available outside of large urban areas. Although this discussion has focused on the systematic independent training of a post graduate student in forensic psychiatry, it is important that the physician interested in psychiatry and the law keeps up with the progress in general psychiatry and in relevant areas of medicine. Forensic psychiatry builds upon the foundation of clinical competence. Unless that basic foundation is maintained, no amount of training and education in forensic psychiatry will produce a credible and creditable doctor.

FELLOWSHIP TRAINING PROGRAMS
IN FORENSIC PSYCHIATRY

The great advantage of a full-time fellowship training program in forensic psychiatry over systematic independent study is that all of the components of didactic education and closely supervised psychiatric-legal "hands-on" experiences have been pre-assembled and organized into a timed, efficient, and effective opportunity for ready learning. Thus, although it might take 4 to 6 years to acquire the necessary practical, on-the-job training on a part-time basis, a full-time training program might offer essentially the same range of experience within a single year. The range of experiences would not be duplicated, and more efficient and effective learning would be possible because of the close supervision and integrated didactic curriculum that a fellowship would provide. One can get from New York to London by ship in several days or one can make the same trip by supersonic Concorde jet in a few hours. One can take several years to become competent in forensic psychiatry through independent study, or one can enroll in a full-time fellowship training program. In each case, one would have to weigh the relative advantages and disadvantages.

A major warning is indicated to those who are considering fellowship training programs in psychiatry and the law: the programs are not identical.[5] One may be looking for a Concorde, but may have to make do with a Boeing 747. The wise airline traveler makes careful inquiry before purchasing a ticket, and the wise postgraduate fellow makes a similarly careful inquiry before signing a contract for training. Each of the fellowship programs in forensic psychiatry is unique, each offers a mixture of resources derived from the guiding educational philosophy of its director(s), the staff, and the facilities that it has available. Some programs may stress correctional experiences, others will emphasize liaison-consultation experiences in hospitals or Court settings. Some will focus primarily on criminal law issues, others will offer relatively more experiences in civil law cases. For the prospective fellow, the important consideration is that a comprehensive and balanced training program be chosen.

Until recently, it was difficult for a fellow to determine whether or not a given training program was sufficiently well designed to offer good training. There were no reliable criteria against which a program could be measured, unlike determining whether a given residency program in general psychiatry was reliable. The Accreditation Council on Graduate Medical Education has developed uniform criteria regarding what should comprise an acceptable program in a general psychiatry residency. The prospective general psychiatrist can compare any given program in general psychiatry with the standards of the ACGME and ascertain whether the program will be worthwhile. The standards for evaluation of a competent fellowship training program in forensic psychiatry have recently been developed by a joint committee of the American Academy of Psychiatry and the Law and the Psychiatry Section of the American Academy of Forensic Sciences.[6] The prospective forensic psychiatrist can now compare any individual fellowship program in forensic psychiatry with the AAPL/AAFS standards and determine if the program under consideration is likely to provide good training.

The value of fellowship training in psychiatry and the law has been recognized by The American Board of Forensic Psychiatry. Although the Board requires 5 years of substantial experience in forensic psychiatry as one of the criteria for eligibility for its examination, graduates of fellowship programs in forensic psychiatry are permitted to count 1 year of fellowship training as 2 years of experience toward the 5 years required by the Board.

In general, a fellowship training program in psychiatry and the law should be built upon the foundation of a residency program in general psychiatry that is accredited by the ACGME. The unaffiliated, free-standing training programs are not likely to have the academic resources and depth of consultative support staff that can be found in programs directly linked to accredited residency programs in general psychiatry. The Director of the fellowship program should be certified by the American Board of Forensic Psychiatry. One of the purposes of that Board is to distinguish among persons who *assert* their competence in forensic psychiatry and persons who have *demonstrated* their competence in forensic psychiatry. If one is going to enter a training program for 1 year, full-time, one wants to be certain that the head of the program has demonstrated knowledge of the field of forensic psychiatry. The Director should have been recognized as competent by the medical school at which he or she holds an appointment; should be possessed of at least initial professorial-level rank, (assistant clinical professor or higher). There should be at least one other forensic psychiatrist on the program's staff, although that person need not have the same degree of demonstrated expertise and academic rank as the Director. Among the faculty resources available to the program should be an attorney, a forensic psychologist, a child psychiatrist, and a family-systems therapist.

The psychiatric-legal experiences, the "hands-on" training, should be designed as learning experiences, rather than as a means of meeting the service needs of the field placements used in the course of the program. In a standard 40-hour work week, approximately half the time should be devoted to practical, on-the-job training. The fellow's role should be an active one, rather than that of a passive observer of other doctors' work. In any one year, a fellow should have been responsible for at least 30 cases, a minimum of 10 having been in the area of criminal law and another 10 related to civil law issues. These are minimal figures, any less substantial experience will be overly theoretical and lacking in adequate preparation for the real world. The types of cases to be experienced are parallel to those outlined earlier in the discussion of systematic independent study.

The didactic core curriculum of the fellowship program should include training in basic issues in law, landmark cases in forensic psychiatry, correctional psychiatry, legal regulation of psychiatry, criminal law issues, civil law issues, and special topics that relate to the clinical, methodologic and historical aspects of psychiatry and the law.

Although all the introductory books, procedural manuals, case-and-materials texts, major journals, legal publications, and research monographs can be obtained by inter-library loans, a well-designed fellowship training program in forensic psychiatry should have the majority readily available. These reading materials are particularly germane to the fellow acquiring skills needed to do independent research and to being an educator. A good fellowship training program will aim at helping the fellow to make the transition from a passive student of others' work into a contributor to the basic knowledge of the field; training in research in forensic psychiatry fellow must be trained to move from the passive role of student to the active role of teacher. Throughout a career, the competent forensic psychiatrist will be teaching psychiatry to lawyers, judges, and jurors and will be teaching general psychiatrists about psychiatric-legal problems. Training to be an educator is an integral part of a fellowship program.

The forensic psychiatrist must have some basic background in the law as it pertains to the practice of the medical sub-specialty of forensic psychiatry. Such training should be provided by the attorney who is on the faculty of the fellowship program. At minimum, the fellow should learn about the historical and philosophic foundations of our legal system, the organization of the courts, the nature of criminal and civil procedure, applications of the concepts of responsibility, mens rea, due process, jurisdiction, and the rationale for punishment of offenders. The use of a law library should be explained and demonstrated, so that the fellow will know how to use that resource effectively.

Even after the successful completion of a fellowship training program in forensic psychiatry, the task of learning is not complete. In fact, the ideal fellowship program should provide the grounding for a lifetime of further study and practice in the same way that an ideal residency in general psychiatry is merely the beginning of the postgraduate education of the practicing psychiatrist.

SYSTEMATIC INDEPENDENT STUDY
VS. FELLOWSHIP TRAINING

The decision of whether to pursue a career in forensic psychiatry through systematic independent study or through a full-time fellowship training program will be an individual one. For the busy practitioner of general psychiatry, part-time, systematic independent study may be the most convenient route. Fellowship training in a full-time program may be a more realistic option for physicians emerging from their residency training in general or child and adolescent psychiatry. It is easier to continue in the student's role than to return to it after many years' absence. Both types of education and training in psychiatry and the law are valid and will produce competent forensic psychiatrists if pursued diligently.

REFERENCES

[1]Pollack, S: Forensic psychiatry—a specialty. *Bull. Am. Acad. Psychiatry Law, 2:*(1), 1974.
[2]Examples of such books that present an overview of issues are: Slovenko, R: Psychiatry and Law. Boston, Little, Brown & Co., 1973; and Rosner, R: Critical Issues in American Psychiatry and the Law. Springfield, Illinois, Charles C Thomas Co., 1982.
[3]Examples of books that emphasize procedures, techniques, and are guides to the actual application of psychiatry to legal ends are: Gutheil, T, and Appelbaum, P: Clinical Handbook of Psychiatry and the Law. Hightstown, New Jersey, McGraw-Hill Book Co., 1982; and Sadoff, R: Forensic Psychiatry, Springfield, Illinois, Charles C Thomas Co., 1975.
[4]Examples of compilations of cases-and-materials includes: Brooks, A: Law, Psychiatry and the Mental Health System. Boston, Little, Brown & Co., 1974, with a 1980 Supplement to the book; and Allen, R, Ferster, E, and Rubin, J: Readings in Law and Psychiatry, revised edition. Baltimore, Johns Hopkins University Press, 1975.

[5]Rosner, R: Accreditation of fellowship programs in forensic psychiatry: A preliminary report. *Bull. Am. Acad. Psychiatry Law. 8:*(4), 1980.

[6]Joint committee on accreditation of fellowship programs in forensic psychiatry: Standards for fellowship programs in forensic psychiatry. *Bull. Am. Acad. Psychiatry Law, 10:* (4), 1982.

[7]Rosner, R: Accreditation of fellowship programs in forensic psychiatry: The development of the final report on standards. *Bull. Am. Acad. Psychiatry Law, 10:*(4), 1982.

[8]Rosner, R: Summary report: Committee on accreditation of fellowships in forensic psychiatry. *J of Forensic Sci,* January 1983.

17

Standards for Fellowship Programs in Forensic Psychiatry

A Report by The Joint Committee on Accreditation of Fellowship Programs in Forensic Psychiatry

RICHARD ROSNER

ACADEMIC AFFILIATION

The Fellowship Program in Forensic Psychiatry should be built upon the foundation of a residency program in psychiatry that has been accredited by the Accreditation Council for Graduate Medical Education.

DIRECTOR OF THE PROGRAM

The Director of the Fellowship Program in Forensic Psychiatry should be an experienced forensic psychiatrist. By the year 1983, the Director must be certified by the American Board of Forensic Psychiatry. The Director should hold a faculty position at the medical school that operates the underlying residency program in general psychiatry;

Reprinted from the *AAPL Bulletin,* Vol. 10, No. 4 © 1982 by the American Academy of Psychiatry and the Law.

RICHARD ROSNER • Medical Director, Forensic Psychiatry Clinic for the New York Criminal and Supreme Courts (First Judicial Department) 100 Centre St. — Room 124, New York, NY 10013.

his or her rank in that program should be at the level of Assistant Professor or Clinical Assistant Professor at the minimum.

FACULTY OF THE PROGRAM

It is important that Fellows have exposure to more than one perspective in forensic psychiatry, so that at least one member of the faculty (i.e., in addition to the Director) should be an experienced forensic psychiatrist. It is not necessary, although it is highly desirable, that this person be certified by the American Board of Forensic Psychiatry. It is necessary that this person is also on the faculty of the medical school that operates the underlying residency program in general psychiatry, but he or she need not be of professorial rank.

An attorney must be part of the faculty of the Fellowship Program in Forensic Psychiatry, although (in deference to the requirements for medical school faculty appointments) that attorney need not be a formal member of the faculty of the medical school that operates the underlying residency program in general psychiatry.

An experienced forensic psychologist should be a member of the consultants available to the Fellowship Program, although that person need not be a formal member of the faculty of the Fellowship Program. It is desirable, but not required, that the forensic psychologist be certified by the American Board of Forensic Psychology.

An experienced child and adolescent psychiatrist should be a member of the consultants available to the Fellowship Program, although he or she need not be a formal member of the faculty of the Fellowship Program. It is desirable, but not required, that the consultant be certified by the American Board of Psychiatry and Neurology in the subspecialty of Child and Adolescent Psychiatry.

It is recommended, but not required, that a family systems therapist, preferably a psychiatrist, be available as a consultant to the Fellowship Program. It is not necessary that the therapist be a formal member of the faculty of the Fellowship Program.

MANAGEMENT BY OBJECTIVES

The Fellowship Program should have a clear statement regarding the desired outcome of its training. A formal statement should be made of the goals, the objectives, the methods, and the mechanism for the assessment of the effectiveness of the training program. An assessment of the effectiveness of the program in meeting its own objectives, and the relevance of those objectives for the goals of the program, should be made annually. Based on that assessment, the program's goals, objectives, and methods should be reviewed annually by the Director and the program faculty, with the aim of increasing the program's effectiveness, if necessary by the modification of those goals, objectives, and methods.

DIDACTIC CORE CURRICULUM

The didactic core curriculum represents that body of information and skills that is to be communicated to the fellow by means of lectures, seminars, demonstrations, and formal teaching. The subjects to be included are:

Civil Forensic Psychiatry including, at minimum, conservators and guardianships, child custody determinations, parental competence, termination of parental rights, child abuse, child neglect, psychiatric disability determinations (e.g., for social security, workers compensation, private insurance coverage), testamentary capacity, psychiatric negligence and malpractice, personal injury litigation issues.

Criminal Forensic Psychiatry including, at minimum, competence to stand trial, competence to enter a plea, testimonial capacity, voluntariness of confessions, insanity defense(s), diminished capacity, sentencing considerations, release of persons who have been acquitted by reason of insanity.

Legal Regulation of Psychiatry including, at minimum, civil involuntary commitment, voluntary hospitalization, confidentiality, right to treatment, right to refuse treatment, informed consent, professional liability, ethical guidelines.

Special Issues in Forensic Psychiatry including, at minimum, the history of forensic psychiatry, assessment of dangerousness, amnesia, organic brain syndromes, neuropsychiatric assessment, forensic uses of hypnosis/amytal/polygraphy, psychopathic or sociopathic or antisocial personalities, the role and responsibilities of forensic psychiatrists.

Correctional Psychiatry including, at minimum, approaches to the treatment of incarcerated persons, administrative considerations in the operation of a treatment program in a secure setting, rape and sexual problems in a secure setting, gradations of security within the correctional system, psychological aspects of inmate riots, history of correctional psychiatry, ethical issues in a secure setting.

Basic Issues in Law including, at minimum, the nature of law and its foundations in case law/common law/statutes/administrative regulations, the structure of the federal and state court systems, use of a law library, theory and practice of punishment, basic civil procedure, basic

criminal procedure, jurisdiction, mens rea, responsibility, tort law, legislative processes, equal protection.

Landmark Cases including, at minimum, the cases specifically listed in
the syllabus of the American Board of Forensic Psychiatry.

SUPERVISED CLINICAL EXPERIENCES

The fellow should spend a minimum of 15 hours, but not more than
a maximum of 25 hours, each week in supervised clinical experiences.
Emphasis should be placed on meeting the educational needs of the
fellow, rather than on the service needs of the constituent clinical components of the Fellowship Program.

In the course of the fellowship year, each fellow should have performed a minimum of thirty clinical case assessments in the areas of civil
and criminal forensic psychiatry, at least ten of those assessments in the
civil area and at least ten in the criminal area. A written case report
should be required in at least twenty-five of those thirty assessments.
Related to these thirty assessments the fellow should have the responsi-
bility/opportunity of testifying in court on at least five cases. In addition,
the fellow should have an opportunity to witness at least ten in-court
appearances by a forensic psychiatrist. Among the written reports that
the fellow prepares in the course of the training year there should be, at
the minimum, three assessments related to aiding the court in the sentencing of criminal offenders, one assessment in a domestic relations
case, one civil commitment assessment, one personal injury assessment,
and one civil competency assessment.

Criminal Forensic Psychiatry experiences should include male and
female adolescents and adults covering a variety of ages. Incarcerated
defendants and defendants on bail, i.e., persons seen both as inpatients
and outpatients, should be available for assessment. Evaluations should
encompass such issues as the competence of the defendant to stand trial,
competence to confess, criminal responsibility, and post-conviction reports in aid of sentencing by the Court. Opportunities should be provided for consultation with lawyers, probation officers, judges. Written
reports should be drafted to conform to the special requirements of
forensic psychiatry and training should be provided in report writing.

Civil Forensic Psychiatry experiences should include such cases as
child custody, termination of parental rights, child abuse, child neglect,
spouse abuse, assessment of psychiatric impairment in cases for Social
Security/Workers Compensation/private insurance coverage, civil commitment.

Legal Regulation of Psychiatry experiences should provide the fellow
with a minimum of ten cases for assessment. Preferably the fellow

should do the assessments himself or herself. However, if that is not possible, intensive seminar case review, averaging two hours per case for ten cases, may be substituted. The cases should include civil commitment, and it is recommended that such other cases as confidentiality, patients' rights, professional liability, and ethical issues also be included (if need be, by the use of seminar case reviews). It would be desirable for the fellow to assess patients who are refusing their medication, are contesting their involuntary hospitalization, and whose capacity to provide competent/voluntary/informed consent is at issue.

Special Issues in Forensic Psychiatry should provide the fellow with a minimum of five cases for assessment including examples of potential or present dangerousness, psychopathy, organic brain syndromes, neuropsychiatric testing, and double-agent ethical problems. While it is preferable for the fellow to examine the cases, if that is not possible, then an intensive seminar case review may be substituted, averaging two hours per case for five cases.

Correctional Psychiatry experiences, at minimum should occupy twenty-five hours in the course of the training year. Among the clinical settings that are appropriate for the fellow to experience are state and federal prisons, municipal and federal and state detention centers, court detention areas for persons awaiting arraignment/hearing/trial, secure court clinics, secure areas for persons contesting involuntary hospitalization, secure units for persons who have been acquitted by reason of insanity.

Clinical Supervision should be in addition to the didactic program. It should be scheduled weekly and be provided by a forensic psychiatrist. Where appropriate to the case material, supplemental supervision (in addition to that provided by the forensic psychiatrist) may be provided by a forensic psychologist, child psychiatrist, or family systems therapist.

TRAINING IN LAW

Included in the core didactic curriculum in forensic psychiatry, the fellow must be provided with a minimum of twenty-five hours of formal training devoted to acquisition of legal information. Among the essential elements to be addressed are foundations and sources of law, the structure of the court systems, use of a law library, criminal procedure, civil procedure, theory and practice of punishment, responsibility, jurisdiction, due process, and mens rea.

The attorney on the faculty of the training program should have particular responsibility in the development and presentation of the legal segment of the formal educational program. Elective opportunities for legal learning are recommended as a supplement to the training provided by the attorney on the faculty. Such opportunities may be found in law school courses, consultation with Public Defenders and Prosecutors, consultation with the law departments of hospitals, governmental agencies, and guest lectures from visiting private practitioners of law.

TRAINING IN RESEARCH

The training program should provide the fellow with basic skills in research in forensic psychiatry, such that the fellow learns to obtain and critically evaluate published research findings in the sub-specialty and such that the fellow is equipped to make some contribution to the scholarly or scientific development of forensic psychiatry.

The fellowship training program must include a research requirement for completion of its course. Suitable research projects include a scholarly review or a clinical study suitable for publication in a refereed journal, participation in ongoing externally funded research at a level of effort equivalent to at least two months of full-time work, production of a videotape or film suitable for presentation at a major national meeting, production of a practice manual in some selected area of forensic psychiatry, preparation of an annotated bibliography on some topic in the sub-specialty.

The training program must include the resources that would make such research possible. These include, at minimum, accessibility to a major medical library, accessibility to a major law library and accessibility to at least one behavioral science research resource (e.g., computer processing, a programmable calculator, a one-way mirror observation room, videotape equipment, endocrine assays, psychotropic drug assays, electroencephalography, computerized tomography, polygraphy, penile plethysmography, or a medical examiner's office).

TRAINING IN TEACHING

The training program must provide opportunities to foster the fellow's development as a teacher of forensic psychiatry. Such opportunities should be consistent with the fellow's acquisition of the essential knowledge and skills of the sub-specialty, so that the bulk of the fellow's teaching should be scheduled after the fellow has received basic training in forensic psychiatry. It is recommended that the fellow have exposure to senior teachers in the field, who can provide effective role models.

Among the suitable teaching opportunities are: teaching basic psychiatry to lawyers, probation, and correction officers; teaching residents in general and child psychiatry; teaching forensic psychiatry to parole and police officers; teaching relevant topics to non-psychiatric physicians (e.g., professional liability, informed consent, confidentiality).

ACKNOWLEDGMENTS

The Joint Committee on Accreditation of Fellowship Programs in Forensic Psychiatry is co-sponsored by The American Academy of Forensic Sciences (Psychiatry Section) and The American Academy of Psychiatry and the Law. Committee members are:

David Barry	Seymour Pollack
Elissa Benedek	Joseph Palombi
Harvey Bluestone	Jonas Rappeport
John Bradford	Phillip Resnick
James Cavanaugh	Richard Rosner
J. Richard Ciccone	Robert Sadoff
Park Dietz	Selwyn Smith
Mark Mills	Henry Weinstein
Thomas Mould	Howard Zonana

For further information about the Joint Committee on the Accreditation of Fellowship Programs in Forensic Psychiatry, contact either The American Academy of Forensic Sciences (Psychiatry Section), 225 South Academy Blvd, Colorado Springs, CO 80910 or The American Academy of Psychiatry and the Law, 1211 Cathedral St, Baltimore, MD 21201.

LIBRARY RESOURCES

The following publications should be part of the core library.

Textbooks

American Psychiatric Association: *Clinical Aspects of the Violent Individual*. Washington, DC, American Psychiatric Association, 1974.

Bromberg, W: *The Uses of Psychiatry in the Law: A Clinical View of Forensic Psychiatry*. Westport, CT, Quorum Books, 1979.

Brooks, A: *Law, Psychiatry and the Mental Health System*. Boston: Little, Brown and Co, 1974. Also, obtain the *1980 Supplement* to the text, by the same author, same publisher, with the same title.

Cleckly, H: *The Mask of Sanity: An Attempt to Clarify Some Issues about the So-called Psychopathic Personality*. St. Louis, C. V. Mosby Co, 1976.

Goldstein, A: *The Insanity Defense*. New Haven, Yale University Press, 1967.

Goldstein, J, Freud, A, Solnit, A: *Beyond the Best Interests of the Child*. New York, MacMillan

Publishing Co., 1973. Also obtain the companion volume, *Before the Best Interests of the Child*, by the same authors and the same publisher.

Halleck, S: *Law in the Practice of Psychiatry: A Handbook for Clinicians*. New York, Plenum Publishing Co., 1980.

Keiser, L: *Traumatic Neurosis*. Philadelphia, J. L. Lippincott Co.

Leedy, J: *Compensation in Psychiatric Disability and Rehabilitation*. Springfield, IL, Charles C Thomas Co, 1971.

Rosner, R: *Critical Issues in American Psychiatry and the Law*. Springfield, IL, Charles C Thomas Co, 1982.

Sadoff, R: *Forensic Psychiatry*. Springfield, IL, Charles C Thomas Co, 1975.

Schetky, D and Benedek, E: *Child Psychiatry and the Law*. New York, Brunner/Masel, 1980.

Slovenko, R: *Psychiatry and Law*. Boston, Little, Brown & Co., 1973.

Stone, A: *Mental Health and Law: A System in Transition*. New York, Jason Aronson.

Ziskin, J: *Coping with Psychiatry and Psychological Testimony*, 3rd ed. Venice, CA, Law and Psychology Press.

Reference Books

Allen, Ferster, Rubin: *Readings in Law and Psychiatry*, rev. ed., Baltimore, Johns Hopkins University Press, 1975.

American Medical Association: *Guides to the Evaluation of Permanent Impairment*. Chicago, American Medical Association, 1971.

Curran, WJ, McGarry, AL, Petty, CS (eds.): *Modern Legal Medicine, Psychiatry, and Forensic Science*. Philadelphia, F. A. Davis Co., 1980.

Curran, WJ, Shapiro, ED: *Law, Medicine, and Forensic Sciences*, 2nd ed. Boston, Little, Brown and Co., 1970.

Glaser, D (ed.): *Handbook of Criminology*. Chicago, Rand-McNally, 1974.

Holder, AR: *Medical Malpractice Law*. New York, John Wiley & Sons, 1975.

Laboratory of Community Psychiatry, Harvard Medical School: *Competency to Stand Trial and Mental Illness*. New York, Jason Aronson, 1974.

Rada, RT (ed.): *Clinical Aspects of the Rapist*. New York, Grune & Stratton, 1978.

Radzinowicz, L, Wolfgang, ME (eds.): *Crime and Justice* (3 vols.). New York, Basic Books, 1971.

Spitz, WU, Fisher, R (eds.): *Medicolegal Investigation of Death: Guidelines for the Application of Pathology to Crime Investigation*. Springfield, IL, Charles C Thomas, 1973.

Wadlington, W, Waltz, JR, Dworkin, RB: *Cases and Materials on Law and Medicine*. Mineola, NY, Foundation Press, 1980.

Waltz, JR, Inbau, FE: *Medical Jurisprudence*. New York, The Macmillan Co., 1971.

Research Monographs

Gunn, J, Robertson, G, et al.: *Psychiatric Aspects of Imprisonment*. New York, Academic Press, 1978.

Guze, SB: *Criminality and Psychiatric Disorder*. New York, Oxford University Press, 1976.

Lewis, DO, Balla, DA: *Delinquency and Psychopathology*. New York, Grune & Stratton, 1976.

Mednick, S, Christiansen, KO: *Biosocial Bases of Criminal Behavior*. New York, Gardner Press, 1977.

Mohr, JW, Turner, RE, Jerry, MB: *Pedophilia and Exhibitionism*. Toronto, University of Toronto Press, 1964.

Monroe, RR: *Episodic Behavioral Disorders*. Cambridge, Harvard University Press, 1970.

Robins, LN: *Deviant Children Grown Up*. Baltimore, Williams and Wilkins Co., 1966.

Roesch, R, Golding, SL: *Competency to Stand Trial*. Urbana, IL, University of Illinois Press, 1980.

Simon, RJ: *The Jury and the Defense of Insanity*. Boston, Little, Brown and Company, 1967.

Steadman, HJ: *Beating a Rap? Defendants Found Incompetent to Stand Trial*. Chicago, University of Chicago Press, 1979.

Steadman, HJ, Cocozza, JJ: *Careers of the Criminally Insane: Excessive Social Control of Deviance*. Lexington, MA, Lexington Books, 1974.

Thornberry, TP, Jacoby, JE: *The Criminally Insane: A Community Follow-up of Mentally Disordered Offenders*. Chicago, University of Chicago Press, 1979.

West, DJ: *Murder Followed by Suicide*. Cambridge, Harvard University Press, 1967.

Index